Textbook of

# Practical Physiology for Dental Students

SECOND EDITION

Textbook of

# Practical Physiology for Dental Students

SECOND EDITION

G K Pal

MBBS, MD, PhD, DSc, BNYT (Yoga Therapy), MD (Yoga), MD (AM), MABMS, FABMS, FABAP, FSAB
Dean, JIPMER (Karaikal), Puducherry, Nodal Officer to Ministry, Professor of Physiology
Program Director, Advance Center for Yoga
JIPMER, Pondicherry

Pravati Pal

MBBS, MD, BNYT, MD (AM), MABMS
Professor, Department of Physiology,
Jawaharlal Institute of Postgraduate Medical Education and Research (JIPMER), Pondicherry

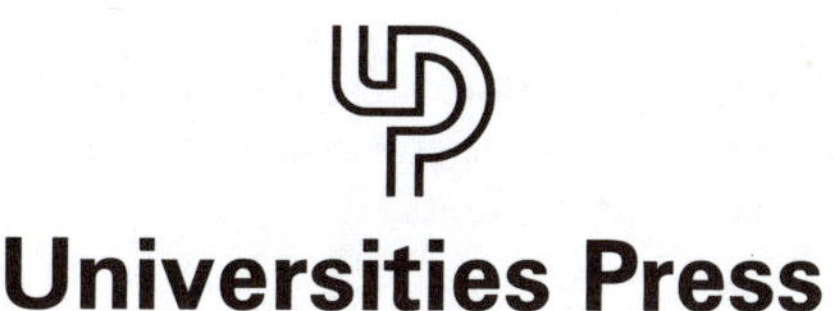

Universities Press

Textbook of Practical Physiology for Dental Students (Second Edition)

UNIVERSITIES PRESS (INDIA) PRIVATE LIMITED

*Registered Office*
3-6-747/1/A & 3-6-754/1, Himayatnagar, Hyderabad 500 029, Telangana, India
info@universitiespress.com; www.universitiespress.com

*Distributed by*
Orient Blackswan Private Limited

*Registered Office*
3-6-752 Himayatnagar, Hyderabad 500 029, Telangana, India

*Other Offices*
Bengaluru, Bhopal, Chennai, Guwahati, Hyderabad,
Jaipur, Kolkata, Lucknow, Mumbai, New Delhi,
Noida, Patna, Vijayawada



First published 2007
Second edition 2017

ISBN 978 93 86235 00 8



*Cover and book design*
© Universities Press (India) Private Limited 2017

*Typeset in* Minion Pro 11/13.5 pt *by*
OSDATA, Hyderabad 500 029

*Illustrations by*
RK Majumdar
New Delhi 110 092

*Printed in India at*
Ashwin Printing Agency, Chennai

*Published by*
Universities Press (India) Private Limited
3-6-747/1/A & 3-6-754/1 Himayatnagar, Hyderabad 500 029, Telangana, India
email: info@universitiespress.com

# Contents

# Acknowledgements

The second edition of Textbook of Practical Physiology for Dental Students was long pending. Due to my heavy administrative, academic and research responsibilities at the institute, I was not able to take up the revision of the book, which I knew is a tough task. However, with the repeated requests and full encouragement and support of Mr Madhu Reddy, Director, Universities Press and President, Orient Blackswan, I had no other option but to initiate and complete the job. I sincerely thank Mr Reddy for his consistent efforts in getting this work done through me in spite of my very hectic schedules. I profusely thank Dr Sudha Ganesan, Managing Consultant, Medical Publishing and the editor Ms Parvath Radha for providing their full cooperation throughout this endeavour. It was a pleasure working with them. I am grateful to my friends from Sri Aurobindo Ashram, Mahapatra Babu and Chandramani Bhai, for becoming subjects of our clinical examinations.

We have no words to express our appreciation to Auroprakash, Auroprajna, Nivedita, Sabita and Anupama of our family who have been our constant sources of inspiration. We are always indebted to the Grace of the Divine Mother, without which nothing can be achieved.

**G K Pal**
**Pravati Pal**
E-mail: drgkpal@gmail.com

*All sincere prayers are granted, every call is answered. With my blessings.*

—The Mother (of Sri Aurobindo Ashram)

# Preface to the Second Edition

In recent years, rapid advancements have taken place in dental science. Dentistry as a subject of human health has wider application in preventive and promotive medicine. Though practice in dental science is limited to the diseases of teeth and oral cavity, this branch of medicine directly or indirectly has link with all major systems of the body. Moreover, dental pathology and dental pharmacology are close to medical pathology and pharmacology. Therefore, physiology as the mother subject in medicine has equal relevance in dentistry as applicable in modern medicine. A dental surgeon must have basic knowledge in neurophysiology, cardiorespiratory physiology, endocrine physiology, blood physiology, gastrointestinal and musculoskeletal physiology, as the diseases affecting buccal cavity might have association with or influence on any systemic physiology. Therefore, 'Physiology' is a core subject in dentistry.

The Dental Council of India has recommended learning of human or medical physiology as an integral part of the dental curriculum. A student must learn and develop basic skills in all human physiology practicals starting from preparation and examination of a blood smear to the examination/recording and interpretation of clinical findings or parameters such as pulse, heart sounds, blood pressure, sensations, reflexes and so on. Therefore, all human practicals have been included in physiology curriculum of BDS course. In this revised and enlarged edition of the practical book for dental students, we have included all relevant human and clinical practicals, in addition to updating the practicals on hematology. The core concepts and principles of experimental physiology have been described very briefly. We are sure this new edition will be quite useful to physiology students and teachers of dental colleges in understanding the principles and practice of dentistry as a whole and dental physiology in specific.

**G K Pal**
**Pravati Pal**
E-mail: drgkpal@gmail.com

*Whatever work you do, do it as perfectly as you can. That is the best service to the Divine in Man.*
—The Mother (of Sri Aurobindo Ashram)

# Preface to the First Edition

In recent years, the importance of physiology in medical sciences has increased enormously. Practical physiology, especially, has become more applicable and relevant to present-day medical practice; its contribution to learning in clinical medicine is being realised.

Dentistry is considered a surgical branch of medical science. Contrary to the common view, dental science is vast in its approach. Dentistry is linked with orofacial surgery, ophthalmic surgery, otorhinolaryngology and plastic surgery. A good dental surgeon can perform surgery on head and neck, thyroid gland, sinuses in the face, nasal and paranasal pathologies and diseases of oral cavity in addition to his regular dental surgeries. Hence, the study of dentistry is interlinked with many branches of medicine. A student in this speciality should have adequate practical and theoretical knowledge of the various aspects of physiology. Therefore, study of dental practical physiology lays emphasis on practicals related to the physiology of many systems including cardiovascular and respiratory physiology, hematology, endocrinology and neurophysiology.

This book covers all aspects of practicals in the subject. The experiment and its principle are presented in a very precise though comprehensive form. The book contains not only details of practicals, but also adequate theoretical aspects of the practical: therefore, this is a complete textbook of practical physiology. We have made special efforts to emphasise the application of practical knowledge in clinical medicine. The book contains all essential underlying principles of practical physiology as per latest recommendations of Dental Council of India (DCI) and Medical Council of India (MCI). The instruction of DCI to lay emphasis on applied aspects of physiology practicals has been adequately taken care of in this book. Therefore, details of hematology and human clinical practicals, and basic principles of experimental practicals have been described in the book. The student should read the chapter from the beginning to the end, from the learning objectives and introduction to the discussion on applied physiology, to gain an understanding of the concepts and an integrated knowledge of practical physiology.

We hope this book will be very useful to all students. We look forward to receiving feedback, constructive criticism and suggestions to make the book more useful in its subsequent editions.

**G K Pal**
**Pravati Pal**

# General Introduction

Education is the process that brings about desirable changes in the behaviour of the learner in the form of acquisition of knowledge, proficiency in skills and development of attitudes. Knowledge and skill should grow simultaneously and harmoniously. Knowledge without skill is useless and skill without knowledge is dangerous. Therefore, to become a good physician, a medical student should have knowledge, skill and proper attitude.

Physiology is a vast subject. Knowledge of physiology is used in all branches of medicine, from biochemistry and pharmacology to gynecology and medicine. A good physician is a good physiologist and vice versa. Knowledge of practical physiology is applied in clinical medicine to understand the pathophysiology of the disease, to explain the clinical manifestation of the disease, to provide the physiological basis of the diagnosis and treatment of the disease, and to assess the prognosis. In this book, we have tried to explain the clinical significance of the practicals, in addition to detailed descriptions of various physiological aspects of the topics. *This introduction will help you extract maximum benefit from the book.*

Each topic of this book has most of these sections: learning objectives, introduction, methods (including observation and result), discussion, OSPE and viva.

## Learning objectives

Objectives are to a student (or teacher) what blueprints are to an architect. Learning objectives give the student an idea of the desired competence in the form of acquisition of knowledge and skill. Unless these competencies are clearly stated, it cannot be known whether they are properly acquired. Objectives help the students organise their efforts to obtain the desired knowledge and skill. Therefore, each topic, whether theory or practical, must have learning objectives. The objectives should be relevant, unequivocal, observable, measurable and feasible.

A set of 'Learning Objectives' has been given at the beginning of each topic. The student should go through these objectives before performing the practical. The objectives are intended to inform the students what they must know and what is desirable for them to know. Accordingly, the learning objectives are divided into two categories. The first set of objectives provides what students must learn *(the minimum that they should learn)* by performing that practical and the second set of objectives describes what they may know *(it is better to learn this too, though it is not mandatory)*. In the latest recommendation by the Medical Council of India, it has been emphasised that teaching should be clinically based with clearly outlined objectives of what students must know and what is desirable for them to know. For physiology practicals, the students should read the objectives *before* starting the practical and should again look at them *after* completing the practical, to assess whether they have achieved the required skill and knowledge. The objectives that are described in this book are basic in nature. The teacher can modify these objectives according to the needs and the instructions of the university teaching curriculum.

## Introduction

It is desirable that the students have a basic knowledge of the topic before they perform the practical. It helps them understand the scientific basis and the importance of the practical. Every effort has been made to give a clear and concise theoretical explanation in this section. It introduces the topic and describes the important points of the methods. Therefore, the students should read this before they perform a practical.

## Methods

Under "Methods", a detailed description has been given of the different methodologies that are used widely in different laboratories. Each method contains four to five sub-sections—Principle, Requirements, Procedure, Precautions, Observation and Result. A brief description of the "Principle" of the method is given at the beginning. In "Requirements", the equipment and chemicals required to perform the test are listed and a brief description is given about the important equipment and chemicals. A short description is also given about the *use* of the equipment. In "Procedure", a detailed and stepwise description of how to perform the practical is given. Important steps are followed by a "Note", which describes the significance of that particular step. A list of important "Precautions" are given following the procedure. The methods that are usually not used but are important from the examination point of view (likely to be asked in the viva voce) are described briefly. A practical, unless done properly following the proper procedure and precautions, is likely to yield erroneous results. Therefore, the student should read and understand the procedure and precautions thoroughly before performing the practical.

## Discussion

"Discussion" gives details of the physiological and clinical significance of the practical. Only points that are pertinent to the practical have been included. Discussion of the result, merits and demerits of different methods, and practical implications of a specific test should be undertaken by the teacher only **after** the student has completed the practical and got the result. Therefore, the student should not read this section before performing the practical. However, *there must be discussion at the end of the practical* because only after a thorough and complete discussion does one gain complete practical knowledge.

## Viva

The questions that are usually asked in viva voce are described under 'Viva'. Answers to many of the questions are already given in the text; therefore, the answers are not repeated in this section. Answers to a few questions for which answers may not be found in the text are given in the viva section. Therefore, students must read all the questions and answers in the viva section, otherwise they may miss some important points.

# General Laboratory Instructions

A medical laboratory is the workshop that provides the knowledge and experience to develop practical skills and attitudes. To achieve this, the working atmosphere in the laboratory should be congenial to the teachers and students. For smooth and harmonious conduct of laboratory work, cooperation from the technical staff, attendants, students and teachers is of utmost importance.

## Instructions for students

Desire to learn, dedication to study, sincerity and cooperation in work, and a caring attitude are essential qualities in a medical student. The student should keep in mind the following:

1. Wear a clean and well-ironed white coat while working in the laboratory.
2. Bring the necessary equipment for hematology (disposable lancets, etc.), amphibian or experimental (dissecting instruments) and human practicals (stethoscope, knee hammer, etc.).
3. Have a basic theoretical knowledge of the concerned practical (the practical of that day). For this, read the introduction to each topic, before attending the instruction of the demonstrator or before performing the practical.
4. Pay due attention to the demonstration of the practical given by the instructor or teacher.
5. Check to see if the apparatus is working properly before starting the experiment.
6. Do not disturb the instruments that are not assigned to you or are not required for the practical.
7. For any technical assistance, take help from the appointed technician or the instructor without disturbing other students.
8. Handle the apparatus gently and carry out the experiment without damaging it.
9. Perform the practical step by step following the proper procedure and precautions. For this, refer to the method described for each practical.
10. After obtaining the observation, discuss with the teacher about the accuracy of the result, and about the physiological and clinical utility of the practical. For this, read the discussion section given under each topic.
11. Enter the observation and result in your practical record, and note the physiological and pathological variation in the parameters and also write the answers to the questions given.
12. After completing the practical, check whether you have achieved the minimum knowledge and skill prescribed. For this, refer to the list of learning objectives given for that practical.
13. Get the practical record checked by the teacher regularly.
14. Return the apparatus to the laboratory staff before leaving the laboratory.
15. Keep the practical record and book in good condition.

## Instructions for demonstrators

A medical educator has a dual ethical obligation: to produce competent health professionals for the society, and to improve the standard of the student under care. Teachers of practical physiology have two important roles to play. First, they should familiarise themselves with the objectives (both essential and desirable objectives) and select what the student should learn, and second, they should help facilitate the learning of the student. Teachers (demonstrators) should:

1. Wear a white coat while taking practical classes for the students.
2. Give proper direction to the students to follow the laboratory discipline.
3. Practise, read and understand the practical, before taking classes for the students.
4. Do the demonstration confidently and clearly, without confusion.
5. Emphasise and explain the important steps of the practical.
6. Pay equal attention to all the students.

7. Not be seen sitting idle in the laboratory.
8. Encourage students to express their difficulties without fear.
9. Try to detect and solve the individual practical problems of the students.
10. Explain the physiological and clinical importance of the practical.
11. Check and evaluate the practical record of the students regularly.
12. Give feedback to the students for their improvement.

CHAPTER 1

# Introduction to Hematology

## LEARNING OBJECTIVES

After studying this chapter, you will be able to:

- Define hematology.
- State the components of blood.
- Explain the functions of each component.
- Name the routine hematologic tests.
- List the source of collection of specimens used in a hematology laboratory.

You may also be able to:

- Describe the appearance of a blood specimen after centrifugation.
- Explain the significance of buffy coat.

## INTRODUCTION

Hematology is defined as the branch of science that deals with the study of blood. The word "hematology" is derived from the Greek words haima, meaning blood, and logos, meaning study. It is primarily concerned with the study of formed elements of blood. Blood is the fluid constituent of the body that flows through the vascular channels. The total volume of blood in a 70 kg adult is about 5.5 litres or 8 per cent of the body weight. About 45 per cent of this amount is composed of formed elements. Plasma constitutes about 5 per cent of the body weight.

## BLOOD COMPONENTS AND THEIR FUNCTIONS

Blood has two major components: cells and fluid (plasma).

### The Cellular Component

The cellular component consists of red blood cells (erythrocytes), white blood cells (leucocytes) and platelets (thrombocytes). The thrombocytes are the smallest (2–4 μm), the erythrocytes are medium-sized (7–8 μm), and the leucocytes are the largest of all the cells with a wide range (8–20 μm) of size. The red blood cells constitute the highest number of formed elements in the circulation (4.5–6 million /mm$^3$ of blood) followed by platelets (1.5–4 lakhs/mm$^3$ of blood) and leucocytes (4–11 thousand/mm$^3$ of blood). The **erythrocytes** help in transport of gases, that is, they carry oxygen from the lungs to the tissues and carbon dioxide from the tissues to the lungs. The **leucocytes** assist in the defence processes of the body. The **thrombocytes** assist in stoppage of bleeding (hemostasis). Development of blood cells is called *hemopoiesis*. In post-natal life (after birth), hemopoiesis occurs in the bone marrow.

### The Fluid Component

The fluid component of the blood is known as **plasma** which consists of a soluble protein called **fibrinogen**. During the process of coagulation of blood, fibrinogen is removed from plasma as fibrin, and the clear fluid left behind is called **serum**. Therefore, to obtain plasma for diagnostic tests, blood should not be allowed to clot.

**Plasma** Plasma is the principal medium for transportation of materials from one part of the body to another through the blood vessels. Plasma carries various substances: nutrients, metabolites, waste products, hormones, chemicals, and other substances. Plasma contains clotting factors that participate in blood coagulation.

**Serum** The serum contains most of the chemicals present in the plasma except fibrinogen and some clotting factors. Therefore, many investigations like estimations of glucose, proteins and lipids, are performed in serum, which is collected by clotting the blood.

## HEMATOLOGIC TESTS

Several hematologic tests are regularly performed as part of every patient's initial laboratory investigations.

Many of these tests are considered routine and can be done by a technician with limited training. These routine hematologic tests include estimation of hemoglobin, total RBC count, total leucocyte count, ESR and differential count of leucocytes. These tests are performed mainly to study the patient's ability to fight diseases. These tests also aid in diagnosis of diseases and help in assessing the prognosis.

Performing accurate hematologic tests, however, requires repeated practice. Many of the techniques require adequate skill and experience, especially for using instruments. In recent years, especially in advanced laboratories, many of these tests are performed by automated methods. However, in most clinical and medical college laboratories, tests are performed mainly by manual techniques.

A student should acquire enough knowledge about the formed elements of blood, their enumeration and their characteristics, to perform and analyse these tests accurately. They should therefore be knowledgeable about the formation, structure and functions of blood cells, the basic principle of determination, the use and care of equipment, the preparation of reagents, and the calculation and interpretation of results.

## SPECIMEN

Blood samples for hematologic study are usually obtained by finger puncture (capillary blood) or venipuncture (venous blood).

### Capillary Blood

Capillary blood can be used with good results for morphologic studies in hematology. Capillary blood is obtained from the finger tip, ear lobe, heel or big toe. In newborns and infants, blood is usually obtained by heel puncture because blood supply is limited in finger-tips and removing blood by venipuncture would deplete too much of their blood. In adults, the tip of any of the middle three fingers is punctured to obtain a sample.

### Venous Blood

It is not always advisable to obtain capillary blood, especially when a large quantity of blood is needed for hematologic tests. Venous blood is used for this purpose. Coagulation should be prevented as clotted blood cannot be used. For most hematologic studies, the anticoagulant used is EDTA (ethylenediamine tetra-acetic acid). This preserves the morphology of the cellular elements. It is important that the blood be mixed well with the anticoagulant immediately after it is collected to ensure proper anticoagulation. White cell count, microhematocrit, platelet count and sedimentation rates can be measured up to 24 hours after blood is collected in EDTA if it is refrigerated at 4°C. Immediately after collecting the blood, the sample should be gently mixed with anticoagulants by repeated inversion to ensure thorough contact of blood with the anticoagulant. The presence of even a tiny clot in a specimen may affect the result.

**Appearance** When the blood specimen has been properly drawn and preserved, the plasma will have its natural colour, a very light yellow or the colour of straw. In some diseased states, the plasma may have altered colour. But this can also result from improper handling of the specimen.

Two types of blood samples are *unsuitable for hematologic investigations*: (1) clotted samples and (2) samples that are hemolysed in the process of collection or handling.

If blood is collected, anticoagulated and allowed to settle or centrifuged, three layers will be observed (Fig. 1.1). The bottom layer will consist of packed red blood cells which make up 40–47 per cent of the total blood volume. On top of this layer is a thin whitish layer called **buffy coat**. This consists of leucocytes and platelets, and makes up about 1 per cent of the total volume. Abnormal cells like LE cells as found in SLE, and atypical mononuclear cells as found in malignant

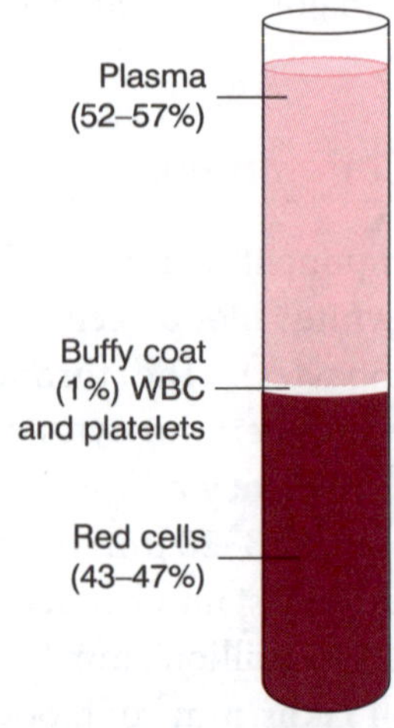


Fig. 1.1 Layers of normal blood after centrifugation.

conditions are detected in smears made from buffy coat. Buffy coat preparation is also useful for detection of bacteria, fungi and parasites within the circulating leucocytes. The uppermost layer is the colloidal liquid called plasma, which makes up 52–57 per cent of the total blood volume.

## VIVA

1. What is blood and what are its components?
2. What are the formed elements of blood and what are their functions?
3. What is the difference between plasma and serum?
4. How is the serum prepared in the laboratory?
5. What is the purpose of performing routine hematologic tests?
6. What are the types of specimens collected for hematologic tests?
7. Why are the middle three fingers preferred for skin puncture?
8. Why is venipuncture not used for collecting blood samples in newborns and infants?
9. Which is the ideal site for collecting blood in newborns and infants, and why?
10. Why is EDTA commonly preferred for collecting venous blood?
11 What is buffy coat and what is its significance?
12. Why should blood be properly mixed with anticoagulants immediately after collection?
13. What types of blood samples are unsuitable for hematologic tests and why?

Chapter 2

# Collection of Blood Samples

**Learning Objectives**

After completing this practical, you will be able to:

- List the general precautions for collecting blood.
- List the methods of collection of blood sample.
- Collect peripheral blood by finger prick method.
- List the precautions observed during collection of blood by finger prick method.
- Name the specific uses of commonly used anticoagulants in hematological procedures.

You may also be able to:

- Collect blood by the venipuncture method.
- List the precautions for the venipuncture method.
- List the steps of collection of blood by the earlobe puncture and heel puncture methods.
- Explain the mechanism of action and uses of various anticoagulants.

## INTRODUCTION

Blood is one of the most common specimens used in laboratory determinations. Venous blood is preferred for most hematological examinations. Peripheral samples (capillary blood) can be used satisfactorily for many purposes if a free flow of blood is obtained, but this procedure should be avoided in patients who may be possible carriers of transmissible diseases. Capillary blood is used commonly for hemoglobin estimation, cell counts, blood grouping, bleeding and clotting time determination, and other investigations that use less blood, whereas venous blood is preferred for a comprehensive hematological investigation.

### General Precautions

Because of the increasing risks of fatal transmissible diseases, the following precautions must be taken while collecting a blood sample from a patient.

1. Care must be taken to prevent injuries while handling syringes and needles.
2. Disposable rubber gloves should always be used while collecting blood samples. The operator must wear disposable plastic/rubber gloves, especially if the patient is uncooperative and if the operator has any cuts, abrasions or skin breaks on the hands.
3. It should be ensured that there is no leakage from the specimens (if collected in bottles or bags).

## METHODS OF COLLECTION

For physiology practicals, blood is often collected by pricking the tip of the finger. Therefore, collection of peripheral blood by finger puncture method (with details of steps and precautions) is described clearly in this chapter.

### Principle

There are two general sources of blood for clinical laboratory tests: peripheral (capillary) blood and venous blood. For small quantities of blood for hematologic investigations, the specimen is obtained from the capillary bed by puncturing the skin. The tip of the finger is the most common site for puncture. For larger quantities of blood, a puncture is made directly into a vein (phlebotomy) using a sterile syringe-and-needle collection system.

### Collection of Capillary (Peripheral) Blood

Capillary blood is often used for bedside investigations. But this blood is likely to give erroneous results if not collected properly; therefore, it should only be used when it is not possible to obtain venous blood. Free flow of blood is essential and only the very gentlest squeezing is permissible. Ideally, large drops of blood should exude slowly but spontaneously.

### Source

Blood can be obtained from the ear lobes or the finger tips of adults and older children, and from the heel or plantar surface of the big toe of infants. The ear lobe is not ideal for puncture as the flow of blood is slow and the concentration of cells and hemoglobin is more in ear lobe.

> Note: The blood obtained from the ear lobe contains a higher concentration of hemoglobin and more cells than from the finger tips or venous blood. Hence, it is not reliable for hemoglobin estimation and total leucocyte count. However, blood from the ear lobe is preferred for preparing blood films for differential count and to study leucocyte abnormalities, since larger cells are frequently trapped in the capillary bed of the ear lobe due to its slow circulation.

### Requirements

- Disposable sterile lancet (or 24G needle)
- Alcohol
- Dry gauze
- Slides or pipettes

Various types of disposable lancets are used for skin puncture. Non-disposable lancets are not recommended because of the risk of transmission of infectious pathogens. 24G disposable needles can be used if lancets are not available. The lancet is preferred to a needle because the puncture (depth and size of the wound) is effectively performed and well controlled with lancets.

## Procedure for Finger Puncture

1. Assemble the necessary equipment (lancet device, alcohol, dry gauze, slides).
2. Make the subject sit comfortably.
3. Put on disposable rubber gloves.
4. Select the finger tip suitable for puncture.

> Note: A finger tip free from calluses, infection, edema or cyanosis is ideal for puncture.

5. Warm the puncture site by rubbing it.

> Note: Warming the skin before puncturing improves circulation and ensures free flow of blood. This must always be done if the finger tip is cold.

6. Clean the skin of the tip of the finger by using cotton or a gauze piece touched with alcohol.

> Note: This removes dirt and makes the area relatively sterile.

7. Allow the area to dry. The subject can shake his finger in air to hasten drying.

> Note: The finger should not be punctured until the tip of the finger is completely dry, because of the following reasons.

   i) A blood drop does not form on the finger tip if it is not dry. Blood spreads sideways along with spirit. Formation of a spherical blood drop is essential for many procedures, especially for pipetting (sucking blood into the RBC, WBC or hemoglobin pipette).
   ii) Sterilisation by alcohol is effective only after it dries on the finger tip.
   iii) Blood cells are hemolysed when they come in contact with alcohol. Therefore, drying of the finger tip must be ensured for any investigation that requires study of cells.

8. Hold the finger firmly and make a quick puncture about 3–5 mm deep with the lancet.

> Note: The puncture should be at the middle of the tip, not too far down on the finger nor too close to the nail.

9. Wipe the first drop of blood using sterile dry gauze.

> Note: The first drop is diluted with tissue fluid and interferes with laboratory results, therefore it should be discarded. The succeeding drops are used for tests.

10. Allow the blood to flow slowly and freely. If it does not come out spontaneously, apply pressure gently so that a spherical drop is formed.

> Note: Squeezing (milking) the tip of the finger to draw blood must be strictly avoided, as it causes exudation of tissue fluid that dilutes the blood.

11. Rapidly collect blood and use immediately for laboratory study to prevent coagulation.
12. Once the blood sample is collected, give the subject a sterile, dry piece of gauze or cotton to hold over the puncture site until the bleeding stops.
13. Remove gloves and wash hands.

### Precautions

1. Always use sterile gloves if you are collecting blood from unknown subjects or patients.

2. Warm the portion by rubbing slightly as this improves circulation.
3. Disposable lancets should be used.
4. The tip of the lancet should not touch anything until it punctures the skin of the subject.
5. Do not squeeze, because this dilutes the blood with tissue fluid.
6. The first drop of blood should be discarded as it is diluted with tissue fluid.
7. It is preferable to puncture any of the middle three fingers, because the venous bursa (palmar fascia) of the thumb and the little finger are continuous with that of the limb, whereas the venous bursa of the middle three fingers are limited to the hand only. Therefore, if infection occurs following puncture it will be limited to the hands.

## Procedure for Ear Lobe Puncture

1. Select and warm (by gentle rubbing) the puncture site.
2. Clean the ear lobe with a cotton swab touched with spirit.
3. Make a quick puncture (to a depth of about 2 mm) of the ear lobe with the help of a sterile lancet.
4. Collect blood as it drops down spontaneously.
5. Apply pressure to stop bleeding.

## Procedure for Heel Puncture

1. Select, warm and clean the puncture site (Fig. 2.1).

> Note: Perform puncture only if the heel is really warm, otherwise it may need to be warmed in warm water.

2. Hold the heel firmly and puncture on the most medial or most lateral portions of the plantar surface.

> Note: The central plantar area and the posterior curvature should not be punctured in infants as this may cause injury to the underlying tarsal bones. The puncture should not be more than 2–4 mm deep.

3. Apply pressure to stop bleeding.

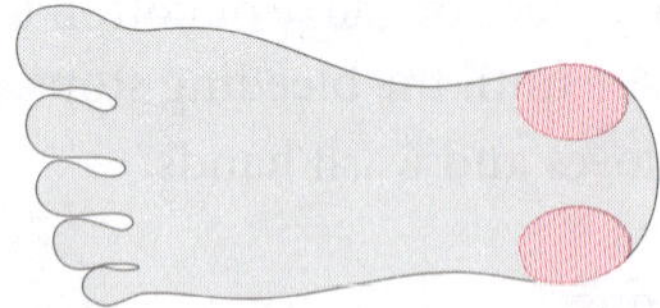

Fig. 2.1 Sites of heel puncture (striped areas). Middle of the heel is spared.

## Collection of Venous Blood

### Source

Venous blood is generally obtained by performing venipuncture of the veins of the forearm, wrist or ankle. This is best withdrawn from an antecubital (forearm) vein because the veins are larger and fuller than those in the wrist, hand or ankle. The wrist, hand and ankle veins are used only if the forearm site is not available. The median cubital vein is usually chosen for venipuncture because it does not roll or slip beneath the skin (Fig. 2.2).

### Requirements

1. Disposable syringe and needle
2. Alcohol
3. Sterile gauze or cotton
4. Collection bottle containing anticoagulant
5. Disposable gloves

### Procedure

Venipuncture should be performed with proper care and skill. The veins have to be made prominent by applying a tourniquet in the arm just above the elbow and just tight enough to stop blood flow. The subject should also be instructed to clench the fist to aid in building up the blood pressure in the area of the puncture.

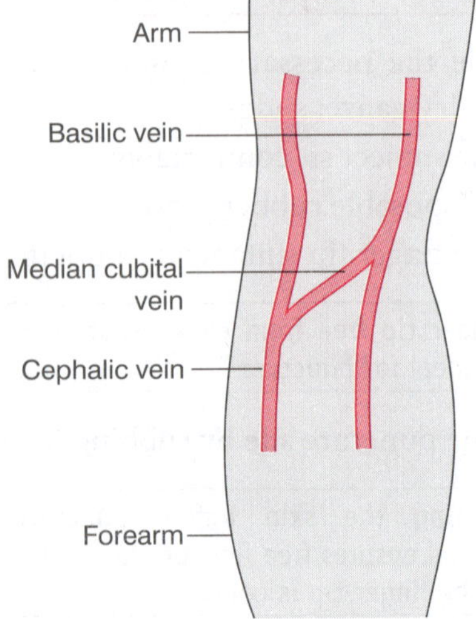


Fig. 2.2 Forearm veins. Median cubital vein is used for venipuncture.

1. Assemble all the materials required for blood collection, like disposable syringe and needle, alcohol, gauze or cotton, collection bottle, and so on.
2. Decide on the total amount of blood to be collected; for example, if a total hemogram is required, 2 ml of blood will be sufficient. Keep the required anticoagulant (details described below) in the collection bottle.
3. Wash your hands and put on sterilised/disposable gloves.
4. Reassure the subject. Ask him to sit alongside the table, keeping his arm on the table with palm facing upwards.

> **Note:** Never draw blood from a standing patient.

5. Select the puncture site carefully after inspecting the arm. Using the index finger of your left hand, feel for the vein where you will introduce the needle.
6. Make the vein prominent by asking the subject to clench his fist. If necessary, apply a tourniquet above the elbow.
7. Clean the area with cotton touched with alcohol.
8. Remove the syringe and needle from the protective wrap. Assemble them and see that the needle is fixed tightly with the syringe. Do not touch the needle.

> **Note:** Ensure that the needle is not blocked and the syringe does not contain air.

9. Grasp the elbow of the subject with your left hand and hold his arm fully extended. Anchor the vein with your thumb, drawing the skin tight over the vein to prevent it from moving.
10. Hold the syringe in the right hand and position the needle to keep the bevel upward, and then push it firmly and steadily into the centre of the vein. First enter the skin and then the vein, at a 30°– 40° angle.
11. Push the needle along the line of the vein to a depth of 1–1.5 cm.

> **Note:** As the needle enters the vein, there occurs a sudden loss of resistance.

12. Look for blood appearing in the barrel. Slightly pull back the piston and fill the syringe with the required amount of blood.
13. Ask the subject to relax and release the tourniquet.

> **Note:** Always remove the tourniquet before taking the needle out of the vein to prevent the formation of a hematoma.

14. Withdraw the needle from the vein in one rapid movement.
15. Ask the patient to press the site firmly with a cotton wool swab for 3–5 minutes.
16. Remove the needle from the syringe and gently expel the blood into the container. Mix the blood immediately and thoroughly but gently with anticoagulant to prevent clotting.
17. Immediately dispose the set (if disposable) or rinse the syringe and needle with water.
18. Before the subject leaves the laboratory, ascertain that the bleeding has stopped. Otherwise, ask him to continue to apply pressure until the bleeding stops.

### Precautions

1. The collection bottle containing anticoagulant should be kept ready before collecting blood.
2. The subject should be seated comfortably and should be reassured.
3. Disposable gloves should always be used to prevent contamination.
4. A disposable syringe and needle should be used to draw the blood.
5. The puncture site should be cleaned with alcohol.
6. The vein should be made prominent before making a puncture.
7. The needle should be held at an angle of 30°–40° and introduced into the vein steadily and firmly.
8. The tourniquet if applied should be removed before taking the needle out of the vein to prevent hematoma formation.
9. The patient should be instructed to press the puncture site for 3–5 minutes with cotton wool to prevent bleeding.
10. To prevent clotting, the blood from the syringe should be immediately transferred to the bottle containing anticoagulant.

## DISCUSSION

### Causes of Misleading Results Related to Specimen Collection

It is essential to have standard procedure for collection and handling of blood specimen, as the constituents of

Table 2.1 Factors that may alter the results due to improper collection procedure.

| |
|---|
| A. Precollection factors |
| 1. Physical activity like fast walking within 20 min |
| 2. Smoking within 1 hour |
| 3. Drugs within 8 hours or dietary supplement |
| 4. Food or water intake within 2 hours |
| 5. Urination within 30 min |
| 6. Stress |
| B. Factors during collection |
| 1. Excessive negative pressure when drawing blood into the syringe |
| 2. Incorrect type of tube |
| 3. Hemoconcentration due to prolonged application of tourniquet |
| 4. Time of collection (Morning/Day/Evening/Night): diurnal variation |
| 5. Posture (Standing/Sitting/Lying) |
| 6. Capillary blood versus venous blood |
| C. Improper handling of specimen |
| 1. Improper quantity (less or excess) of anticoagulant |
| 2. Inadequate mixing of blood with anticoagulant |
| 3. Delay in dispatch to laboratory |
| 4. Inadequate specimen storage condition |
| 5. Error in identification of patient |
| 6. Error in identification of specimen |

blood may alter due to faulty procedure of collection (Table 2.1).

## Differences Between Capillary and Venous Blood

The constituents of capillary and venous blood are not identical (Table 2.2). Though the blood obtained by skin puncture (capillary blood) is mainly the capillary blood, it also contains some quantity of a mixture of blood from arterioles and venules, and also the interstitial and intracellular fluid, whereas the blood of venipuncture is only the venous blood.

## Anticoagulants

Anticoagulants prevent blood from clotting. They are added to the blood sample, especially when blood is collected by venipuncture, and sent to the laboratories for investigation. Several anticoagulants are available, but some of the standard and commonly used anticoagulants in hematology are EDTA, trisodium citrate, double oxalate, sodium fluoride and heparin. EDTA is usually used in hematology while citrated blood is used for coagulation studies and in blood banks. Use of heparin and fluoride (oxalated) is limited to testing of blood gases (and pH) and plasma glucose respectively.

### EDTA (Ethylenediamine Tetra-acetic Acid)

This is also known as sequestrene or versene. The sodium and potassium salts of EDTA are powerful anticoagulants.

*Preparation*

Prepare a 10 per cent solution of dipotassium salts of EDTA. Dissolve 10 g of salt in about 80 ml of water in a 100 ml volumetric flask and then make up the volume of the solution to 100 ml. Dipotassium salts of EDTA are preferred over disodium salts of EDTA as the former are more soluble.

*Mechanism of Action*

EDTA acts by its chelating effect on the calcium molecules of the blood. Calcium is one of the important factors required in the coagulation process.

Table 2.2 Differences between capillary and venous blood.

| | Capillary blood | Venous blood |
|---|---|---|
| 1. Collection procedure | Skin puncture of finger tip, ear lobe, etc. | Venipuncture of superficial veins |
| 2. Type of specimen | Capillary blood mixed with small quantity of blood from arterioles and venules | Venous blood |
| 3. Contamination with tissue fluid | May contain tissue fluid, especially if the finger is squeezed to collect blood | Does not contain tissue fluid |
| 4. Difference in counts | PCV, RBC and Hb concentration of capillary blood are slightly less than that of venous blood. TLC and neutrophil counts are higher by 8%, and monocyte count by 12%, especially in children. | Platelet count is higher in venous blood than in capillary blood. This may be due to adhesion of platelets to the site of skin puncture. |
| 5. Preferred | When individual count or less number of counts are done | When more number of counts or complete hemogram is needed that requires more blood |

### *Effective Concentration*

To achieve the chelating effect, a concentration of 1.2 mg of the anhydrous salt per ml of blood is required. Excess of EDTA, irrespective of its salts, affects both red cells and leucocytes causing shrinkage and degenerative changes. If the concentration of the anticoagulant is high, it causes distortion of cells. EDTA in excess of 2 mg/ml of blood may result in a significant decrease in packed cell volume (PCV) by centrifugation and increase in mean cell hemoglobin concentration (MCHC). The platelets are also affected. They swell and then disintegrate causing an artificially high platelet count, as the fragments are large enough to be counted as normal platelets. Therefore, care must be taken to ensure that the correct amount of EDTA is added, and by repeated inversions of the container, the blood is thoroughly mixed with the anticoagulant.

### *Uses*

EDTA is suitable for all routine hematological investigations except coagulation studies.

## Sodium Citrate

Trisodium citrate (32 g/l, $Na_3C_6H_5O_7 \cdot 2H_2O$) is the anticoagulant of choice in coagulation studies.

### *Preparation*

It is prepared as a 0.106 M solution of trisodium citrate in distilled water and then sterilised.

### *Mechanism of Action*

Sodium citrate prevents coagulation by inactivating calcium ions (chelating effect).

### *Concentration*

Nine volumes of blood are added to one volume of sodium citrate (9 : 1) solution for anticoagulation studies. If it is used in estimation of ESR (erythrocyte sedimentation rate), four volumes of venous blood are added to one volume of the sodium citrate (4 : 1) solution.

### *Uses*

It is used for coagulation studies, including prothrombin times and partial thromboplastin tests, in blood banks, in the estimation of ESR, especially by the Westergren method.

## Double Oxalate

This is an anticoagulant containing ammonium oxalate and potassium oxalate. Therefore, it is called double oxalate. Potassium oxalate alone causes shrinkage of red cells whereas ammonium oxalate increases their volume. So, double oxalate is also called **balanced oxalate** as it preserves cell morphology.

### *Preparation*

Double oxalate is prepared as a solution containing 1.2 per cent ammonium oxalate and 0.8 per cent potassium oxalate. Double oxalate solution 0.25–0.5 ml is delivered into penicillin bottles and evaporated in an oven (60°C) or incubator (37°C) and then kept for collecting blood.

### *Mechanism of Action*

The oxalates in the anticoagulant form an insoluble complex with the calcium in the blood, and thereby inhibit coagulation. When calcium ions are combined with oxalate and are therefore not available to participate in clotting, the blood does not clot.

### *Uses*

This is used for estimation of ESR, PCV or investigations in which the volume of the cells should not be affected.

## Sodium Fluoride

This anticoagulant is used mainly for preparing blood specimens for plasma glucose estimation. Fluoride is an inhibitor of glycolytic enzymes and thus prevents loss of glucose. However, fluoride is not a strong anticoagulant, and hence, it is mixed with the oxalate.

## Oxalates

Oxalates of sodium, potassium, ammonium or lithium as dry additives act as anticoagulants. They form insoluble complexes with calcium and therefore calcium is not available to participate in clotting.

## Heparin

Heparin is, theoretically, the best anticoagulant because it is a natural constituent of blood and introduces no foreign contaminants into the blood specimen.

### *Preparation*

Sodium, lithium, potassium and ammonium salts of heparin are commercially available. Suitable concentration of stock solution is prepared and the required amount is taken in a penicillin bottle and dried at room temperature.

### *Mechanism of Action*

It prevents coagulation for approximately 24 hours by inhibiting the action of thrombin, thus preventing formation of fibrin from fibrinogen.

### *Concentration*

Heparin is used at a concentration of 10–20 IU/ml of blood. In this concentration, it does not alter the size of red cells.

### *Uses*

It is used for blood gas determination and pH assays. It is the best anticoagulant for the osmotic fragility test. It is inferior to EDTA for general use and should not be used for leucocyte count as it promotes clumping of the leucocytes. It is also not used for differential count as it gives a blue colour to the background.

## VIVA

1. Name the methods of blood collection.
2. Name the sites of skin puncture for collecting capillary blood.
3. What are the important precautions for finger-tip puncture?
4. Why are middle three fingers preferred for finger-tip puncture?
5. What are the advantages and disadvantages of ear lobe puncture?
6. What are the indications for heel puncture?
7. What are the veins that are preferred for venipuncture?
8. List the precautions for venipuncture.
9. List the factors that may alter the results of blood counts due to improper procedure of blood collection.
10. List the differences between capillary blood and venous blood.
11. Name different anticoagulants; give their mechanism of action and specific uses.

CHAPTER 3

# Estimation of Hemoglobin Concentration

## LEARNING OBJECTIVES

After completing this practical, you will be able to:

- Describe the clinical importance of estimation of hemoglobin.
- Estimate hemoglobin by Sahli's acid hematin method.
- List the precautions and sources of error of estimation of Hb.
- List the advantages and disadvantages of Sahli's method.
- Name the other methods for estimation of Hb.
- Give the normal values of Hb in males and females and in different age groups.
- List the functions of Hb.
- List the common conditions of decreased and increased Hb concentration in the blood.
- Define anemia.
- List the common causes of anemia in developing countries.

You may also be able to:

- Describe the synthesis and structure of Hb.
- Classify Hb.
- Describe different complexes and derivatives of Hb.
- Explain the principle of other methods of Hb estimation.
- Compare the merits and demerits of different methods.
- Explain the variation of Hb concentration in different conditions.
- Briefly describe different types of anemia.

## INTRODUCTION

Hemoglobin (Hb) is a conjugated protein present in red blood cells. It carries $O_2$ from the lungs to the tissues, and $CO_2$ from the tissues to the lungs. It is made up of heme and globin. The heme group is an iron complex containing one iron atom. Iron is essential for the primary function of hemoglobin, i.e., the transport of oxygen. When reduced hemoglobin is exposed to oxygen at increased pressure, oxygen is taken up at the iron atom until each molecule of hemoglobin has bound four oxygen molecules, one molecule at each iron atom. This is not a true oxidation–reduction reaction, and therefore, the combination of hemoglobin with oxygen is known as **oxygenation**. When the Hb molecule is fully saturated with oxygen, that is, when four oxygen molecules combine with one hemoglobin molecule, it is called **oxyhemoglobin**. One gram of hemoglobin carries 1.34 ml of oxygen. Hemoglobin returning with carbon dioxide from the tissues is called **reduced hemoglobin.**

### Synthesis and Structure of Hemoglobin

Hemoglobin is made up of two components: heme and globin. It is synthesised in the precursors of red cells during their development in the bone marrow. It appears in the early normoblast stage and attains maximum concentration in the late normoblast stage (for details, refer Chapter 7).

#### Heme

Heme is a complex molecule, made up of a series of **tetrapyrrole** rings, terminating in **protoporphyrin**, with a central iron atom. After their normal lifespan (120 days), the red cells are destroyed by the reticuloendothelial cells especially in the spleen, and the components of hemoglobin undergo metabolic degradation. The iron part of heme is recycled and used up again in hemoglobin synthesis. The only component of Hb that cannot be recycled is protoporphyrin, which forms *bilirubin*. Bilirubin is finally converted to various bile salts and pigments.

#### Globin

Globin is a protein substance that consists of four chains of amino acids (polypeptides). Each polypeptide chain is attached to a heme moiety to form a single hemoglobin molecule. After the degradation of hemoglobin, the globin component breaks down into its amino acid constituents that are recycled for hemoglobin synthesis.

### Types of Hemoglobin

Hemoglobins can be broadly divided into normal and abnormal types.

**Normal Hb** Adult Hb, Fetal Hb and Embryonic Hb.

**Abnormal Hb** HbS, HbC, HbD, HbE and Unstable hemoglobins.

## Normal Hemoglobins

### *Adult Hemoglobins*

**Hemoglobin A (HbA)** About 97 per cent of hemoglobins of adult red cells is HbA. It consists of two $\alpha$ and two $\beta$ chains with the structural formula $\alpha_2\beta_2$. HbA is detected in small amounts in the fetus as early as the eighth week of intrauterine life. During the first few months of postnatal life, HbA almost completely replaces HbF and the adult pattern is fully established in six months.

**Hemoglobin A2 (HbA2)** This is the minor hemoglobin in the adult red cell. It has the structural formula $\alpha_2\delta_2$. HbA2 is present in very small amounts at birth and reaches the adult level of 3 per cent during the first year of life. Its concentration increases in some types of anemia.

### *Fetal Hemoglobins*

**Fetal hemoglobin (HbF)** HbF is the major hemoglobin in intrauterine life. It has the structural formula $\alpha_2\gamma_2$. HbF accounts for 70–90 per cent of hemoglobins at term. It then falls rapidly to 25 per cent in one month, and 5 per cent in six months. The adult level of 1 per cent is not reached in some children until puberty. HbF concentration in adults increases in some types of anemia, hemoglobinopathies and sometimes in leukemia.

**Hemoglobin Bart's (Hb Bart's)** This is the minor hemoglobin present in fetal life. It consists of four gamma ($\gamma$) chains, $\gamma_4$. Hb Bart's concentration increases in fetal life in thalassemia.

### *Embryonic Hemoglobins*

These hemoglobins are confined to the very early stages (the embryonic stage) of development. There are three embryonic hemoglobins:

1. **Hb Gower 1** (consisting of two zeta and two epsilon chains: $\zeta_2\varepsilon_2$),
2. **Hb Gower 2** (consisting of two alpha and two epsilon chains: $\alpha_2\varepsilon_2$), and
3. **Hb Portland** (consisting of two zeta and two gamma chains: $\zeta_2\gamma_2$).

## Abnormal Hemoglobins

There are four clinically important abnormal hemoglobins: HbS, HbC, HbD and HbE. These are present in different hereditary hemoglobinopathies. The most commonly encountered hemoglobin is HbS, which consists of $\alpha_2\beta_2$, but in the beta chain, valine is substituted for glutamic acid at the sixth position. HbS is present in sickle cell anemia.

**Unstable hemoglobins** are hemoglobin variants that undergo denaturation and precipitate in the red cells as *Heinz bodies*. Unstable hemoglobins are present in a type of congenital non-spherocytic hemolytic anemia.

# Hemoglobin Complexes

Hb can combine with other substances besides oxygen, some normally and some abnormally.Some of these commonly encountered complexes are carbaminohemoglobin, carboxyhemoglobin, methemoglobin, sulfhemoglobin and cyanmethemoglobin.

## Carbaminohemoglobin

When $CO_2$ combines with Hb, carbaminohemoglobin is formed. $CO_2$ combines with amino groups in the polypeptide chains of globin, not with heme. It helps in the transport of $CO_2$ from tissues to lungs.

## Carboxyhemoglobin

When hemoglobins combine with carbon monoxide (CO), carboxyhemoglobin is formed. Hemoglobin has a much greater affinity for CO than for oxygen. Therefore, it readily combines with CO even when CO is present in low concentration. Fortunately the formation of carboxyhemoglobin is reversible, so, once CO is removed from the blood, the hemoglobin combines with oxygen. Carboxyhemoglobin is found in very low concentrations in normal persons, but in smokers, its concentration is in the range of 1–10 g/dl, which impairs transport of oxygen from lungs to tissues.

## Methemoglobin

Methemoglobin is an abnormal Hb in which iron is oxidised from its ferrous state to ferric state. Therefore, it is incapable of carrying oxygen. Normally, it is present in low concentration, but its formation increases in the presence of certain chemicals or drugs. The formation of methemoglobin is also reversible.

## Sulfhemoglobin

This is an abnormal Hb complex formed by the action of some drugs and chemicals such as sulphonamides.

Once it is formed, it is irreversible and remains in the carrier RBC. It is incapable of transporting oxygen.

### Cyanmethemoglobin (Hemiglobincyanide)

This is formed by the action of a chemical called cyanide (for example, potassium cyanide, KCN). The combination is reversible. Hemiglobin is the hemoglobin in which the iron has been oxidised to the ferric state. Hemiglobincyanide is the methemoglobin bonded to cyanide ions.

> **Note:** To accurately measure the total Hb in the blood, it is essential to prepare a stable derivative that will contain all the Hb forms (complexes) that are present in the blood. All forms of circulating hemoglobin are readily converted to hemoglobincyanide (cyanmethemoglobin), except for sulphhemoglobin which is normally not present in the blood. Therefore, the *cyanmethemoglobin method is the most accurate method* for the determination of hemoglobin.

## Hemoglobin Derivatives

When red blood cells are destroyed in the tissue macrophage system, hemoglobin is degraded into heme and globin. Globin returns to the body's metabolic pool where its amino acids are subsequently reutilised. The porphyrin ring of heme is cleaved by the microsomal enzyme, heme oxidase, yielding *biliverdin*. The biliverdin is further reduced to form *bilirubin* by biliverdin reductase.

## Normal Values

Adult males : 14–18 (16 ± 2) g/dl of blood
Adult females : 12–16 (14 ± 2) g/dl of blood

In newborns, hemoglobin concentration is normally 16–22 g/dl. It decreases to 9–14 g/dl by about two months of age. By ten years of age, the normal hemoglobin concentration will be 12–14 g/dl. There may be a decrease in hemoglobin level after 60 years of age.

## Functions of Hemoglobin

Hemoglobin serves two important functions: the transport of gases and pH homeostasis. However, Hb also contributes to tissue blood flow.

1. It transports oxygen from the lungs to the tissues by forming oxyhemoglobin, and carbon dioxide from the tissues to the lungs by forming carbaminohemoglobin. When fully saturated, *1 g of hemoglobin carries 1.34 ml of oxygen*.
2. Hemoglobin acts as an important buffer in maintaining blood pH. In fact, Hb is an important non-bicarbonate buffer system of the body.
3. Hb to some extent contributes to regulation of tissue blood flow. Hb has sufficient affinity for another gas in the blood, nitric oxide (NO), which is a strong vasodilator. In the tissue, as Hb picks up NO, vasoconstriction occurs due to relative decrease in NO concentration, which in turn decreases tissue blood flow. In the lungs, Hb picks up super nitric oxide (SNO) and by altering SNO level, controls pulmonary blood flow. However, the role of Hb in the regulation of systemic blood volume, peripheral resistance and blood pressure is negligible.

# METHODS

The different methods of estimation of hemoglobin can be classified under the following categories:

**I. Visual methods**
1. Sahli's method
2. Dare's method
3. Haden's method
4. Wintrobe's method
5. Haldane's method
6. Tallquist's method

**II. Gasometric method**

**III. Spectrophotometric method**
1. Oxyhemoglobin method
2. Cyanmethemoglobin method

**IV. Automated hemoglobinometry**

**V. Non-automated hemoglobinometry**

**VI. Other methods**
1. Alkaline-hematin method
2. Specific gravity method
3. Comparator method

Visual methods are more commonly used than photometric methods. In Sahli's method, hemoglobin in the blood sample is converted to acid hematin which gives a brown colour. Since brown is more easily *matched* by the human eye than red (the colour of Hb), Sahli's method for testing hemoglobin is one of the most acceptable visual methods. However, the error in visual methods is higher. Therefore, visual methods are usually not recommended for hemoglobin estimation in research. But, because visual methods (especially Sahli's) are convenient and the cost of estimation is less, they are usually practised in clinical hematology laboratories and by students performing physiology practicals in medical colleges.

## Sahli's Acid Hematin Method

### Principle

Hemoglobin is converted to acid hematin by the action of HCl. The acid hematin solution is further diluted until its colour exactly matches that of the permanent standard of the comparator block. The hemoglobin concentration is read directly from the calibration tube.

### Requirements

1. **Sahli's hemoglobinometer** This contains a comparator, hemoglobin tube, hemoglobin pipette and stirrer.

   *Comparator* At the middle there is a slot which accommodates the hemoglobin tube. Non-fading, standard, brown-tinted glass pieces are provided on either side of the slot for colour matching. An opaque white glass is fitted at the back to provide uniform illumination (Fig. 3.1).

   *Hemoglobin tube* It is graduated on one side in gram per cent (g%), from 2 to 24, and on the other side as percentage (%), from 10 to 140. This tube is called the Sahli–Adams tube.

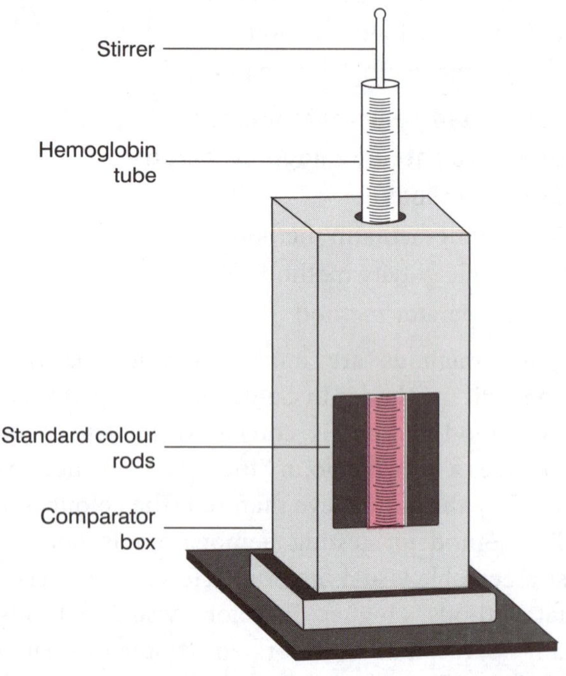


Fig. 3.1 Hemoglobinometer.

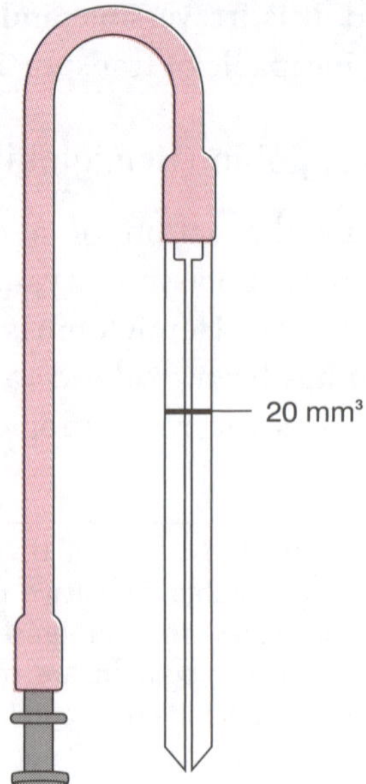


Fig. 3.2 The hemoglobin pipette.

   *Hemoglobin pipette* The pipette bears only one mark indicating 20 mm$^3$ (0.02 ml) (Fig. 3.2). There is no bulb in this pipette.

   *Stirrer* It is a thin glass rod used for stirring the solution.
2. N/10 HCl
3. Distilled water
4. Dropper
5. Materials for a sterile finger prick

### Procedure

1. Clean the hemoglobinometer tube and pipette and ensure that they are dry.
2. Fill the hemoglobinometer tube with N/10 HCl up to its lowest mark (10 per cent or 2 g%) with the help of a dropper.
3. Prick the finger observing all aseptic precautions, and discard the first drop of blood.

> **Note:** The prick should be deep enough to enable spontaneous flow of blood. Do not squeeze the finger to bring out the drop of blood.

4. Allow a large drop of blood to form on the finger tip, then dip the tip of the hemoglobinometer pipette into the drop and suck blood up to the 20 cu. mm mark of the pipette.

> Note: While sucking blood into the pipette, care should be taken to prevent entry of air bubbles. This is done by not lifting the tip of the pipette out of the blood drop during pipetting. If an air bubble enters, remove and discard the blood and obtain another drop of blood to re-pipette. If blood is sucked above the 20 mm$^3$ mark of the pipette, bring the blood column down to the mark by tapping the pipette against the finger, but not by using any absorbent material like cotton wool.

5. Wipe the tip of the pipette. Immediately transfer the 0.02 ml of blood from the pipette into the hemoglobinometer tube containing N/10 HCl by immersing the tip of the pipette in the acid solution and blowing out blood from the pipette. Rinse the pipette two to three times by drawing up and blowing out the acid solution. Withdraw the pipette from the tube.

> Note: Make sure that no solution remains in the pipette.

6. Leave the solution in the tube in the hemoglobinometer, for about ten minutes (for maximum conversion of hemoglobin to acid hematin, which occurs in the first ten minutes).
7. After ten minutes, dilute the acid hematin by adding distilled water drop by drop. Mix it with the stirrer. Match the colour of the solution in the tube with the standards of the comparator.

> Note: After addition of every drop of distilled water, the solution should be mixed and the colour of the solution should be compared with the standard. While matching, take care to hold the stirrer above the level of the solution. However, remember that at no stage should the stirrer be taken out of the tube.

8. If the colour of the test solution is darker, continue dilution till it matches that of the standard.
9. Note the reading when the colour of the solution exactly matches the colour of the standard and express the hemoglobin content as g%.

> Note: The reading of the lower meniscus of the solution should be noted as the result. One more drop of distilled water should be added and the colour should be observed to check the result. The colour will be lighter than the standard if the previous reading was accurate.

## Precautions

1. Do not take a large volume of N/10 HCl (not above the 20 per cent mark) in the tube. This is because, in cases of severe anemia, the final colour produced will be lighter than that of the standard if more HCl is taken, and there is no way to concentrate the colour.
2. The pricking should be done boldly; do not squeeze the finger as the tissue fluid comes out with the blood and gives a false low result.
3. The first drop of blood should be discarded as it is mixed with tissue fluid.
4. Suck blood exactly up to the 20 mm$^3$ mark.
5. Wipe the tip of the pipette before transferring blood from the pipette to the hemoglobinometer tube. Otherwise the extra blood adhering to the tip of the pipette will give a false high result.
6. Blood should be immediately transferred from the pipette into the tube containing HCl to prevent clotting in the pipette.
7. While transferring the blood, the pipette should be rinsed several times to remove all blood from the pipette.
8. Wait for a minimum of ten minutes after mixing blood with HCl, for complete conversion of hemoglobin into acid hematin.
9. The colour of the acid hematin solution should be checked frequently (preferably after addition and mixing of every drop of distilled water), to prevent overdilution.
10. When you compare the colour of the solution in the tube with that of the standard, keep the stirrer above the solution, but do not take it out of the tube. If the stirrer is taken out of the tube, the solution sticking to the stirrer will be lost and will give a false low result. If the stirrer remains in the solution, the colour of the solution becomes lighter.
11. Comparison should always be done by holding the hemoglobinometer at eye level, at full arm length and against good light. The tube should be placed in the comparator in such a way that the graduations on it do not lie directly in front, which may interfere with the matching of colour.

## Sources of Error

### *A. Technical Errors*

i) Blood should be taken up exactly to the 20 mm$^3$ mark and the tip of the pipette should be wiped off before introducing the blood into the HCl taken in the hemoglobinometer tube.

ii) Ten minutes should be allowed for complete conversion of Hb into acid hematin.
iii) The solution should be diluted till the colour exactly matches that of the standard.

*B. Errors Inherent in the Method*

i) As it is a visual method, the matching of the colour may vary.
ii) It may not detect all types of hemoglobins in the blood.
iii) The colour of the standard may fade.

### Reporting

As the hemoglobinometer tube has % markings on one side and g% markings on the other, the hemoglobin estimated can be reported as either of the values, that is, % of normal or g%. Usually, hemoglobin is reported as grams of hemoglobin per 100 ml of blood (g/dl or g%). Reporting hemoglobin as a percentage of the normal value is not satisfactory, because there are many methods and each method has its own standard of normal value. For example, 80 per cent of normal of one method may be 98 per cent of normal of another. The values for 100 per cent hemoglobin in five different testing methods are as follows:

| | |
|---|---|
| Sahli | 16.3 g/dl |
| Dare | 16.0 g/dl |
| Haden | 15.6 g/dl |
| Wintrobe | 14.5 g/dl |
| Haldane | 13.8 g/dl |

Therefore, if it is reported as a per cent of the normal, the method by which it is estimated should also be mentioned.

### Advantages

1. Sahli's method is easy to perform and convenient.
2. The cost is minimal.
3. It is not very time-consuming (maximum fifteen minutes).

### Disadvantages

1. Being a visual method, error is very likely (about 5–10 per cent). Error can be reduced by taking the average of three readings; first, when the colour is slightly darker than the standard; second, when the colour exactly matches the standard; and the third, when the colour is slightly lighter than the standard.
2. The colour of the standard may not always be reliable, especially if an old apparatus was used.
3. Sahli's acid hematin method does not estimate all the hemoglobins. It estimates only oxyhemoglobin and reduced hemoglobins, but not the carboxyhemoglobin, methemoglobin and sulfhemoglobin.
4. The acid hematin is not a true solution. Some degree of precipitation may be present at times, which may interfere with colour matching.

## Other Methods

### Gasometric Method

The gasometric method of estimation of hemoglobin by using van Slyke apparatus is the *most accurate* method. But it is not used routinely in clinical laboratories because it is time-consuming and the process of estimation is complex. It is used as a reference method to obtain the hemoglobin concentration in blood samples used for standardisation of hemoglobin estimation procedures. This is the preferred method for research.

### Spectrophotometric Method

These methods are rapid and give accurate results.

*a) Oxyhemoglobin Method*

Ammonium hydroxide (0.04 ml/dl) is used to hemolyse the red cells and convert the hemoglobin to oxyhemoglobin for measurement in the spectrophotometer. This conversion is complete and immediate and the resulting colour is stable.

*b) Cyanmethemoglobin Method*

Modified Drabkin's reagent is used in this method. Drabkin's reagent contains sodium bicarbonate, potassium ferricyanide and potassium cyanide. This reagent takes at least ten minutes for complete conversion of hemoglobin to cyanmethemoglobin. It also produces turbid solutions caused by protein precipitation or incomplete hemolysis. In modified Drabkin's reagent, potassium phosphate is used for sodium bicarbonate, which shortens the conversion time to three minutes, minimises turbidity and enhances red cell lysis.

### Automated Hemoglobinometry

Various automated techniques have been employed to measure hemoglobin. Automatic pipettors and dilutors are used for pipetting and diluting blood in many procedures. Hemoglobin estimation by an automated instrument applies the same principle as that described for manual methods.

### Non-automated Hemoglobinometry

Disposable, self-filling, self-measuring dilution micropipettes are commercially available for the determination of hemoglobin. One such system is the Unopette. These systems are easy to use and are available with a series of different diluting fluids for different purposes.

The **Unopette system** for hemoglobin determination consists of a self-filling, self-measuring pipette attached to a plastic holder. The pipette is filled with blood automatically by capillary action. A plastic container called a reservoir is filled with modified Drabkin's reagent. The pipette containing blood is inserted into the reagent reservoir, emptied and rinsed according to the manufacturer's instructions. The blood is mixed well with the reagent and is then ready to be read in the spectrophotometer.

### Alkaline Hematin Method

The alkaline hematin method is a useful ancillary method, used under special circumstances as it gives a true estimate of total hemoglobin including methemoglobin and sulfhemoglobin. A true solution is obtained, and plasma proteins and lipids have little effect on the colour. The principle is to convert hemoglobin into alkaline hematin, which is in the true solution. There are two methods: the standard method, and the acid-alkaline method.

### Specific Gravity Method

This method uses the principle that when a drop of whole blood is dropped into a solution of copper sulphate, which has a given specific gravity, the drop will maintain its own density for approximately 15 seconds. The density of the drop is directly proportional to the amount of hemoglobin in that drop. If that drop is denser than the specific gravity of the solution, the drop will sink to the bottom; if not, it will float on the surface. It is not a quantitative test. However, it is a quick, easy and reasonably accurate technique to screen blood donors for possible anemia. It is also used to detect hematocrit.

### Comparator Method

This is a visual method similar to that of the acid hematin method, except that the diluent used is an alkali solution (ammonia solution 0.04 per cent). After mixing with dilute ammonia solution, the intensity of the colour of the hemolysed solution of red blood cells is compared against a standard colour disc in the comparator. This method carries all the disadvantages of Sahli's acid hematin method.

### Tallquist Method

This method involves direct visual matching of the red colour of a drop of whole fresh blood on a filter paper with colour standards on a paper. This technique is totally unsatisfactory with a high degree of error, though it is one of the quickest methods.

### Haldane Method

In this method, hemolysis of red cells is produced by mixing blood with a hypotonic solution like distilled water. Carbon monoxide is added to the mixture. The colour of the solution is compared with the standard one.

## DISCUSSION

### Physiological Significance

Hemoglobin is present in red blood cells and it forms more than 90 per cent of the dry weight of these cells. Erythrocytes appear red due to the presence of hemoglobin, which is a red pigment. The primary function of hemoglobin is to carry oxygen from the lungs to the tissues. Therefore, in conditions of hemoglobin deficiency, the tissues suffer from hypoxia. When hemoglobin is released into the plasma, as seen in hemolysis, it is filtered through the renal tubules and appears in the urine (hemoglobinuria). Hemoglobin casts block the renal tubules and cause acute tubular necrosis (acute renal failure). Hemoglobin in the blood (hemoglobinemia) exerts an osmotic effect and increases blood viscosity that affects cardiac output and alters the dynamics of blood flow.

## Clinical Significance

Estimation of hemoglobin is the most frequently ordered laboratory test in clinical practice. It is done as part of routine investigation in outpatient departments and also as a bedside test in hospital patients. It is mandatory to check the hemoglobin status of a patient prior to any surgical intervention. Estimation of hemoglobin is usually done to detect anemia because it is convenient and less time-consuming than the total RBC count. Anemia is said to be present when the hemoglobin level in the blood is below the lower limit of the normal range for the age and sex of the individual. The value of hemoglobin must always be in the normal range appropriate for the age and sex of the individual.

## Conditions that Alter Hemoglobin Concentration

### Conditions that Decrease Hb Concentration

**I. Physiological**

1. Pregnancy (due to hemodilution).
2. Children have lower values than adults.
3. Women have lower values than men because the total RBC count is less in women. This is because estrogen inhibits erythropoiesis in females and there is cyclical loss of blood in women in the reproductive age group, while testosterone stimulates erythropoiesis in males.

**II. Pathological**

1. Different types of anemia
2. Relative decrease in Hb concentration occurs in different pathological conditions that produce hemodilution as for example, excess ADH secretion as seen in pituitary tumours.

### Conditions that Increase Hb Concentration

**I. Physiological**

1. High altitude (due to hypoxia)
2. Newborns and infants
3. Excessive sweating (due to hemoconcentration)

**II. Pathological**

1. Conditions that produce hemoconcentration (due to loss of body fluid); for example, severe diarrhea, vomiting
2. Conditions that produce hypoxia; for example, congenital heart disease, emphysema
3. Polycythemia vera

## Types of Anemia

Anemia is defined as decreased Hb content or RBC count below the range that is normal for the age and gender. Anemia is classified in two ways, morphologically (according to red blood cell indices) and etiologically (according to the cause).

### Morphological Types

#### *1. Hypochromic Microcytic Anemia*

The values of MCV, MCH and MCHC are below normal. Such subnormal red cell indices correspond to microcytosis and hypochromia of red cells in the blood film. This is due to a defect in red cell formation in which hemoglobin synthesis is impaired to a greater extent than the synthesis of other cellular components. The most important examples are *iron deficiency anemia* in which there is inadequate iron for formation of the heme component of the hemoglobin, and *thalassemia* in which the formation of the globin component of hemoglobin is defective.

#### *2. Normochromic Normocytic Anemia*

MCV, MCH and MCHC are within the normal range. The size and hemoglobin concentration of the red cells are normal in the blood film. It usually occurs:

i) In substantial blood loss (*blood loss anemia*),
ii) In hemolysis (*hemolytic anemia*) and
iii) When red cell production is impaired by bone marrow failure, chronic kidney failure, chronic inflammation or infection (*aplastic anemia*).

#### *3. Macrocytic Anemia*

The MCV is above the upper limit of the normal. It corresponds to macrocytosis of red cells in the blood film. The red cells are usually normochromic. A classical example of this type of anemia is **megaloblastic anemia**, which occurs due to deficiency of vitamin $B_{12}$ or folic acid.

### Etiological Types

1. Blood loss
2. Impaired red cell production

- Inadequate supply of nutrients (deficiency of iron, vitamins and proteins)
- Aplastic anemia
- Anemia associated with chronic diseases
- Anemia associated with renal failure
- Anemia due to inherited diseases (for example, thalassemia)

3. Excessive red cell destruction (hemolysis)

## VIVA

1. What is the normal value of hemoglobin in an adult?
2. Why is the hemoglobin content of blood lower in women?
3. What is the principle of hemoglobin estimation in Sahli's acid hematin method?
4. What difference would it make if N/10 HCl is taken above the 20 per cent mark?
   Ans. If more HCl is taken, the colour of the undiluted solution may be lighter than the standard, especially if there is severe anemia.
5. Can N/10 HCl be used for dilution?
   Ans. Yes, because it will not change the colour of the solution. However, tap water should not be used as it causes turbidity and interferes with the colour of the solution.
6. Why is the result preferably expressed in g/dl rather than in per cent?
7. What are the precautions to be observed during hemoglobin estimation?
8. Why should the stirrer be kept above the solution, but not taken out of the tube while matching the colour?
9. Why should the tip of the pipette be wiped before transferring blood from the pipette into the N/10 HCl in the tube?
10. Why should absorbent material not be used for adjusting the level to the 20 $mm^3$ mark, if more blood is sucked into the pipette?
11. Why should ten minutes be allowed before diluting the solution of blood and HCl?
12. What are the advantages and disadvantages of Sahli's acid hematin method? What are the possible errors in this method?
13. What are the other methods of hemoglobin estimation?
14. What is the quickest method of hemoglobin estimation?
    Ans. The quickest method is Tallquist's method as it only compares the colour of the blood with that of the standard. However, it is not an accurate method.
15. Which method is more accurate for hemoglobin estimation, and why?
    Ans. The most accurate method is the gasometric method using van Slyke apparatus. But because it is time-consuming and complicated, it is not routinely used in laboratories. Of the routinely used tests, the most accurate method is the cyanmethemoglobin method, because it detects all forms of hemoglobin including sulfhemoglobin and methemoglobin.
16. What are the functions of hemoglobin?
17. What is the oxygen-carrying capacity of hemoglobin?
18. What are the types of hemoglobins?
19. What is the structure of normal adult hemoglobin (HbA)?
20. At what stage in erythropoiesis does hemoglobin appear in the red cells?
    Ans. Hemoglobin appears in the early normoblast stage of erythropoiesis; then the concentration increases and attains its maximum in the late normoblast stage.
21. What is the fate of hemoglobin in the body?
22. What is anemia? What are the types of anemia?
23. What is the most common cause of anemia in developing countries like India and why?
24. Give a physiological cause for anemia. What is the physiological basis of anemia in this condition?
25. What is megaloblastic anemia and how is it produced?
26. What is pernicious anemia?
27. What is aplastic anemia?

Chapter 4

# Determination of Hematocrit

## Learning Objectives

After completing this practical, you will be able to:

- Explain the importance of determination of hematocrit in clinical medicine.
- Name the methods of determination of hematocrit.
- Identify the Wintrobe tube.
- Fill the Wintrobe tube properly with the blood provided.
- Determine PCV by the Wintrobe method.
- List the possible sources of error in this method.
- List the normal values of PCV in men and women.
- Name the common conditions in which PCV is altered.

You may also be able to:

- Describe the microhematocrit method for determination of PCV.
- State the principle and advantages of determination of hematocrit by automated methods.
- List the physiological bases of alteration.

## INTRODUCTION

Hematocrit literally means "blood separation." It measures the percentage of volume of packed red cells. Therefore, hematocrit is also known as packed cell volume (PCV). Hematocrit is a reliable index of the red cell population in the blood. The manually estimated PCV is more reliable than the manually performed red cell count, because much less error is associated with determination of hematocrit. It provides valuable information about the red cells. Therefore, it should always be correlated with the number of red cells and their hemoglobin content. The hematocrit is used in the detection and classification of various types of anemias along with other parameters (hemoglobin and red cell count) of red cell indices.

**Normal Values**

| | |
|---|---|
| Adult male | : 46% (40–50%) |
| Adult female | : 42% (37–47%) |

## METHODS

Two manual methods are used for determining hematocrit: the macrohematocrit method and the microhematocrit method. The microhematocrit method has the advantages of using less time and labour, and requiring less blood. The macrohematocrit method is known as the Wintrobe method. Hematocrit is also measured by automated techniques; these have virtually replaced the manual methods in advanced laboratories.

### Macrohematocrit Method (Wintrobe Method)

Since a large volume of blood is needed in this procedure, only venous blood can be used.

#### Principle

Anticoagulated blood is taken in a Wintrobe tube, filled to the graduation mark and then centrifuged for the prescribed length of time. The volume of packed cells is read directly from the graduation mark on the Wintrobe tube.

#### Requirements

**I. Apparatus**

1. *Wintrobe tube* This is a 110-mm-long, narrow, thick-walled test tube with a 3 mm internal bore, graduated from 0 to 10 cm (100 mm) with graduations both in ascending and descending order on the two sides of the tube (Fig. 14.2). Thus, at the top, 0 and 10 cm coincide. The scale with the markings 0–10 from above downwards is used in ESR determination, while the scale with 0–10 from below upwards is used for hematocrit determination. It holds about 1 ml of blood.
2. *Centrifuge machine* The centrifuge should be capable of producing a force of 2300 *g*. A force of less

than 2300 *g* will give a false high hematocrit reading; conversely, an excessive force may lead to false low values. The centrifuge should be standardised for speed and time by taking a reference blood sample and determining the time and speed necessary to obtain the reference value.

3. *Pasteur pipette* It is a 22-cm-long glass tube with a long thin nozzle about 13 cm in length. It is used to transfer blood from the container to fill the Wintrobe tube.

**II. Blood sample** A sample of venous blood to which EDTA or double oxalate anticoagulant has been added is taken for the study.

## Procedure

1. Carefully mix the blood specimen by repeated inversion.
2. Fill the Wintrobe tube with blood with the help of the Pasteur pipette to the 10 cm mark (which represents 100 per cent). If the level of blood crosses the mark, use a dropper to remove the extra blood. Do not use a cotton swab or blotting paper or any other absorbent material for this purpose. Otherwise, note the error from the top of the blood column, which can be deducted from the final result.

> Note: Filling the Wintrobe tube requires special care since air bubbles may be trapped and cause damage to the red blood cells. To avoid this, place the tip of the pipette at the bottom of the Wintrobe tube and fill from the bottom, gradually withdrawing the pipette as the blood goes in. Try to keep the tip of the pipette under the rising column of blood to avoid foaming.

3. Place the Wintrobe tube in one of the cups of the centrifuge, and place a Wintrobe tube containing water in the opposite cup of the centrifuge, to balance it.
4. Turn the centrifuge on to slow speed, then increase the speed gradually, and finally bring it up to the required speed.
5. Centrifuge for 30 minutes at 3000 rpm.
6. After 30 minutes, switch off the centrifuge and allow it to stop by itself. Do not use the brake.Take out the Wintrobe tube and read the PCV directly off the graduation given on the tube. If, for example, the red cell column is one division above the graduation mark of 4, the reading is 41, or the hematocrit is 41 per cent.

> Note: A buffy coat (Fig. 1.1, Chapter 1) is the thin grey-white layer of white cells at the top of the red cell column. Do not include this while reading the height of the red cell column.

## Precautions

1. Hematocrit should be determined ideally within six hours of collection of blood.
2. Mix the blood thoroughly before taking the sample for hematocrit determination.
3. Do not use a hemolysed specimen. It will yield false low results.
4. A suitable anticoagulant should be used in proper concentration. The anticoagulant should not affect the size and shape of red cells.
5. If the blood is present above the graduation (10 cm) mark, do not remove the excess blood by cotton swab or blotting paper. Use a dropper for this purpose.
6. If air bubbles enter the tube while filling the tube with blood, the preparation should be discarded (blood should be removed totally) and the tube should be refilled.
7. Blood should be centrifuged for an adequate time.
8. While taking the reading, exclude the buffy coat.

## Advantages

1. ESR (by Wintrobe method) can be determined simultaneously by using the same sample. For this, first the Wintrobe tube filled with blood is kept vertically in the Wintrobe rack for one hour (*see* Chapter 14) to record the ESR, following which the tube is centrifuged to determine the hematocrit.
2. It is not an expensive method.

# Microhematocrit Method

This method requires only a small volume of blood. Therefore, it is ideal for a small specimen (for example, sample collected from pediatric patients and burn patients). It can be done with either free-flowing capillary blood from a finger puncture or EDTA anticoagulated venous blood. Since the test is done with a high-speed centrifuge, it takes less time.

## Principle

Anticoagulated blood is centrifuged in a sealed capillary tube, and the volume of packed red cells and percentage of whole blood (level of plasma) are determined by a special hematocrit reader.

### Requirements

1. *Capillary hematocrit tubes* These tubes are approximately 75 mm in length, and have an internal diameter of approximately 1 mm. For anticoagulated venous blood, simple capillary tubes can be used. For blood collected by skin puncture, heparinised tubes should be used.
2. *Microhematocrit centrifuge* This is a special centrifuge that runs at high speed and is capable of producing a force of 12,000 *g*, and runs at a speed of about 12,000 rpm.
3. *Hematocrit reader* There are several hematocrit readers available. The simplest one is the card reader, which can be made by hand.
4. *Modelling clay* This is used to seal the end of the hematocrit tubes.
5. *Sterile skin puncture equipment* Disposable lancet, spirit and needle.

### Procedure

1. Perform a sterile skin puncture and draw the blood sample into an appropriate capillary tube by capillary action.

> Note: Use a plain tube for anticoagulated venous blood, or a heparinised tube for skin puncture. The blood should flow freely in this case. Fill three-quarters of the tube.

2. The dry end of the tube is sealed with a specially manufactured plastic sealing clay. These tubes can also be heat-sealed.
3. Place the two sealed hematocrit tubes in the radial grooves of the centrifuge, with their heads opposite each other.
4. Turn the centrifuge on for 5 minutes at 12,000 rpm. Stop the centrifuge, take out the tubes, and read the PCV from the microhematocrit reader.

### Precautions

1. The blood sample must be properly collected.
2. Anticoagulated venous blood should be used within six hours of collection.
3. The blood must not be clotted or hemolysed.
4. Centrifugation must be sufficient to yield packing of red cells.

### Advantages

1. This procedure needs very little blood, so it can easily be done in pediatric patients and patients suffering from hemoconcentration or blood loss, like burns.
2. It is not a time-consuming test.
3. It can be used in mass surveys, because a large number of specimens can be handled simultaneously.
4. Capillary tubes are easy to fill.
5. The tubes are cheap and the replicates are easily obtainable.

## Automated Method

Measurement of hematocrit by automated technique is done by using electronic cell counters. This result is computed from individual red cell volumes and not affected by the trapped plasma left in the red cell column of the manual hematocrit methods. Therefore, the hematocrit value obtained by automated cell counters is accurate and lower than the value obtained by manual methods.

## DISCUSSION

Hematocrit or PCV is the percentage of packed red blood cells, following centrifugation. When blood is centrifuged in a tube, the red cells are packed together at the bottom of the tube by centrifugal force, as cells are heavier than the plasma. However, if the cells are deformed as in hereditary spherocytosis or sickle cell disease, more plasma remains between the packed cells, giving a false high result.

## Physiological and Clinical Significance

1. Hematocrit is a reasonable index of red cell population or Hb content of blood (Fig. 4.1). Therefore, it is used to detect conditions in which red cell count increases (polycythemia) or decreases (anemia). The hematocrit measurement is more useful and reliable than the red cell count performed manually because less error is associated with it.
2. The value of hematocrit is used in determination of blood indices, especially MCV (mean corpuscular

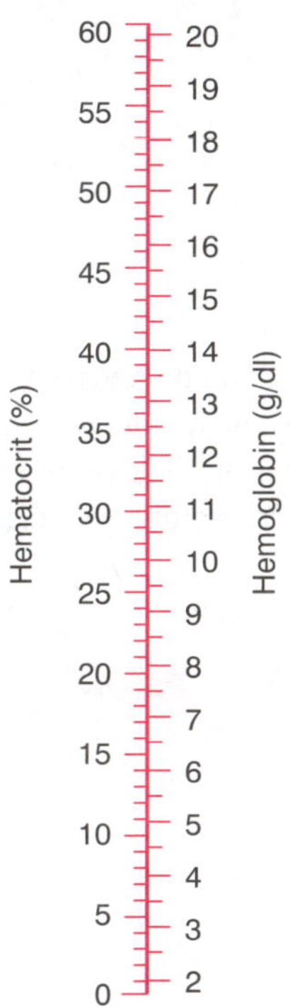


Fig. 4.1 Relationship between hematocrit and hemoglobin.

volume) and MCHC (mean corpuscular hemoglobin concentration). Blood indices help in the diagnosis and classification of various types of anemia.

3. Hematocrit is an important factor that determines viscosity of blood. Increase in hematocrit increases blood viscosity, as observed in polycythemia. This increases peripheral resistance, which in turn decreases cardiac output as the afterload on the heart increases. Conversely, decrease in hematocrit as seen in anemia, decreases the peripheral resistance that increases cardiac output. This also makes circulation hyperdynamic.

## Conditions that Alter Hematocrit

### Conditions that Decrease Hematocrit

**Physiological**

1. Pregnancy (due to hemodilution)
2. Excess water intake
3. Gender (lower in women)

**Pathological**

1. Various types of anemia
2. Conditions in which there is hemodilution and expansion of plasma volume; for example, hyperaldosteronism

### Conditions that Increase Hematocrit

**Physiological**

1. High altitude (due to hypoxia)
2. Newborns and infants
3. Excessive sweating (due to hemoconcentration)

**Pathological**

1. Decreased oxygen supply to the tissues (hypoxia), for example, congenital heart disease and emphysema
2. Polycythemia
3. Conditions in which there is hemoconcentration, for example, severe vomiting and diarrhea (due to dehydration)

## VIVA

1. What is hematocrit? What is the significance of hematocrit?
2. What are the different methods of estimation of hematocrit?
3. What are the precautions and sources of error of the microhematocrit method?
4. What is the ideal anticoagulant to be used for hematocrit determination and why?
5. Why is an anticoagulant used in a recommended concentration for estimation of hematocrit?

   Ans. The use of higher concentration of anticoagulant gives false low result, because excess EDTA may cause hemolysis.
6. Why should the hematocrit ideally be determined within six hours of collection of blood?

   Ans. If blood is kept for longer time, the change in metabolism of the red cells may cause a change in size and shape of the cells. Hemolysis starts after six hours of collection. Therefore, if the estimation of hematocrit cannot be done within six hours, the blood should be preserved in the refrigerator.
7. What are the sources of error in the Wintrobe hematocrit method?

   Ans.

   i) Improper mixing of blood

   ii) Improper anticoagulant and improper concentration of anticoagulant
   iii) Inadequate centrifugation
   iv) Reading of hematocrit with buffy coat
8. What is the normal value of hematocrit in adults?
9. Why is the value lower in women?
10. What are the physiological and pathological conditions that alter hematocrit value?
11. Why is the hematocrit value of venous blood slightly higher than that of arterial blood?

   Ans. Hematocrit value of venous blood is normally 3 per cent more than that of arterial blood because:

   i) Venous blood carries the blood that comes from tissues to the lungs. At the tissue, when one $CO_2$ molecule is added to the blood (to the red cell), there is an increase in one osmotically active particle that is either a bicarbonate ion or a chloride ion (because of chloride shift). Consequently, the red cells take up water and increase in size. This is the main cause of higher hematocrit in venous blood.
   ii) A small amount of fluid in arterial blood returns via the lymphatics, instead of the veins.

# CHAPTER 5

# Study of the Compound Microscope

## LEARNING OBJECTIVES

After completing this practical, you will be able to:

- Identify different parts of the compound microscope.
- List the uses of different parts of the microscope.
- Make microscopic adjustments for viewing the object under low-power, high-power, and oil-immersion objectives.
- List the precautions to be taken while using the microscope.
- Handle the microscope carefully.

You may also be able to:

- Describe the principle of microscopy.
- Explain the physical principles of construction of the compound microscope.
- Provide the solutions for common problems encountered in microscopy.
- Explain the basic principles of working of other types of microscopes.

## INTRODUCTION

The microscope is usually used in physiology to study the morphology of blood cells and for making different cell counts. Therefore, a physiologist should be competent in microscopy and a student of physiology should learn the basic principles of microscopy. To obtain the best performance from a microscope, one needs to understand the optical principles, the basics of the construction of the microscope, and the scientific basis of routine care and maintenance of the instrument.

A microscope magnifies the image of an object and in simple terms, it is a magnifying glass. The modern compound microscope (light microscope) is one of the most frequently used equipment in medical laboratories for students. Improper use of the microscope leads to loss of clarity of the image, which results in loss of definition. Therefore, it must be kept in excellent condition, optically and mechanically.

Microscopes designed by different manufacturers differ greatly in details of their construction and mode of operation. Therefore, the manufacturer's manual and instructions for operating the microscope must be followed properly before using the instrument.

### Physical Terms

The compound microscope consists of two magnifying lenses: the objective and the eyepiece. It is used to magnify an object to a point where it can be seen with the human eye. Before a student learns microscopy, he should understand a few physical terms fundamental to microscopy—the resolution, the working distance and the numerical aperture.

**1. Resolution** The limit of useful magnification of a microscope is set by its resolving power, that is, its ability to reveal closely adjacent structural details as separate and distinct. Resolution, therefore, describes how small individual objects can lie close to each other and still be recognisable. Generally, the human eye can separate (or resolve) dots that are 0.25 mm apart; the light microscope can separate dots that are 0.25 mm apart; and the electron microscope can separate dots that are 0.5 nm apart.

| Note: 1 nanometre (nm) | = 0.001 micrometre (μm) |
|---|---|
| | = 0.000 001 mm |

The resolving power is expressed quantitatively as the microscope's *limit of resolution* (LR), that is, the minimum distance between two visible bodies at which they are seen as separate and not in contact with one another. The LR is determined according to the following formula:

$$LR = \frac{0.61 \times W}{NA}$$

where, *W* is the wavelength of the light rays, and NA is the numerical aperture of the objective in use.

For example, if green light (wavelength 0.55 mm) and oil-immersion objective (NA 1.3) are used, the LR will be 0.25 μm (0.61 × 0.55 / 1.3 = 0.25 μm).

**2. Working distance** Working distance is the distance between the objective and the objective slide. The working distance decreases with increasing magnification. It is 0.15–1.5 mm in the case of the oil-immersion objective, 0.5–4 mm in the case of high-power, and 5–15 mm in the case of low-power objective.

**3. Numerical aperture (NA)** The numerical aperture of a lens is the ratio of the diameter of the lens to its focal length. Any particular lens has a constant numerical aperture and this value is dependent on the radius of the lens and its focal length (the distance from the object being viewed to the lens or the objective).

NA of a lens is an index of the resolving power. As the NA increases, the resolution (or distance from each other at which objects can be distinguished) decreases. That means the greater the NA, the greater is the resolving power. The NA for low-power, high-power and oil-immersion objectives are 0.30, 0.65 and 1.30 respectively. The NA is also described as an index of the light-gathering power of a lens, that is, the amount of light entering the objective. The NA can be decreased by decreasing the amount of light that passes through a lens. Therefore, the illumination has also to be increased in the same order when the objectives are changed from low-power to high-power.

## PARTS OF THE COMPOUND MICROSCOPE

There are two commonly used compound microscopes: monocular and binocular. Basically, they are the same except that the monocular microscope has one eyepiece (ocular) whereas the binocular microscope has two eyepieces. The structure of the compound microscope can be discussed under four main systems:

1. The support system (the framework)
2. The illumination system
3. The magnification system
4. The adjustment system

### The Support System

The support system is the framework of the microscope that holds its components. The framework consists of several units (Fig. 5.1).

1. **Base** The base supports the microscope and is horseshoe-shaped to provide maximum stability.
2. **Pillars** Two upright pillars project upwards from the base, and the handle of the microscope is hinged to the pillars.

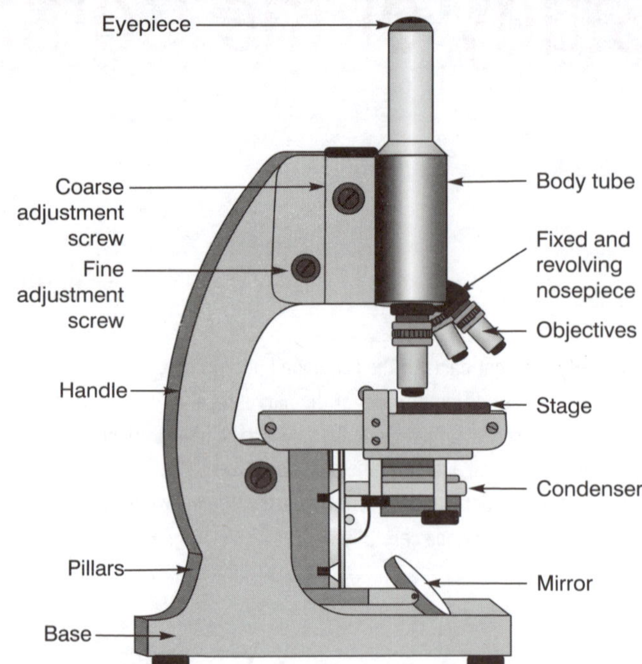


Fig. 5.1 Parts of the compound microscope.

3. **Handle (arm)** The arm supports the magnifying and adjusting systems. It is also the handle by which the microscope can be carried without damaging the delicate parts. It is curved and the microscope can be tilted at the hinged joint when desired.
4. **Body tube** The body tube is the part through which the light passes to the eyepiece. The length of the tube is usually 160 mm. This is the tube that actually conducts the image.
5. **Stage** The *fixed stage* is the horizontal platform on which the object being observed is placed. The centre of the stage has an aperture centre through which the converging cone of light passes. Most microscopes have a *mechanical stage* which makes it much easier to manipulate the objects being observed. It is calibrated and fitted on the fixed stage. There is a spring-mounted clip to hold the slide or the counting chamber in position, and two screws for moving these transversely, or forwards and backwards.
6. **Nosepiece** The *fixed nosepiece* is attached to the lower end of the body tube and the *revolving nosepiece* is mounted under it. The revolving nosepiece carries the objective lenses of different magnifying powers.

### The Illumination System

A microscope cannot function optimally without proper illumination. The illumination system provides uniform and soft-bright illumination of the entire field viewed under the microscope. The illumination system is, therefore, an important part of the compound light microscope.

There are six types of illumination systems based on which the microscopes work:

1. **Bright-field or light microscope** This uses white light, either external sunlight or internal tungsten filament lamp, as the source of illumination. When viewed under the microscope, objects look dark or coloured, contrasted against a lighted background.
2. **Dark-field microscope** A special dark-field condenser is used that lights up the object, like stars against a dark sky.
3. **Fluorescent microscope** This uses a special ultraviolet lamp as the source of illumination. A fluorescent dye is attached to the object through laboratory procedures; this glows when exposed to ultraviolet radiation.
4. **Polarising microscope**
5. **Phase-contrast microscope**
6. **Interference-contrast microscope**

The illumination system of a compound microscope consists of a light source, condenser and iris diaphragm.

### Light Source

The illumination system begins with a source of light. This may be internal or external.

**Internal source** In most modern compound microscopes there is a built-in light source with an electric lamp, which provides better control of illumination. The lamp housing has a frosted tungsten lamp, which is placed directly under the stage.

**External source** In the students' compound microscope there is no in-built light source. These microscopes use an external source of light. This can be from an electric lamp housed in a lamp box with a window, or from the sun. The rays of light are reflected by a mirror towards the object. The **mirror** is located at the base of the microscope. It has two surfaces, plane and concave. The ***plane mirror*** is used for the oil-immersion objective whereas the ***concave mirror*** is used for the low- and high-power objectives.

### Condenser

The condenser focuses the rays of light reflected from the mirror onto the object under examination and also helps in resolving the image. It is mounted below the stage of the microscope with a rack and pinion mechanism for adjusting its focus. Microscopes generally use a substage **Abbe-type condenser**. This Abbe condenser is composed of two lenses uncorrected for spherical and chromatic aberration. Therefore, for better microscopic examination, a good quality *achromatic condenser* should be used. The condenser can be raised and lowered beneath the stage by means of an adjustment knob. It must be correctly positioned to focus the light properly on the object being viewed, because, being a lens, it has a fixed numerical aperture. The numerical aperture of the condenser should be equal to or slightly less than the numerical aperture of the objective being used. Changing the position of the condenser can vary its numerical aperture. Therefore, the position of the condenser must always be adjusted with each objective used, to get the maximum focus of light and the accurate resolving power of the microscope.

When a low-power objective is used, the condenser is positioned at the lowest level; with a high-power objective, it is raised optimally; and with an oil-immersion objective it is raised fully. Most modern microscopes do not need a condenser adjustment; the condenser is placed at the highest position and the illumination is adjusted primarily by opening or closing the iris diaphragm.

### Iris Diaphragm

The iris diaphragm regulates the amount of light that passes through the material under observation. It is located at the bottom of the condenser. It has a central aperture, which can be opened for more light or closed for less light, according to necessity, by means of a lever provided with a shutter. The size of the aperture regulates the amount of light that passes to the field under observation. Regulation of the light by such means affects the numerical aperture of the condenser. By reducing the field size with the help of the iris diaphragm, the numerical aperture of the condenser is decreased. Thus, proper illumination procedure includes a combination of light intensity regulation, light source position, condenser position, and field size regulation.

## The Magnification System

The magnification system plays an extremely important role in the use of a microscope because it magnifies the image of the object under view. The compound microscope consists of two magnifying lenses, the eyepiece and the objective. The total magnification provided by a compound microscope is the product of the magnification contributed by the objective and that by the eyepiece. The eyepiece forms a virtual magnified image of the real magnified image formed by the objective.

## Eyepiece

The eyepiece or the ocular is a lens that magnifies the image formed by the objective. It fits into the top of the body tube. Most microscopes are provided with two eyepieces, 5× and 10×, with magnifying powers of 5 and 10 respectively. However, 2×, 8× and 20× eyepieces are also available. Most microscopes have a provision to fit one eyepiece and these are called **monocular microscopes**, whereas some microscopes have a provision for fitting two eyepieces at a time and these are called **binocular microscopes**. The magnification produced by the eyepiece multiplied by the magnification produced by the objective gives the total magnification of the object being viewed.

## Objectives

Objectives are the most important part of the magnification system. Usually, three objectives are screwed into the revolving nosepiece in a compound microscope. The nosepiece is a pivot that ensures a quick change of objectives. The three objectives are (a) 10×: low-power objective, (b) 40× or 45×: high-power objective, and (c) 90× or 100×: oil-immersion objective.

**Low-power objective** The low-power objective is usually 10×, which magnifies the image 10 times. This objective is used for initial focusing and observation. Some microscopes also have very low-power objectives (3× or 4×), the **scanning objectives.** These are used in initial scanning of histologic sections.

The numerical aperture (NA) of the low-power objective is always less than that of the condenser in most microscopes. Therefore, to achieve focus, the numerical apertures must be more closely matched by reducing the light to the specimen. This can be achieved by lowering the condenser and by closing the iris diaphragm (iris slightly opened). NA of objectives is related to the magnification capacity of microscope (Table 5.1).

**High-power objective** It is usually a 40× or 45× magnification lens. It magnifies the image 40 or 45 times. This objective is used for more detailed study, as the total magnification (with a 10× eyepiece) is usually

Table 5.1 Relation of NA of objectives to the magnification.

| Objective | NA | Magnification | | |
|---|---|---|---|---|
| | | Objective | Eyepiece | Total |
| Low-power | 0.30 | 10 | 10 | 100 |
| High-power | 0.65 | 45 | 10 | 450 |
| Oil-immersion | 1.30 | 100 | 10 | 1000 |

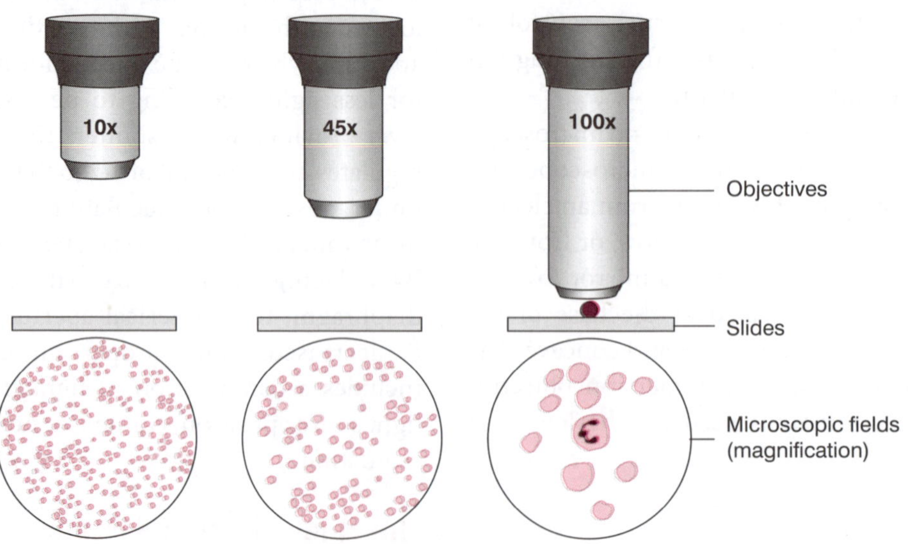


Fig. 5.2 Distance (working distance) between the objective lenses and the object in the three types of objectives. Note the magnification obtained under the three objectives.

Table 5.2 Microscopic adjustments for use of different types of objectives.

| Objective | Mirror | Condenser position | State of iris diaphragm |
|---|---|---|---|
| Low-power | Concave | Lowest | Partially closed |
| High-power | Concave | Slightly raised | Partially opened |
| Oil-immersion | Plane | Fully raised | Fully opened |

400 or 450 times. It is used for a broad view of blood films or histologic sections prior to their examination under the oil-immersion objective. The numerical aperture of the high-power objective is almost close to (or slightly less than) that of most commonly used condensers. Therefore, the condenser should be slightly raised and the iris be partially opened to achieve maximum focus.

**Oil-immersion objective** The oil-immersion objective is generally a 90 × or 100 × lens, which magnifies the image 90 or 100 times. The objective lens almost rests on the slides when in use (Fig. 5.2). It requires a special type of oil called immersion oil, which is placed between the objective and the slide. The most commonly used immersion oil is cedar wood oil. Oil is used to increase the numerical aperture and thus the resolving power of the objective. Light travels through air at a greater speed than through glass; through the immersion oil, light travels at the same speed as through glass. Therefore, the oil is used to decrease the speed at which light travels to increase the effective numerical aperture of the objective. It also decreases the defraction of light rays.

Since the numerical aperture of the oil-immersion objective is always greater than that of the condenser, the condenser should be placed at the highest position and the iris diaphragm should be fully open (Table 5.2). The oil-immersion lens gives a total magnification of 1000 times or 900 times with a 10× eyepiece. Therefore, it is generally used for detailed morphologic examination of blood films or histologic slides.

## The Adjusting System

The adjusting system consists of two adjustment systems: the coarse adjustment system and the fine adjustment system. The coarse adjustment system is used to obtain an approximate focus whereas the fine adjustment system is used to obtain the exact focus of the object after prior coarse adjustment.

### Coarse Adjustment System

Two *coarse adjustment screws* are used for making coarse adjustments. These screws are mounted on the top of the handle by a double-sided micrometer mechanism, one on each side. If one screw is rotated, its member on the opposite side also rotates at the same time. Therefore, there is no need to operate the adjustment screws from both sides simultaneously. If the left hand is used for handling the adjustment screw, the right hand can be used for manipulating the body tube or the mechanical stage. The body tube or stage can be raised or lowered quickly with the coarse adjustment screw.

### Fine Adjustment System

Two *fine adjustment screws* are used for making fine adjustments. Usually these screws are mounted on the handle below the coarse adjustment screws by double-sided micrometer mechanisms, one on each side. These screws are operated for fine adjustment and exact focusing of the object.

# METHODS

## Method of Use of the Microscope

### Principle

In the compound microscope, a focused beam of light scans the specimen or object placed on a glass slide on the stage of the microscope. Parts of the specimen that are optically dense, have a high refractive index or are coloured with a stain, cast a potential image like a shadow which is magnified in different stages as it passes up the microscope to the eye.

### Requirements

1. Microscope
2. Light source
3. Blood film

### Procedure

The microscope should be handled carefully. Before using the microscope, examine it thoroughly. The student should follow the steps given below while using a compound microscope.

1. Place the microscope on the working table in the upright position and adjust the height and position

of your chair so that you are comfortable and prepared for prolonged viewing. The eyepieces of the microscope should level with and be close to your eyes while you are sitting upright. Keep your forearms on the table so that you can easily handle the adjustment screws. You need not remove your glasses if you use them constantly.

> Note: Observers who wear glasses may be able to dispense with them when using a microscope; if not, they must take care to prevent their spectacles touching and scratching the lenses of the eyepieces.

2. Check that the eyepieces and objectives are free from dust and oil. Use a fresh lens tissue for this purpose.

> Note: Only benzol or xylol should be used to remove hardened oil.

3. Provide adequate illumination. If you have to use the external lamp, place it about 20 cm away from the microscope, switch on the lamp and allow the light to fall on the mirror. If you have to use natural light, place the microscope near the window for maximum illumination.
4. Select and adjust the mirror for optimal illumination according to the objective to be used. Direct the path of light to pass through the hole of the stage with maximum intensity while setting the mirror (look from the side to check illumination).
5. Place the slide with the object on the stage, such that it is held by the stage clips and pressed at both ends so as to be in close contact with the surface of the stage.
6. Make various microscopic adjustments to view the object under low-power objective (the correct procedure is first to view the object in low-power). The steps are:
   - Bring the low-power objective (10×) into position by revolving the nosepiece (the objective must click into place).
   - Adjust the illumination to improve contrast. Use the concave mirror, place the condenser at the lowest position, and slightly open the iris.

> Note: For low-power, the illumination is cut down to the minimum by reducing the aperture size.

   - Use the coarse focusing adjustment to focus the specimen on the slide.

> Note: Never use fine focusing adjustment until the specimen has been made visible and brought nearly into focus with coarse adjustment.

   - Use the fine adjustment only to obtain and maintain exact focus. Put one hand on the focusing knob (coarse or fine, one at a time) and the other on the screw to move the stage.
   - Bring the object of interest to the centre.
7. After preliminary screening under low-power objective, proceed to examine the film under high-power objective. The steps are:
   - Bring the high-power objective (40× or 45×) into position by rotating the nosepiece; make sure that the objective clicks into place.
   - Use the concave mirror, raise the condenser slightly, and check that the iris diaphragm is partially open so that the illumination is properly centred. Increase the illumination as needed.
   - Repeat the process of focusing as described earlier by using the coarse adjustment knob and fine adjustment knob in sequence.

> Note: As the high-power objective does not normally touch the slide (check carefully the distance between the slide and the high-power objective at its lowest position), the use of the coarse and fine adjustment knobs may not be so critical and they can be switched freely.

8. After screening under the low-power and examining under the high-power, use the oil-immersion objective to obtain greater details of the object. The steps are:
   - Swing away the high-power objective and put a tiny drop of immersion-oil on the slide over the path of light.
   - Change the mirror to the plane side.
   - Raise the condenser to maximum (to place below the stage) and open the iris fully to obtain maximum illumination.
   - Turn the nosepiece and set the oil-immersion objective in position; make sure that the objective has clicked into place.
   - Use the fine adjustment knob to get the object in focus. If this fails, look from the side, keep the eye level with the slide and lower the objective carefully with the coarse adjustment knob until the oil-immersion objective touches the oil. Lower the objective further down and

stop when the oil-immersion objective touches the slide (**Caution**: avoid pressing hard on the preparation). First, focus the object with the coarse adjustment knob while increasing the gap between the slide and the objective. Finally, focus the object with the help of the fine adjustment knob.

### Precautions

1. The microscope should be placed on the working table in a stable position.
2. The height of the observer's chair should be raised to a position that allows for comfortable handling of the microscope.
3. Objectives and eyepieces should be free from dust and oil. Xylol or benzol should be used to remove hardened oil. Lenses should never be touched with the fingers.
4. If natural light is used, the microscope should be kept near the window; if the lamp is used, it should be kept about 20 cm from the microscope, to prevent heating of the microscope.
5. The mirror, the position of the condenser and the aperture of the iris should be checked in order to get proper illumination.
6. While changing the objective, it should be noted that the objective clicks into its proper position. Otherwise the objective may not remain in position.
7. Never bring down the objective with the coarse adjustment while looking through the microscope. You should look from the side.
8. Examination of the specimen under low and high power should always precede examination under the oil-immersion objective.
9. The stage of the microscope should always be brought down before bringing the oil-immersion objective into position. Otherwise it may damage the preparation.
10. The distance between the slide and the objective should always be checked while using the coarse adjustment screw, especially for high-power and oil-immersion objectives.
11. Always keep the stage clean. Do not soil the stage with specimen material, stain, oil or water.
12. Keep the microscope covered when you are not using it.

## DISCUSSION

The common difficulties in microscopy and the solutions to these, tips for routine care and maintenance of microscopes, and other types of microscopes are discussed here.

### Common Difficulties in Microscopy

A number of difficulties may be encountered by beginners. The following tips are given to overcome them.

i) *Inability to achieve focus or obtain a clear image*

1. The failure to find focus may be due to the slide not being brought close enough to the objective to remain within its focal distance, or there may be no visible material on that small area of the slide within the field of the objective. First, move the slide so that the focus material is brought into the field. This procedure will ensure that there is visible material to focus on. Then, with the eyes level with the stage, use the coarse adjustment to raise the slide until it again comes as close as possible to the objective without touching it. Finally, apply the eyes to the eyepieces and use the coarse adjustment to move the objective away from the slide until the specimen is seen in focus.
2. Check that no dirt or dried oil has adhered to the objective lens. If so, clean it thoroughly.
3. Check that the slide carrying the object has not been placed upside down on the stage. If so, reverse it.
4. Check that the immersion oil has not become sticky. If so, wipe off the old oil and replace.
5. Check whether the specimen is covered with a layer of dried oil or dirt (left on it by a previous viewer). If so, clean it with a lens paper moistened with benzol or xylol.
6. Check whether the coverslip placed on the specimen is too thick or whether the mountant is so thick that the objective cannot reach close to the specimen to bring it within its focal length.
7. If none of the above steps improve the performance of the microscope, you should consider the possibility that the objective may be faulty. Exchange the objective with one from another good microscope and if a sharp image is obtained, discard the faulty one.

ii) *A dark shadow in the field resulting in loss of definition of the image*
   1. This is usually due to a dirty eyepiece. If the shadow moves when the eyepiece is rotated, remove the eyepiece and clean it.
   2. It may also be due to the presence of an air bubble in the immersion oil. It is better to remove the oil from the slide and put fresh oil on it.

iii) *Poor illumination*
   1. Check whether the condenser is appropriately positioned, that is, racked fully upwards. Sometimes it slips downwards in its mounting ring. It should be pushed up so that it can be racked up to within 1 mm below the specimen slide, for the oil-immersion objective.
   2. Check whether the iris is kept fully open while using an oil-immersion objective.
   3. Check that the illumination is properly centred. Ensure that the concave surface of the mirror faces the light while using the low- and high-power objectives and the plane surface faces the light while using the oil-immersion objective, and that it is in the correct position to reflect light centrally into the condenser.

iv) *Presence of unclear image under the oil-immersion objective*
   1. It suggests a problem in the slide or with the objective. First check the slide to see whether it contains dirt. If so, clean it with benzol.
   2. Check the objective, and if required clean it properly.
   3. Check for air bubbles in the specimen by holding the slide against the light.

v) *Object not coming into focus even when the objective is in the lowermost position (and the fine adjustment screw not bringing the objective any closer to the slide)* This happens when the fine adjustment screw reaches the end of the thread before the object is brought to the focus. To correct this, turn back the fine adjustment screw in the reverse direction for several turns and then focus the object carefully with the coarse adjustment knob to find the focus. Finally, sharpen the focus by turning the fine adjustment knob.

> Note: It is a good practice to keep the fine adjustment knob in the middle position. To check the position, turn the fine adjustment knob to either extreme end, then turn back, counting each turn until the knob reaches the midpoint.

vi) *The field of view looking oval* Check if the objective is placed in the correct position. Note that whenever the objective is changed, it must click into position.

## Routine Care and Maintenance of the Microscope

A microscope if properly maintained can be used for many years. Fungal growth and scratches (caused by dust particles) on the lens damage microscopes in a short time.

The following points must be noted carefully for routine use of the microscope:

1. Whenever the microscope is to be transported, carry it by holding its arm with one hand and keeping the other hand under the base.
2. When not in use during the day, the microscope should be covered, preferably with a plastic cover. At the end of the day, blow off the dust particles from the surface and store the microscope in a warm and dry place. Do not store the microscope in its wooden box.
3. Remove oil from the oil-immersion objective immediately after use by wiping with a clean lens paper.
4. The eyepiece should be cleaned frequently because it is vulnerable to dirt as it is placed at the top of the microscope and usually comes in contact with the observer's eye. An air syringe can be used for this purpose.
5. The eyepiece should not be removed from the microscope for a long duration; otherwise dust will enter the body tube and will be deposited on the rear lens of the objectives.
6. While working with the oil-immersion objective, do not pull out the specimen-slide from the stage without lowering down the stage or swinging out the objective; the slide may scratch the objective. Also remember that you should not push the oil-immersion objective on the slide; it may damage both the slide and the objective.
7. While handling the fine and coarse adjustments to achieve focus, if the screws offer unusual resistance, do not use force to overcome it, as it may damage the screw and the pinion mechanism. It is better to contact the mechanic.
8. Before storing the microscope after work, clean the lenses.

9. **Cleaning of lenses** Lenses should never be touched with fingers. Lenses are cleaned with special care to avoid dust scratch. If the lens is taken out for cleaning (eyepiece or objective), keep it on a clean surface. The eyepiece is pulled out from the tube while the objective is unscrewed from the nosepiece. First, blow off the dust particles from the surface of the lens with the help of an air syringe or a rubber bulb or a paint brush, followed by gentle rubbing with a lens paper. For cleaning the lens, breathe on it through the mouth but do not clean it by spitting or blowing on it. The oil-immersion objective requires proper cleaning. Use clean tissue paper for removing oil by repeated gentle rubbing on the surface. Move the cloth across and not circularly.

> Note: Do not use organic solvents like ethanol and xylene frequently because the solvent may dissolve the cement holding the lens in the socket.

## OTHER TYPES OF MICROSCOPES

There are other types of microscopes that are not routinely used in laboratories but these microscopes are specially designed and have some advantages over compound microscopes. They are based on different illumination systems. The character of light delivered to the specimen in different systems varies.

### Dark-Field Microscope

A special condenser is used in this microscope, which allows light waves to cross on the specimen rather than pass through the specimen. Therefore, the field in view looks dark, as light does not pass from the condenser to the objective. However, if an object is placed on the stage, light is deflected as it hits the object and passes through the objective which is seen by the viewer. Thus, the object under study appears light against a dark background. This microscope is usually used in the microbiology laboratory to study spirochetes in exudates from leptospiral or syphilitic infections.

### Fluorescence Microscope

Certain compounds when irradiated by short wavelengths, say ultraviolet light, absorb the radiation and then re-emit light energy of longer wavelength, that is, visible light. This phenomenon is called fluorescence. In fluorescence microscope, the material in the specimen that fluoresces becomes visible. The fluorescence microscope is a dark-field microscope, which has been modified by incorporating two special filters. The condenser is preceded by an *exciter filter* that allows only shorter wavelength light to pass through the specimen. If the specimen contains an object that fluoresces, it absorbs the short wavelength light and emits light of a longer wavelength. A *barrier filter* is placed in the microscope tube or eyepiece, which filters only the wavelength of emitted light for the particular fluorescent system. The fluorescence microscope is usually used in immunology laboratories to study fluorescent antibodies.

### Polarising Microscope

A polarising microscope differs from an ordinary microscope in that it has two polarising devices, a polariser and an analyser. The polariser (the filter) absorbs light waves radiating in all directions and allows light waves from a particular direction to pass through the filter. The polariser is placed usually between the light source and the specimen and the analyser is placed between the objective and the eyepiece. The polariser and the analyser are rotated until the two are at right angles to each other. This causes disappearance of light through the microscope because light waves are cancelled when they are at right angles to each other. However, some objects have the property of *birefringence*, that is, the ability to rotate (polarise) light. These objects bend light and can be seen in this microscope. They appear light under a dark background.

### Phase-Contrast Microscope

An important property of light is its phase. If two light waves are completely in phase, they show interference, the resultant amplitude is greater and brighter light is seen. When an object is seen without staining, the indirect waves passing through the object are retarded. The principle of phase-contrast microscope lies in further retardation of these indirect waves. This is achieved by inserting a phase plate within the objective lens. Since some diffracted light passes through the grooves of the plate, a halo appears around the object. The advantage of this microscope is that the cells or the organisms in wet preparations (without prior dehydration or staining) can be observed. As the name of the system indicates, the structures observed show added contrast compared with the bright-field microscope. The retardation of the speed of light makes the system sensitive to differences in refractive index. Objects with differences in refractive index show added differences in the intensity and shade of light passing through them. Therefore, one can observe unstained wet preparations with good resolution and detail. This microscope is used in hematology for counting platelets, by using a direct method.

## Interference-Contrast Microscope

This microscope yields a three-dimensional image of the object. A special beam-splitting prism is added to the condenser. The two split beams are then polarised; one passes through the specimen that alters the amplitude of the light wave and the other (which serves as a reference) does not pass through the specimen. The two dissimilar light beams then pass separately through the objective and are recombined by a second prism. This recombination of light waves provides the three-dimensional image. It is very useful for wet preparations such as urinary sediments, showing finer details without the need for special staining.

## Electron Microscope

The electron microscope uses a beam of electrons instead of light rays. The magnified image is visible on a fluorescent screen and can be recorded on a photographic film. The magnification obtained is very high. It gives the image on the photographic plate, at a magnification of about 5000 to 20,000 times. The negative is then enlarged to about 10 times thus enabling a total magnification of about 120,000× or more. In this microscope, electromagnetic fields are used in place of lenses. This is usually used for the study of finer details of organisms, cells or tissues.

## VIVA

1. Who invented the compound microscope?
2. What is the principle of microscopy?
3. What do you mean by resolution?
4. What is the use of the term numerical aperture (NA) and working distance in microscopy?
5. How are different adjustments made in the microscope while using different types of objectives?

Ans.

| Objective | Mirror | Condenser position | State of iris diaphragm |
|---|---|---|---|
| Low-power | Concave | Lowest | Partially closed |
| High-power | Concave | Slightly raised | Partially opened |
| Oil-immersion | Plane | Fully raised | Fully opened |

6. What are the functions of the condenser and iris diaphragm?
7. How is the NA of objectives related to magnification?

Ans.

| Objective | NA | Magnification | | |
|---|---|---|---|---|
| | | Objective | Eyepiece | Total |
| Low-power | 0.30 | 10 | 10 | 100 |
| High-power | 0.65 | 45 | 10 | 450 |
| Oil-immersion | 1.30 | 100 | 10 | 1000 |

8. Why is a special grade of oil (immersion oil) used in the oil-immersion objective?

   Ans. Immersion oil (cedar wood oil or liquid paraffin) is used to increase the NA and thus the resolving power of the objective. Light travels through air at a greater speed than through glass. Thus, to increase the effective NA of the objective, oil is used to slow down the speed at which light travels (speed of light is measured in terms of the refractive index), increasing the gathering power of the lens and decreasing the diffraction of light rays. The refractive indices of air, glass and immersion oil are 1.00, 1.515 and 1.515, respectively.
9. Why should the eyepiece, objective and condenser lenses never be cleaned with paper tissue, gauze or ordinary cloth?

Ans. These optical lenses are softer than ordinary glass. Therefore, cleaning with paper tissue, gauze or ordinary cloth will scratch the lens. To clean the lenses of the microscope, a lens paper is used. Before polishing with a lens paper, care must be taken to see that nothing is present on the surface that will scratch the optical glass in the polishing process. Potentially abrasive dust or dirt is blown away using an air syringe before polishing.

10. Why should the oil be removed from the oil-immersion objective immediately after use?

    Ans. Oil is removed from the oil-immersion objective by wiping with a clean lens paper immediately after use. If it is not removed, it may dry on the outside surface of the objective or may seep inside the lens and damage it.

11. What microscopic adjustments are made when the field of view is not clear?
12. What is the cause of dark shadows in the field of view, and how can this be prevented?
13. What microscopic adjustments are made if the image is not clear in the oil-immersion objective?
14. What is the cause of oval field of view, and how do you correct it?
15. In microscopy, what does the term parfocal mean?

    Ans. It means that if one objective is in focus and a switch is made to another objective, the focus will not be lost. Thus the microscope can be focused under low-power and then switched to the high-power or oil-immersion objective and it will still be in focus except for fine adjustment. Usually, after focusing in low-power if you switch to high-power, one complete rotation of the fine adjustment screw (which adjusts about one micron) brings the object into clear focus.

CHAPTER 6

# Hemocytometry

## LEARNING OBJECTIVES

After completing this practical, you will be able to:

- Identify RBC and WBC pipettes.
- Focus RBC and WBC squares of the chamber under low-power and high-power objectives of the microscope.
- Dilute the blood in the pipette for RBC and WBC counts.
- List the precautions for diluting blood.
- Charge the Neubauer's chamber.
- List the precautions for charging the chamber.
- Calculate the area and volume of RBC and WBC squares.

You may also be able to:

- Explain the possible sources of error and their effects in diluting the blood in pipettes.

## INTRODUCTION

The formed elements of blood are counted by hemocytometry. The apparatus used is called the **hemocytometer**, consisting of diluting pipettes and counting chambers. The procedures used for enumeration of blood cells include the manual method of hemocytometry and the use of electronic counting devices. The cells counted in routine practice are red cells, white cells and platelets. Manual techniques lend themselves to enumeration of all small separate bodies such as spermatozoa, eosinophils and cells in the cerebrospinal fluid. In the manual method, the hemocytometer is used for counting, whereas in electronic methods, automated electronic counting devices are used. The electronic counting device bypasses the element of human error and is also statistically more accurate because it can count many more cells.

### Units for Reporting

Since the enumerated constituents are to be reported in units per litre of blood, the number of cells actually counted must be converted to the number present per litre of blood. The alternative method is units of cells per cubic millimetre ($mm^3$) or microlitre (μl), since 1 μl is essentially equal to 1 $mm^3$. Though the report is usually expressed per cubic millimetre of blood, the reporting unit of choice is cells per litre of blood.

$1\ mm^3 = 1\ \mu l = 10^{-6}\ l$

$1\ \mu l \times 10^6 = 1$ litre

## METHODS

Hemocytometry includes pipetting (diluting the blood in the pipette) and charging (charging the Neubauer's chamber with diluted blood).

### Pipetting

#### Principle

A measured unit of blood is diluted quantitatively with diluents by using special measuring devices (pipettes).

#### Requirements

1. **Pipettes** To ensure proper dilution of the sample to be used for counting blood cells, the blood can be precisely measured and diluted with specially designed pipettes. For counting the blood cells, two types of pipettes are used: RBC pipettes and WBC pipettes. In hematology, the hemoglobin pipette is used for estimation of hemoglobin (not for counting cells).

***RBC pipette*** This is used for counting red cells. It has a stem, bulb, rubber tube and mouthpiece. The stem has two markings, 0.5 and 1. The stem widens into a bulb with a red bead in it. The bead helps in identifying the pipette and mixing the fluid with blood in the bulb of the pipette. The capacity of the bulb is 100 parts (from 1 to 101 mark). The bulb narrows above ('101' is marked just above the bulb) and to this end, a rubber tubing which ends in a mouthpiece is attached (Fig. 6.1). The

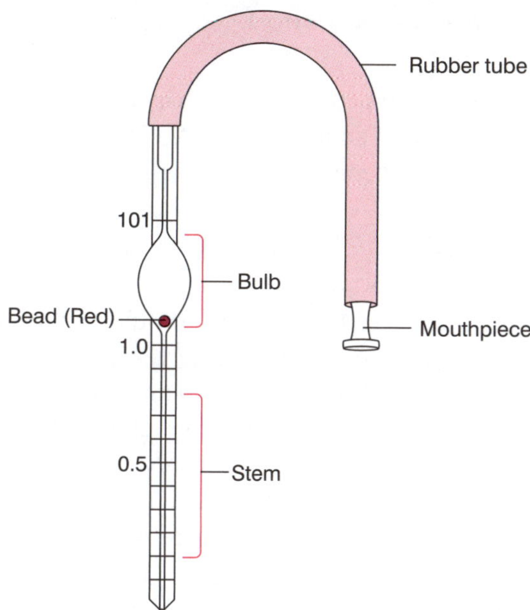


Fig. 6.1 RBC pipette.

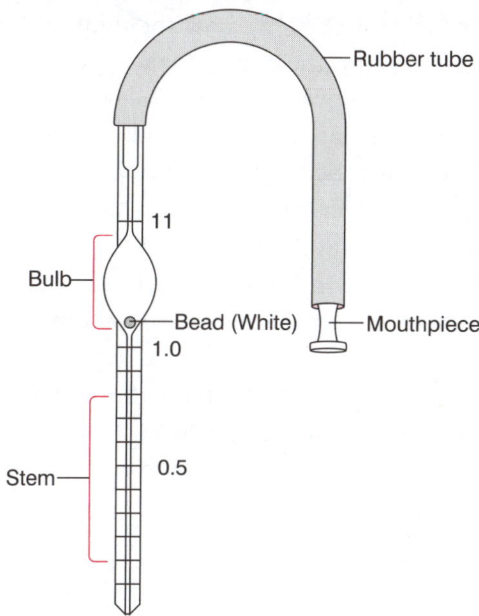


Fig. 6.2 WBC pipette.

mouthpiece is red in colour. As the lumen diameter in the stem of the RBC pipette is less compared to that of the WBC pipette, sometimes the RBC pipette is called a *slow-speed pipette.*

***WBC pipette*** This is used for counting white blood cells. It is similar to the RBC pipette except that the capacity of the bulb is less (10 parts) and the bulb contains a white bead. The marking above the bulb is '11' (Fig. 6.2). The mouthpiece is white in colour. In the WBC pipette, the lumen diameter in the stem is more than that of RBC pipettes (Table 6.1). Hence, sometimes the WBC pipette is called a *fast-speed pipette.*

2. **Diluents (diluting fluids)** Different varieties of diluting fluids are used for counting different types of cells. Diluting fluids are described with each cell count.

Table 6.1 Differences between RBC and WBC pipettes.

| | RBC pipette | WBC pipette |
|---|---|---|
| 1. Calibrations | 0.5 to 1.0 in the stem 101 above the bulb | 0.5 to 1.0 in the stem 11 above the bulb |
| 2. Bulb | Larger, capacity 100 parts, contains red bead | Smaller, capacity 10 parts, contains white bead |
| 3. Mouthpiece | Red | White |
| 4. Stem lumen diameter | Less | More |
| 5. Dilution | 0.5 in 100, or 1 in 200 | 0.5 in 10, or 1 in 20 |

## Procedure

1. Clean the pipette and ensure that it is dry.
2. Collect the diluting fluid in a watch glass from a stock bottle.
3. Prick the finger tip (as described in Chapter 2) with all aseptic precautions to obtain free flow of blood.
4. Discard (wipe off) the first drop of blood.
5. Let a large drop of blood accumulate on the finger tip.
6. Hold the pipette horizontally and dip its end into the drop of blood. Suck gently on the mouthpiece to draw blood up to the required mark (0.5) on the stem of the pipette. If more than the required amount of blood is drawn into the pipette, tap it gently onto the fingernail or palm, or touch the tip with a non-absorbent material keeping the pipette horizontal, in order to bring the blood to the desired mark.

> Note: Do not blow out the extra blood or use absorbent material like cotton wool.

7. Wipe off the tip of the pipette to remove the extra blood sticking to it.
8. Maintain the blood level at the 0.5 mark, and place the tip of the pipette in the diluting fluid well below the surface of the liquid.

> Note: Do not directly draw the fluid from the stock bottle as it may contaminate the solution with the cells.

9. Using constant suction, draw the diluting fluid into the pipette. Draw the mixture exactly to the top mark ('101' or '11') above the bulb. While the bulb is being filled, you may tap the pipette with a finger to knock the bead down below the surface of the solution in the bulb to prevent the formation of bubbles.
10. Maintain the level of the mixture exactly to the mark by closing the pipette tip with the index finger. Holding the pipette in the horizontal position is also important.
11. Mix the contents of the bulb thoroughly for 2–3 minutes by rotating the pipette with its tip pressing against the palm of the left hand (the rubber tube may be removed to facilitate mixing).

> **Note:** The contents may also be mixed by holding and rotating the pipette between the palms, but there is some risk of leakage, especially if it is not held horizontally.

12. Place the pipette on a horizontal surface. The pipette is now ready for charging.

### Precautions

Cell counts are performed by determining the number of cells in the diluted sample, and converting the number of cells counted in the diluted sample to the final result, i.e., the number of cells in 1 litre or in 1 µl of whole blood. Blood cell counts are performed on minute quantities taken from small samples of an individual's blood. Errors are inherent even in the best methods. Therefore, the steps in the procedure must be followed as carefully as possible to reduce the variation of the final result from the actual or true count.

1. Pipettes should be clean, dry and without chipped or broken tips.
2. The puncture should be deep enough for free flow of blood. The first drop should be discarded as it contains tissue fluid.
3. A large drop of blood should have formed on the finger tip to provide adequate blood to fill up to the 0.5 mark of the pipette at a time.
4. The tip of the pipette should dip into the blood drop, otherwise while sucking blood into the pipette, air bubbles also enter along with blood.
5. Blood should be taken exactly up to the 0.5 mark. If blood is present above the mark, absorbent material, such as gauze or cotton, should not be used to adjust the blood level because these materials absorb the water content of the blood and cause blood to concentrate.
6. The tip of the pipette should be wiped off. Otherwise, the extra blood attached to the tip enters the pipette along with diluent when the diluting fluid is sucked in.
7. Blood in the pipette should be diluted immediately, otherwise it will clot.
8. Contaminated diluting fluids should not be used. Blood should not be allowed to get into the diluent because this will affect subsequent cell counts with the same diluent. Therefore, the diluent should not be drawn into the pipette directly from the bottle. Rather, the fluid should be taken in a watch glass from where it should be drawn into the pipette.
9. The tip of the pipette should dip inside the diluting fluid throughout the process of filling the bulb, otherwise air bubbles enter the pipette.
10. The upper dilution mark on the pipette should not be exceeded by more than 1 mm; and the mixture should not be corrected back to the top mark if overdiluted because this would cause the cells from the bulb to be forced to enter into the lower stem of the pipette.
11. If blood is to be used from a blood sample, the preserved blood sample should not be hemolysed nor should it contain a fibrin clot. It should be mixed (preferably by gentle shaking) before use.

## Charging the Chamber

### Principle

A mixture of blood and diluting fluid is released smoothly onto the central platform of the chamber beneath a coverslip.

### Requirements

1. Counting chamber
2. Pipette containing the mixture
3. Coverslip

### Counting Chamber

The counting chamber in common use is the **Improved Neubauer Chamber**. This consists of a thick glass slide divided into two central platforms by an H-shaped groove. The central platform is slightly lower than the sides; i.e., when a coverslip is placed, it covers the central platform and rests on the side platforms. The depth, i.e., the distance between the undersurface of the coverslip and the central platform is 1/10 mm (Fig. 6.3). When the chamber is charged with diluted blood, a thin film of fluid of known volume is spread on the central platform, and this is used for performing the cell counts.

**The counting grid** On the central platforms are engraved ruled squares used for various cell counts. The ruled area on each central platform is called counting grid. The ruled area is a square measuring 3 mm × 3 mm (Fig. 6.4). This area is divided into nine large squares, each having an area of 1 mm$^2$ (1 mm × 1 mm). The four

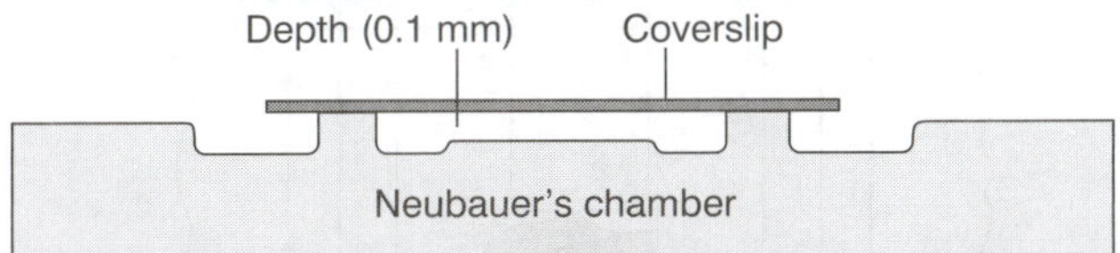


Fig. 6.3 Side view of Neubauer's chamber showing the space between the undersurface of the coverslip and the surface of the platform (0.1 mm deep).

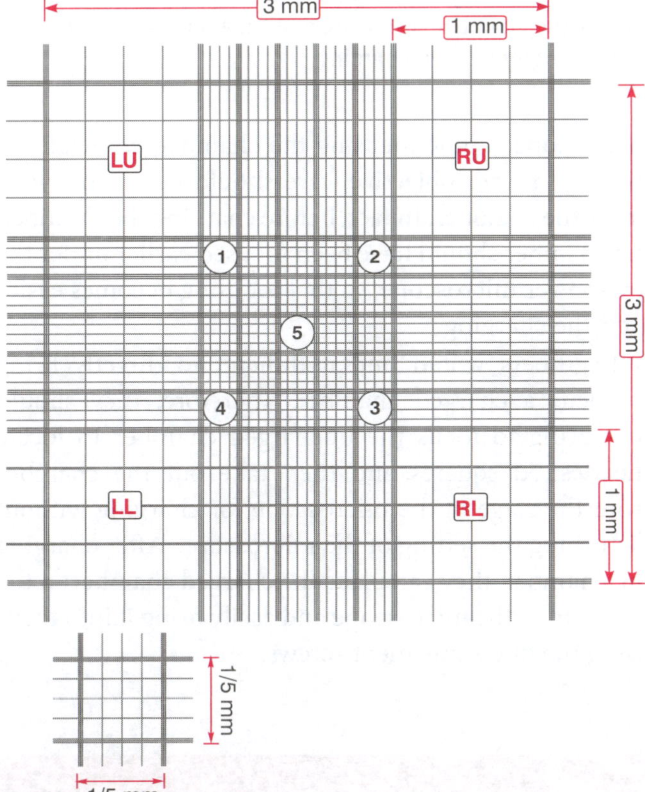


Fig. 6.4 Improved Neubauer's chamber (LU: left upper; RU: right upper; LL: left lower; RL: right lower WBC squares; 1, 2, 3, 4 and 5: RBC squares).

large corner squares are used for WBC count, while the large 1 mm square in the centre is used for RBC count.

Each WBC square is further subdivided into 16 smaller squares, each measuring 1/16 mm$^2$. The 1 mm$^2$ central RBC square is divided into 25 medium-sized squares by means of triple lines. Each medium-sized square measures 1/5 mm in length and has an area of 1/5 × 1/5 = 1/25 mm$^2$. The medium-sized squares of the four corners and the central medium-sized square are used for the RBC count. The area of the five medium-sized squares is 1/25 × 5 = 1/5 mm$^2$. Since the depth of the chamber is 1/10 mm, the volume of the five medium-sized squares is 1/5 × 1/10 = 1/50 mm$^3$ (Fig. 6.4).

Each medium-sized square is further divided into 16 small squares, that is, 25 × 16 = 400 small squares. The side of the smallest RBC square measures 1/20 mm. Therefore, the area of the smallest RBC square is 1/20 × 1/20 = 1/400 mm$^2$. Since the depth under the coverslip is 1/10 mm, the volume of the smallest RBC square is 1/400 × 1/10 = 1/4000 mm$^3$. The red cells are counted in 80 small squares (5 medium-sized squares); the volume of 80 small-sized RBC squares is 1/4000 × 80 = 1/50 mm$^3$.

**Other counting chambers** Other counting chambers are Thoma's chamber and old Neubauer chamber. Presently, both these chambers are not in use. In **Thoma's chamber**, the central platform is depressed and circular. The grid is only 1 mm$^2$, consisting of 25 groups of 16 smaller squares each. The corner 1 mm squares are absent. The **Old Neubauer chamber** has nine 1 mm squares. The four larger corner squares of 16 squares each are meant for WBC counting, and the central 1 mm$^2$ area has 16 groups of 16 squares each, meant for RBC counting. In the improved Neubauer chamber, 25 groups of 16 smallest squares are available for RBC counting. However, in both the chambers, medium squares are separated by triple lines.

## Procedure

1. Clean the Neubauer's chamber and the coverslip.
2. Place the coverslip on the central platform of the chamber.
3. Mix the contents of the bulb thoroughly.
4. Discard the first two drops of fluid from the pipette as it contains only the diluting fluid.
5. Place the tip of the pipette on the surface of the chamber touching the edge of the coverslip at an

angle of 45°. Allow the diluted blood to flow under the coverslip by capillary action. Remove the pipette quickly from the edge of the coverslip as soon as the counting platform is filled with the diluted blood. Take care to avoid entry of air bubbles and overflow of the fluid into the gutters.

> Note: The mixture should completely cover the platform, but should not enter the gutters. If air bubbles enter the platform or fluid enters the gutters, discard the specimen and recharge.

6. Allow the cells to settle for 2–3 minutes before placing the charged chamber on the stage of the microscope for counting.

### Precautions

1. The chamber and the coverslip should be properly cleaned.
2. The contents of the bulb must be thoroughly mixed before charging.
3. Two drops of fluid must be discarded from the pipette before charging as the stem of the pipette contains only diluting fluid.
4. Air bubbles should not enter the platform of the chamber while charging.
5. The chamber should not be overcharged (overflow of fluid into the gutters) or undercharged (fluid does not spread on the entire central platform). If the chamber is overcharged, the cells may enter the gutter and settle there, which gives false low results. If the chamber is undercharged, the cells may not be found in the peripheral squares (Fig. 6.5).

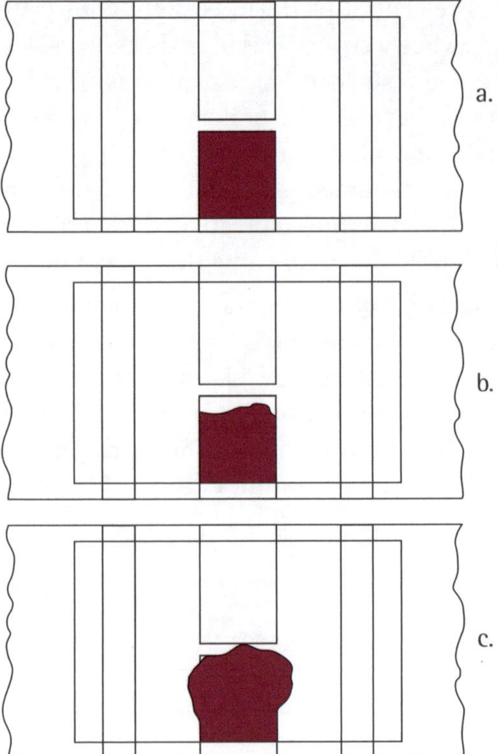


Fig. 6.5 Charging of Neubauer's chamber (only the central part of the chamber is shown). a: normal (ideal) charging; b: undercharging; c: overcharging.

## DISCUSSION

Students should practise pipetting and charging repeatedly. But, before learning this, they should learn to focus the RBC and WBC squares of the chamber under the low-power and high-power objectives of the microscope. While focusing the chamber, especially in the high-power objective, care should be taken not to break the chamber. In fact, before charging the chamber, the chamber should have been focused earlier under the low-power microscope, so that focusing becomes easier after the charging.

Beginners would find it difficult to directly bring to focus a charged chamber. Therefore, they should first bring to focus the uncharged chamber to locate the desired squares and then take out the chamber from the stage of the microscope for charging without disturbing the setting of the microscope. After charging the chamber, they can place the charged chamberon the platform of the microscope and easily bring it into focus using the fine adjustment screws.

## VIVA

1. What are the uses of the hemocytometer in hematology?
2. How do you identify the RBC and WBC diluting pipettes?
3. What are the steps for diluting the blood for various cell counts?

4. What are the precautions taken for pipetting?
5. How do you bring down the level of blood if the blood is sucked above the 0.5 mark of the pipette?
6. Why is the fluid not sucked directly from the stock bottle?
7. How do you prevent the entry of air bubbles into the pipette while diluting the blood?
8. How do you calculate the area and volume of RBC and WBC squares?
9. What are the steps for charging the Neubauer's chamber?
10. What are the precautions taken for charging the chamber with diluted blood?
11. Why are the contents of the bulb mixed thoroughly before charging?
12. Why are the two drops of fluid discarded from the pipette before charging?
13. What do the terms overcharging and undercharging mean and what is their significance?

CHAPTER 7

# Total RBC Count

## LEARNING OBJECTIVES

After completing this practical, you will be able to:
- Describe the importance of performing RBC count in practical physiology.
- Identify the RBC diluting pipette.
- Suck blood up to the 0.5 mark of the pipette.
- Dilute the blood in the pipette.
- Charge the Neubauer's chamber.
- Perform the total RBC count.
- Calculate total RBC count to express the result in $mm^3$ of blood.
- List the precautions taken for performing RBC count.
- Describe the composition and function of each constituent of the RBC diluting fluid.
- List the steps and factors involved in regulation of production of red cells.
- Enumerate the functions of red cells.
- List the normal value of RBC count in adults.
- Define polycythemia and anemia.
- Name the common causes of alteration in RBC count.

You may also be able to:
- State the name, composition and advantages of other RBC-diluting fluids.
- Explain the principle of automated methods of red cell count.
- Classify polycythemia and anemia.
- Explain the physiological basis of alteration of red cell count in different conditions.
- Describe the stages and regulation of erythropoiesis.
- Explain the causes and mechanism of polycythemia and anemia.

## INTRODUCTION

The human red cell is normally a circular, non-nucleated, biconcave disc. The red blood cells (erythrocytes) contain hemoglobin. The surface area of the red cell is much greater than that of a sphere of the same size. Thus the exchange of oxygen and carbon dioxide is maximal with the biconcave configuration. This shape also helps it to withstand osmotic lysis and to easily pass through narrow capillaries.

### Red Cell Dimensions

| | |
|---|---|
| Shape | : Biconcave disc |
| Size | : 7.5 (7 to 8) µm in diameter |
| Thickness | : 2.0 µm |
| Surface area | : 140 $\mu m^2$ |

### Formation

The development of red cells is known as **erythropoiesis.** In postnatal life, erythropoiesis takes place in the bone marrow. In children, cells are produced in the marrow cavities of all the bones. By the age of 20, the marrow in the cavities of the long bones, except for the upper humerus and femur, becomes inactive. The active cellular marrow is called the **red marrow**; the inactive marrow that is infiltrated with fat is called the **yellow marrow**. During fetal life, erythropoiesis occurs in the spleen, liver, thymus and bone marrow. After birth, it is confined to the red marrow.

The stages of erythropoiesis are as follows:

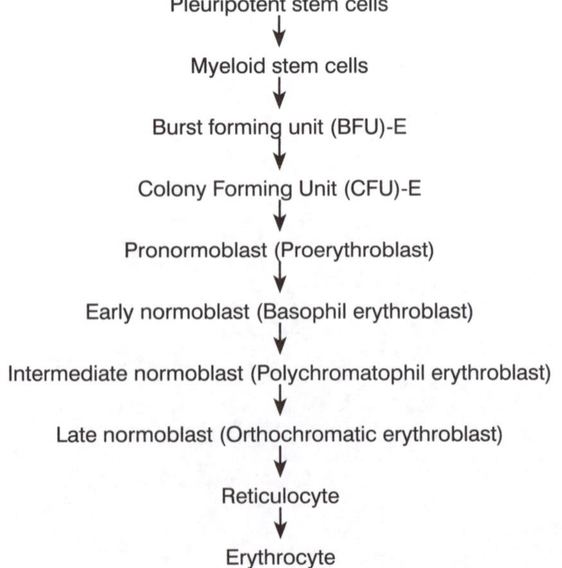


As the cell matures in the bone marrow, its diameter decreases and the nucleus becomes denser and smaller and finally disappears from the cell. While this occurs, the hemoglobin concentration increases and the cytoplasm progressively changes from blue to orange in appearance, on a stained blood film. The whole sequence of maturation from the early precursor to a circulating red cell takes 3–5 days.

Erythropoiesis is subject to feedback control. It is inhibited by a rise in the circulating red cells and is stimulated by decreased red cell count. This alteration is mediated by a number of factors that influence the secretion of *erythropoietin*, a hormone secreted by the kidney. Interleukins ($IL_1$, $IL_3$, $IL_6$) and GM-CSF also affect the development of red cells.

## Functions

The main function of RBCs is to carry oxygen from the lungs to the tissues of the body. Red cells also transport carbon dioxide from the tissues to the lungs. Red cells contribute to blood viscosity and therefore to peripheral resistance of blood. Viscosity of blood is less in anemia and more in polycythemia.

## Lifespan and Fate

The average lifespan of red cells is about 120 days. The bone marrow releases new red cells into circulation every day. The dead red cells are broken down by the reticuloendothelial system. They break down globin to amino acids which are returned to the protein storage pool of the body. They are also essential for the retention and reuse or storage of iron, which is needed for hemoglobin synthesis.

## Normal Values

In adults:

Males : 5.2 (4.5–6.0) million per $mm^3$ of blood

Females : 4.7 (4.0–5.5) million per $mm^3$ of blood

RBC count is higher in newborns (6–8 million per $mm^3$ of blood). The count rapidly decreases thereafter, and is lowest at about two to four months of life (3–4 million per $mm^3$). The count slowly increases from one year of life to reach 5 million per $mm^3$ at about ten years.

# METHODS OF COUNTING

Red cells are counted by two methods: non-automated (manual) and automated. Manual cell count is less accurate but is still widely used in developing countries as automated counting is expensive.

## Manual Method

### Principle

The blood specimen is diluted (usually 200 times) with the diluting fluid, which does not remove the white cells, but allows the red cells to be counted in a known volume of fluid. Finally, the number of cells in undiluted blood is calculated and reported as the number of red cells per $mm^3$ of whole blood.

### Requirements

**I. Apparatus**

1. Microscope
2. Hemocytometer (RBC diluting pipette and counting chamber)
3. Equipment for sterile finger prick
4. Watchglass
5. Coverslip

**II. RBC diluting fluid**

The red cell diluting fluid is isotonic; therefore, it prevents hemolysis. Of the different diluting fluids used for red cell count, the most frequently used is Hayem's fluid.

1. ***Hayem's fluid***

   *Composition*

   Sodium chloride : 0.5 g
   Sodium sulphate : 2.5 g
   Mercuric chloride : 0.25 g
   Distilled water : 100 ml

   Dissolve thoroughly with a stirrer, in a beaker.

   *Function of each component*

   Sodium chloride maintains osmolarity.
   Sodium sulphate prevents aggregation of RBC.
   Mercuric chloride acts as a preservative (it is antifungal and antibacterial)
   Distilled water acts as a solvent.

2. ***Dacie's fluid***

   This is an alternative to Hayem's fluid.

   *Composition*

   Trisodium citrate : 3.13 g
   Commercial formaldehyde

(37% formalin) : 1.0 ml
Distilled water : 100 ml
Dissolve thoroughly with a stirrer, in a beaker.

*Caution*

Formaldehyde is corrosive, and should be handled carefully.

*Advantages*

Dacie's fluid is preferred in some laboratories because of the following advantages:

- It is simple to prepare.
- It keeps well and does not need to be sterilised.
- Red cells maintain their normal disc-like form and do not agglutinate.

Cells are well-preserved and counts may be performed several hours after the blood has been diluted.

3. ***Isotonic saline***

If the above two diluting fluids are not available, isotonic saline may be used. The counting should commence immediately following dilution as it does not contain any agent to prevent aggregation of red cells.

## Procedure

1. Assemble all equipment needed for the practical and ensure that the pipettes, coverslip and Neubauer's chamber are thoroughly clean and dry.
2. Take adequate RBC diluting fluid in a watchglass.
3. Prick the finger under aseptic conditions (as described in Chapter 3) and suck blood into the pipette and dilute it following the procedure step by step as described in Chapter 6 (procedure of pipetting).
4. Hold the pipette horizontally and close both ends, then gently mix the contents of the bulb. For mixing, shake the pipette at right angles to its long axis for a few seconds. The red bead in the pipette should move from one side to the other during the mixing.
5. After mixing, keep the pipette in a horizontal position to prevent any loss of its contents until the cell count is performed.
6. Discard the first two drops of fluid from the pipette.
7. Charge the Neubauer's chamber as described in Chapter 6 and allow two minutes so that the cells settle down.
8. Place the charged chamber on the stage of the microscope and adjust the microscope for observation under low power.
9. Focus the central square of the Neubauer's chamber under the low-power objective, and check for uniform distribution of cells. If the cells are not uniformly distributed (Fig. 7.1), clean the Neubauer's chamber and recharge it.
10. Focus the RBC squares under the high-power objective. Count the cells in five medium RBC squares in sequence as described in Fig. 7.2a (four corner and the central medium-sized RBC squares) that is 16 × 5 = 80 small RBC squares.

> Note: Care should be taken not to count the same cells again. To avoid this, Rules of Counting should be followed, according to which the red cells present in the square and on its left and lower lines are counted, and those on its right and upper lines are ignored. This is called 'L pattern' counting, as demonstrated in Fig. 7.2b. However, '(inverted L) pattern', i.e., counting cells present on the left and upper lines of the square, and avoiding those present on the right and lower lines, can also be followed. But, 'L pattern' for few squares and 'inverted L pattern' for other squares should not be practised. Only one pattern should be followed for the entire counting, and preferably the same should be practised by all the students of the class to maintain uniformity and to avoid confusion.

11. Draw the RBC squares in your notebook and enter the observation. Calculate the final result.

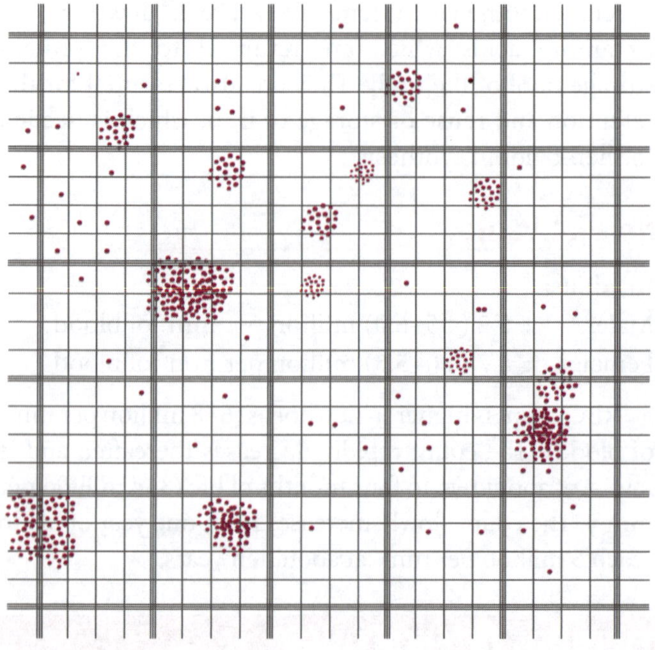

Fig. 7.1 Non-uniform distribution of red cells (as seen under low power). Note that cells are clumped at a few places and sparse at other places.

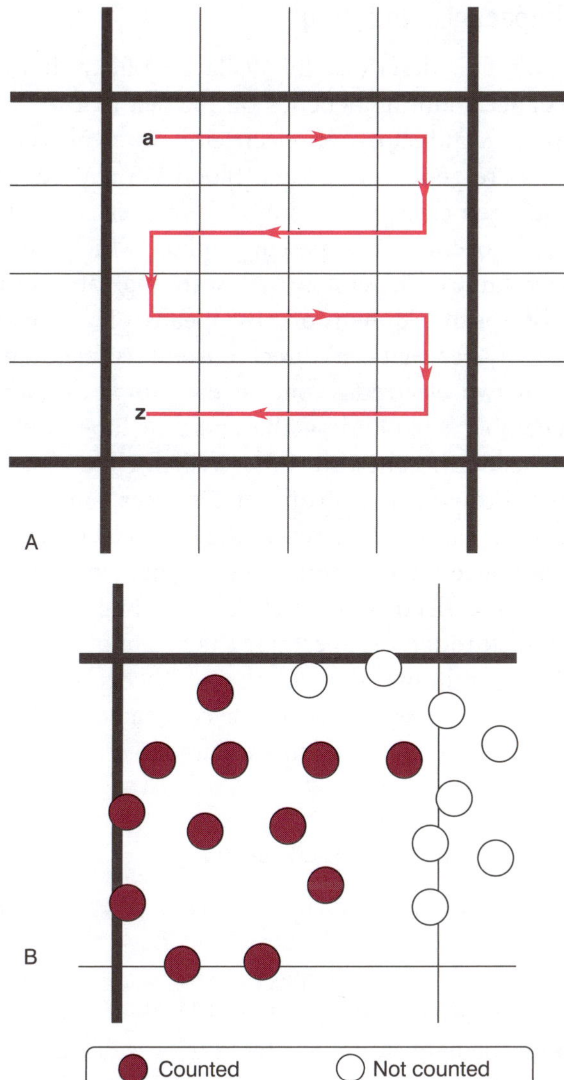


Fig. 7.2 Pattern of counting red cells in a medium RBC square. Arrow indicates the direction of counting (A); cells to be counted (B) as shown in a small square.

## Dilution Obtained

The volume of the bulb is 100 (101 – 1 = 100). The stem of the pipette (from the tip of the pipette to mark 1) contains diluting fluid that does not take part in dilution. Dilution (mixing of blood with diluting fluid) occurs only in the bulb. Thus 100 volumes of diluted blood (in the bulb) contain 0.5 volumes of blood and 99.5 volumes of diluting fluid, resulting in a dilution of 0.5 in 100. Thus, the dilution obtained is 1 in 200 or 200 times.

## Calculation

Area of 5 medium-sized squares = $1/25 \times 5 = 1/5$ $mm^2$.

Volume of 5 medium-sized squares = $1/5 \times 1/10 = 1/50$ $mm^3$ (1/10 is the depth).

Dilution factor = 1 : 200

Let us say the cells in 1/50 $mm^3$ volume of diluted blood is $n$.

Therefore, cells in 1 $mm^3$ volume of diluted blood $= n \times 50$

Therefore, cells in 1 $mm^3$ volume of undiluted blood $= n \times 50 \times 200$

$= \mathbf{n \times 10{,}000}$ where $n$ is the total number of cells counted in 5 medium-sized RBC squares.

## Precautions

1. The pipette, coverslip and Neubauer's chamber should be thoroughly clean and dry.
2. The puncture should be deep enough to allow spontaneous flow of blood. Do not squeeze, as squeezing expresses tissue fluid. If blood is taken from a sample, it should be mixed properly prior to pipetting.
3. Wipe off the first drop of blood as it is mixed with tissue fluid.
4. Draw blood exactly up to the 0.5 mark. The blood column (from the tip of the pipette to the 0.5 mark) should not be fragmented, nor should it contain air bubbles. If blood is drawn above the mark, gently tap against the finger tip or nail bed to bring to the level. Never use absorbent material for this purpose as it absorbs water from the blood and makes the blood concentrated.
5. Wipe the tip of the pipette before diluting the blood. This should always be done; otherwise the extra blood sticking to the tip of the pipette will be sucked into the bulb along with the diluting fluid and will give a false high result.
6. Blood in the pipette should be diluted quickly; otherwise blood clots in the pipette.
7. Suck the RBC diluting fluid exactly up to the 101 mark. If the fluid is drawn much above the mark (more than 1 mm), do not adjust it back to the mark as it forces cells in the bulb to enter into the stem of the pipette. This affects the dilution and cell concentration in the bulb. Therefore, it is better to discard this, clean the pipette and restart the procedure.
8. Before charging the chamber, gently mix the contents of the bulb.

9. Discard the first two drops of fluid as fluid in the stem does not contain cells.
10. Do not overcharge or undercharge. If the chamber is overcharged, discard that, clean the chamber and recharge.
11. If the distribution of cells is not uniform, discard and recharge.
12. Avoid counting the same cells twice.

### Sources of Error

The error in manual total RBC count is 15–30 per cent. It can be reduced by counting more cells. The possible sources of error may be errors inherent in the method or technical errors.

#### A. Errors Inherent in the Method

1. *Error of visual red cell count* Error decreases with increased total number of cells counted. Both sides of the Neubauer's chamber can be charged, and counting can be done on both the chambers. The average of these can be taken for final calculation. This decreases the error.
2. *Error due to distribution of cells* Distribution can never be perfectly uniform even with near-perfect mixing and charging, and therefore gives rise to error.

#### B. Technical Errors

1. *Dilution error* Improper volume measurement of blood and diluent
2. *Pipette error* Use of defective pipettes (improper marking and improper bulb size)
3. *Chamber error* Use of defective chambers (counting grid and depth of chambers may not be accurate)
4. *Charging error* Improper charging of the chamber (overcharging or undercharging)
5. *Counting error* Improper counting (few cells are not counted or few cells are counted twice)
6. *Calculation error* Wrong calculation

## Automated Methods

There are two automated methods: (1) impedance counting and (2) light scattering technology. As these methods are not usually practised in Indian laboratories, only the basic principles of the methods are described here.

### Impedance Counting

This was first described by Wallace Coulter in 1956. Impedance counting depends on the fact that red cells are poor conductors of electricity, whereas certain diluents are good conductors. Blood is highly diluted in a buffered electrolyte solution. An external vacuum initiates movement of a mercury siphon, which causes a major volume of the sample to flow through an aperture tube of specific dimension. By means of a constant source of electricity, a direct current is maintained between two electrodes, one in the sample beaker or the chamber surrounding the aperture tube, and the other inside the aperture tube. When a blood cell is carried through the aperture, it displaces some of the conducting fluid and increases the electrical resistance. This produces a corresponding change in potential between the electrodes which lasts as long as the red cells pass through the aperture. The height of the pulses produced indicates the volume of the cells passing through. The pulses can be displayed on an oscillograph screen. The height of the pulses is used to determine the volume of the red cells.

### Light Scattering Technology

Red cells are counted by means of electro-optical detectors. A diluted cell suspension flows through an aperture so that the cells pass in single file, in front of the light source; light is scattered by the cells passing through the light beam. Scattered light is detected by a photomultiplier or photodiode, which converts it into electrical impulses which are accumulated and counted. The amount of light scattered is proportional to the surface area and therefore, the volume of the cells, so that the height of the electrical pulses can be used to estimate the cell volume.

# DISCUSSION

## Clinical Significance

The total RBC count is performed to assess the red cell mass in the blood. The change in erythrocyte number is frequently detected in clinical practice by ordering estimation of hemoglobin rather than total RBC count, as estimation of hemoglobin is easy and less expensive. Moreover, total RBC count by the manual method is more likely to be erroneous (more than 20 per cent). The total RBC count is still performed in some conditions to detect the red cell population, especially if the count is expected to be very high, as in polycythemia.

## Conditions that Alter Total RBC Count

### Conditions that Decrease RBC Count

**I. Physiological**

1. Pregnancy (due to hemodilution)
2. Children have lower values than adults.
3. Women have lower values than men.

   RBC count is higher in men because male sex hormones stimulate erythropoiesis. It is lower in women because estrogen inhibits erythropoiesis and there is cyclical loss of blood during reproductive life.

**II. Pathological**

1. Different types of anemia.
2. Relative decrease in RBC count occurs in different pathological conditions that produce hemodilution, for example, excess ADH secretion as occurs in posterior pituitary tumours.

### Conditions that Increase RBC Count

**I. Physiological**

1. High altitude (due to hypoxia).
2. Newborns have a high count.
3. Excessive sweating (due to hemoconcentration).

**II. Pathological**

1. Conditions that produce hemoconcentration (due to loss of body fluid), for example, severe diarrhea and vomiting.
2. Conditions that produce chronic hypoxia, for example, congenital heart disease and emphysema.
3. Polycythemia vera.

### Polycythemia

The term polycythemia, strictly speaking, implies elevated levels of all the cellular elements of blood, though it is usually used to describe the increase in the red cell count alone. Polycythemia may result from an increase in the total number of red cells in the body (**true polycythemia**) or from a reduction in the plasma volume relative to the volume of the red cells (**relative polycythemia**). True polycythemia may be due to a primary disorder of the hemopoietic tissue which produces excess of red cells (**polycythemia vera**) or secondary to excessive stimulation of erythropoiesis by erythropoietin (**secondary polycythemia**).

*Causes*

**I. True polycythemia**

1. Polycythemia vera
2. Secondary polycythemia
   a) Secondary to tissue hypoxia
      i) High altitude
      ii) Congenital heart disease
      iii) Chronic pulmonary disease
   b) Secondary to inappropriately increased erythropoietin production
      i) Kidney tumours
      ii) Liver tumours
      iii) Pheochromocytoma
      iv) Virilising ovarian tumour

**II. Relative polycythemia**

1. Dehydration
2. Redistribution of body fluids

### Anemia

Decrease in number of red cells or Hb content below normal is known as anemia (*refer* Chapter 3 *for a detailed account*).

## VIVA

1. What is the composition and function of each component of Hayem's fluid? What other fluid can be used as RBC-diluting fluid?
2. What are the advantages of using Dacie's diluting fluid?
3. What are the precautions to be taken for RBC count?
4. What are the functions of the red bead in the bulb of the pipette?
   Ans. The red bead has two functions. It helps in mixing the contents of the bulb and in quick identification of the RBC pipette.
5. What is the significance of different markings present on the RBC pipette?

Ans. There are three markings on the RBC pipette: 0.5, 1 and 101. The 0.5 mark is the mark up to which blood is sucked and the 101 mark is the mark up to which the diluting fluid is sucked to get a dilution of 1 in 200. In cases of polycythemia, dilution may have to be increased and in case of anemia, dilution may have to be decreased. The 1 mark is used for pipetting blood in conditions of severe anemia where more blood is taken for dilution. In such conditions, blood is sucked up to the 1 mark and then diluted up to the 101 mark, giving a dilution of 1 in 100.

6. When is the RBC pipette used for white cell counting? What are the other uses of the RBC pipette?

   Ans. An RBC pipette is used for counting WBC in leukemia where leucocytes are counted not in thousands but in lakhs or millions per $mm^3$ of blood. In leukemia, blood is sucked up to mark 1 in the RBC pipette and then diluted to 101 mark giving a dilution of 1 in 100. The RBC pipette is also used for sperm count and platelet count.
7. Why are the two drops of the solution from the pipette discarded before charging the Neubauer's chamber?
8. Why is the dilution obtained 1 in 200, not 1 in 202?
9. What are the sources of error in RBC count?
10. What happens to WBCs in the RBC count?

    Ans. WBCs are not lysed, and hence can be seen along with red cells. But the normal ratio of RBC to WBC is 700 : 1. Therefore, hardly any WBC is counted, as total red cells counted in 5 medium RBC squares are usually less than 700. So WBCs do not affect RBC count.
11. How do you remove a blood clot from the pipette?

    Ans. First the clot is dissolved and removed by a strong acid or $H_2O_2$; then the pipette is cleaned with distilled water. The pipette can be rinsed with alcohol or ether for rapid drying.
12. What is the use of coverslip for charging and counting?

    Ans. Coverslip, due to its flat and smooth surface, facilitates uniform spread of diluted blood on the chamber beneath the coverslip. By surface tension, it holds the diluted blood on the platform and prevents its spillage into the gutter.
13. Should both sides of the chamber be charged? Why?

    Ans. Preferably, both sides of the chamber should be charged. If the distribution of cells is not uniform or the counting on one side of the chamber is not successful, counting on the other side can be done immediately. Moreover, counting should ideally be done on both sides to assess the accuracy of the result. Charging both sides simultaneously may keep the chamber in balance and uniformly deep.
14. How do you differentiate red cells from debris or dust particles.

    Ans. Debris particles are irregular, having different shapes and sizes. Red cells are round and uniform, having a central halo-like appearance due to thinness. Therefore, counting is done using high-power objective to distinguish between red cells and debris/dust particles.
15. Why should the 'Rules of counting' be followed?

    Ans. Rules of counting are followed to prevent counting the same cells again. For this, either 'L pattern' (count the red cells present in the square and those present on its left and lower lines and ignore those on its right and upper lines) or '  pattern' (count cells on the left and upper lines and ignore those on the right and lower lines of the square) can be followed. But, 'L pattern' for few squares and 'pattern' for other squares should not be practised. Only one pattern should be followed for the entire counting.
16. What is the value of normal red cell count in adults and why is there a sex difference?
17. What are the functions of red cells?
18. What are the sites of red cell formation before and after birth?

    Ans.

    I. **Before birth (fetal life)** During fetal life, erythropoiesis takes place in three stages:

       i) **Mesoblastic stage** In the early embryo, blood formation takes place first in the mesoderm of the yolk sac (the area vasculosa), and later in the body of the fetus. The mesoderm consists of the syncytium (nucleated mass of protoplasm) which later gives rise to a network of capillary vessels. Erythropoiesis takes place intravascularly. This is the only example of intravascular hemopoiesis.

       ii) **Hepatic stage** After the third month of fetal life, the spleen and the liver are the most important sites of blood formation. Erythropoiesis occurs mainly in the liver. Therefore, it is called the hepatic stage. Red cells develop from the mesenchyme between the blood vessels and the tissue cells.

       iii) **Myeloid stage** From about the middle of fetal life ($5^{th}$ month), the bone marrow begins to form red cells. Slowly, the erythropoiesis in the liver decreases and finally towards term, the marrow becomes the sole region of erythropoiesis.

    II. **After birth** After birth, blood cells are actively produced in the marrow cavities of all the bones. By the age of 20, the marrow in the cavities of the long bones, except for the upper humerus and femur, becomes inactive. In adults, erythropoiesis is limited to the bone marrow of the femur, humerus and membranous bones like the sternum. This is called **medullary hematopoiesis.** Sometimes, because of increased demand, erythropoiesis takes place in the liver and spleen. This is called **extramedullary hematopoiesis.**

19. What are the stages of erythropoiesis?
20. What are the factors that regulate erythropoiesis?

Ans. The factors involved in regulation of erythropoiesis can be classified as follows.

i) Environmental

Hypoxia

ii) Hormonal

Erythropoietin   Androgens   ACTH   Thyroid hormones   TSH   Growth hormone   Estrogen

(All these hormones stimulate erythropoiesis except estrogen, which inhibits it.)

iii) Hemolysates (products of hemolysis)

Products of red cell destruction stimulate erythropoiesis.

iv) Vitamins

Vitamin $B_{12}$   Folic acid   Ascorbic acid

v) Metals

Iron   Cobalt   Copper   Iodine

vi) Proteins

Albumin

21. What are the conditions that alter RBC count?
22. What is anemia?
23. What is the most common cause of anemia in developing countries? What are the types of anemia?
24. What is polycythemia and what are its causes?
25. What is the fate of red cells?
26. What is stem cell therapy and stem cell harvesting?

Ans. Stem cell therapy is the transplantation of stem cells from bone marrow of normal persons to the bone of patients suffering from leukemias or other bone marrow abnormalities. Recently, stem cells are collected (harvested) from umbilical cords or blastocysts of embryos in large numbers, cultured, and used in the treatment of various diseases such as Parkinson's disease, Alzheimer's disease, diabetes, cardiomyopathy, etc.

# CHAPTER 8

# Determination of Red Blood Cell Indices

## LEARNING OBJECTIVES

After completing this practical, you will be able to:

- Explain the importance of calculating red cell indices in clinical hematology.
- Calculate different red cell indices.
- State the normal values of MCV, MCH and MCHC.
- Name the common conditions in which these indices are altered.

You may also be able to:

- Correlate the change in red cell indices in different clinical conditions.
- Explain the physiological basis of these changes.

## INTRODUCTION

From the estimated hemoglobin content, PCV (packed cell volume) and red cell count, it is possible to derive other values which indicate the red cell volume, hemoglobin content and concentration in the red cells. These values are commonly referred to as the red blood cell indices. They are *mean corpuscular volume* (MCV), *mean corpuscular hemoglobin* (MCH) and *mean corpuscular hemoglobin concentration* (MCHC). The MCV defines the volume or size of the average RBC, the MCH defines the weight of hemoglobin in the average RBC, and the MCHC defines the hemoglobin concentration or colour of the average RBC.

Another quantitative measurement of red cells, the mean corpuscular diameter (MCD), is made directly. A derived measurement determined electronically is the red cell distribution width (RDW). This is a measurement of red cell variability.

Determination of these indices is of considerable clinical importance and is widely used in the classification of anemia. When the red cell indices are calculated from manually determined values for hemoglobin, hematocrit and red cell count, the major disadvantage results from the errors associated with manual counts. If electronic counting devices are used, the error is significantly reduced. Indices calculated directly by electronic methods have been found to be more accurate. In recent years, electronic counting of indices is routinely practised in advanced laboratories.

It is important to verify all indices against observations of stained films. When the red cell indices are used in conjunction with an examination of the stained blood film, a clear picture of red cell morphology is obtained. Since red cells are very small and the amount of hemoglobin in a single cell is minute, the units in which the red cell indices are expressed are picograms (pg) and femtolitres (fl).

## METHODS

Red cell indices are determined by two methods: 1) indirectly by calculating the indices from PCV, hemoglobin and red cell count and 2) directly by automated counting.

### Calculation of Red Cell Indices

#### Mean Corpuscular Volume (MCV)

MCV is the average volume of a red cell expressed in femtolitre or cubic micrometre ($1 \text{ fl} = 10^{-15} \text{ l} = 1 \mu\text{m}^3$).

$$\text{MCV (fl)} = \frac{\text{Hematocrit (per cent)} \times 10}{\text{RBC count in millions/mm}^3}$$

where the factor 10 is introduced to convert the hematocrit reading (in per cent) from volume of packed red cells per 100 ml to volume per litre.

For example, if the hematocrit reading is 45 per cent, and the red cell count is 5 million/mm$^3$ of blood, then the MCV will be 90 fl.

$$\text{MCV} = \frac{45 \times 10}{5} = 90 \text{ fl}$$

*Normal value* The MCV in normal adults is 78–96 fl.

### *Derivation of the Formula*

45 percent = 45/100 = 45×10/1000 = $45 \times 10 \times 10^{-3}$
5 million /mm$^3$ = $5 \times 10^6/10^{-6}$ l = $5 \times 10^{12}$/ l [since 1 million = $10^6$, 1 mm$^3$ = $10^{-6}$ l]

$$\text{MCV} = \frac{45 \times 10 \times 10^{-3}}{5 \times 10^{12}/\text{l}} = \frac{45 \times 10}{5} \times 10^{-3} \times 10^{-12}\,\text{l}$$

$$= \frac{45 \times 10}{5}\ 10^{-15}\,\text{l} = 90\ \text{fl}$$

Manual estimation of red cells is less reliable; so is the determination of MCV. Automated electronic counting devices measure the electrical impedance caused by each red cell when it passes through the counting devices. The extent of impedance provides an accurate indication of the volume of each cell. Such machines not only indicate the profile of distribution of the volume of red cells, but also provide a highly reproducible value for the MCV. Therefore, the MCV derived by this means provides a reliable index of the average size of red cells.

## Mean Corpuscular Hemoglobin (MCH)

The MCH is the average weight of hemoglobin content in a red cell expressed in picograms (1 pg = $10^{-12}$ g).

$$\text{MCH (pg)} = \frac{\text{Hb (g/dl)} \times 10}{\text{RBC count in millions/mm}^3}$$

For example, if the hemoglobin content is 14 g/dl, and the RBC count is 5 million/mm$^3$

MCH = 14 × 10/5 = 28 pg

*Normal value* The normal range for MCH is 27–33 pg. It may be as high as 50 pg in macrocytic anemia, or as low as 20 pg or less in hypochromic microcytic anemia.

### *Derivation of the Formula*

14 g/dl = 14 g/100 ml = 14 × 10 g/1000 ml = 14 × 10 g/l
5 million /mm$^3$ = $5 \times 10^6/10^{-6}$ l = $5 \times 10^{12}$/ l [since 1 million = $10^6$, 1 mm$^3$ = $10^{-6}$ l]

$$\text{MCH} = \frac{14 \times 10}{5 \times 10^{12}/\text{l}}\ \text{g/l} = \frac{14 \times 10\ \text{g/l}}{5} \times 10^{-12}\,\text{l}$$

$$= \frac{14 \times 10}{5}\ 10^{-12}\,\text{g} = 28\ \text{pg}$$

## Mean Corpuscular Hemoglobin Concentration (MCHC)

The MCHC is an expression of the average hemoglobin concentration per unit volume of packed red cells. It is expressed as g/dl or per cent.

$$\text{MCHC (per cent)} = \frac{\text{Hb (g/100 ml)}}{\text{PCV/100 ml}} \times 100$$

For example, if the hemoglobin content is 15 g/dl and hematocrit is 45 per cent,

MCHC = 15/45 × 100 = 33.3 per cent.

*Normal value* The normal range of MCHC is 30–37 g/dl (or per cent).

An MCHC above 40 per cent indicates errors in the instrument or in the calculation of the manual measurements used, since an MCHC value of 37 per cent is near the upper limit for hemoglobin solubility. Therefore, this limits the *physiologic upper limit of the MCHC*. MCHC is a more reliable index than other indices as it does not involve RBC count for its calculation. Therefore, the error associated with RBC count is excluded in MCHC.

In hypochromic anemias, the hemoglobin concentration is reduced and values as low as 20–25 per cent are not uncommon.

## Colour Index (CI)

This is the ratio of hemoglobin per cent and RBC per cent.

$$\text{CI} = \frac{\text{Hb per cent}}{\text{RBC per cent}}$$

$$= \frac{\text{Estimated Hb /100 per cent of Hb}}{\text{Calculated RBC count/100 per cent of RBC}}$$

100 per cent of Hb = 14.8 g/100 ml

100 per cent of RBC = 5 million/mm$^3$

For example, if estimated Hb = 12 g/100 ml and calculated RBC count is 4 million/mm$^3$,

$$\text{CI} = \frac{12/14.8}{4/5} = \frac{12}{14.8} \times \frac{5}{4} = 1.01$$

*Normal value* The normal range of CI is between 0.85 and 1.10.

CI less than 0.85 indicates hypochromic anemia.

## DISCUSSION

### MCV

The MCV indicates whether the RBCs are microcytic, normocytic or macrocytic. If the MCV is less than 80 fl, the red cells are microcytic. If it is greater than 96 fl, the red cells will be macrocytic. If it is within the normal range, the red cells will be normocytic. The main source of error in the MCV is the considerable error in the manual red cell count.

#### Microcytosis

**Definition** When the MCV is subnormal, the condition is called microcytosis.

**Causes** Microcytosis occurs due to decreased synthesis of hemoglobin. Hemoglobin deficiency can be caused by either iron deficiency or by a defect in the formation of the globin component of hemoglobin.

1. Iron deficiency (as in iron deficiency anemia)
2. Globin deficiency (as in thalassemia)

Microcytosis frequently occurs in anemia due to hypoproteinemia and iron deficiency.

#### Macrocytosis

**Definition** When MCV is elevated the condition is called macrocytosis.

**Causes** Macrocytosis occurs due to a number of diseases, the most important being megaloblastosis of the bone marrow due to vitamin $B_{12}$ or folate deficiency.

### MCH

MCH indicates the mean amount of hemoglobin per red cell. A subnormal MCH occurs in microcytosis, but MCH is significantly less when microcytosis is associated with hypochromia (decreased concentration of hemoglobin in red cells). This is seen in iron deficiency and thalassemia minor.

### MCHC

MCHC reflects a parameter entirely different from MCH. It indicates the average hemoglobin concentration per unit volume of packed red cells.

#### Decreased MCHC

A subnormal MCHC indicates the abnormality where interference with hemoglobin formation is more than that of other constituents of red cells. This is commonly seen in iron deficiency or thalassemia.

#### Increased MCHC

Increased MCHC reflects dehydration of the red cells. This is commonly seen in spherocytosis.

### Colour Index

CI is the ratio of Hb per cent to the RBC per cent. CI decreases if Hb per cent is low and increases if RBC per cent is low. The CI indicates the Hb content of RBC. It is not a good index of hemoglobin content because when the Hb per cent and the RBC per cent change proportionately, the CI may not change as it is calculated as the ratio of both these parameters.

## VIVA

1. What are the different red cell indices?
2. What is the practical utility of red cell indices in clinical hematology?
3. Define MCV, MCH and MCHC.
4. How do you calculate MCV, MCH and MCHC?
5. What is the significance of calculating MCV?
6. What are macrocytosis and microcytosis? What are their causes?
7. What does MCH indicate? What is the significance of calculating MCH?
8. What does MCHC represent? What is the significance of calculating MCHC?
9. Why is MCHC more reliable than other indices?
10. Why does MCHC have a physiological upper limit?
    Ans. Because red cells cannot possess hemoglobin beyond a limit (metabolic limit), anemia can never be hyperchromic.
11. Why is the colour index not a good indicator of hemoglobin content of the red cells?
12. Classify anemia based on blood indices.
    Ans. Described in Chapter 4.

Chapter 9

# Total Leucocyte Count

## Learning Objectives

After completing this practical, you will be able to:

- Explain the importance of performing total leucocyte count (TLC) in practical physiology.
- Explain the structure and functions of leucocytes.
- Perform TLC by manual method (using the principle of hemocytometry).
- List the precautions and sources of error of TLC.
- State the composition and function of each constituent of Turk's fluid.
- State the normal value of TLC.
- Define leucocytosis, leucocytopenia and leukemia.
- List the common causes of leucocytosis and leucocytopenia.
- Name the types of leukemia.

You may also be able to:

- Describe the steps of leucopoiesis.
- Describe the fate of leucocytes.
- State the principle of automated method of TLC.
- Explain the variation in leucocyte count in different conditions.
- Briefly describe the types of leukemia.

## INTRODUCTION

Leucocytes (white blood cells) are nucleated cells that are involved in the defence mechanism of the body. White cells use the bloodstream primarily for transportation to their place of function in the body tissues. Leucocytes are classified as granulocytes and agranulocytes. Neutrophils, eosinophils and basophils are granulocytes, and lymphocytes and monocytes are agranulocytes.

### Formation of Leucocytes

Development of leucocytes is called **leucopoiesis**. In the embryo, white blood cells develop in the mesoderm and migrate secondarily in the blood vessels. After birth, granulocytes develop exclusively in the bone marrow. The lymphocytes and monocytes also develop from the stem cells in the bone marrow. In adults, lymphocytes are produced primarily in the lymphoid tissue (lymph nodes and spleen) and secondarily in the bone marrow. Leucocytes develop from two types of stem cells: myeloid stem cells forming granulocytes and monocytes, lymphoid stem cells forming lymphocytes (Fig. 9.1).

The number of circulating leucocytes is very precisely controlled. Though there is no definite feedback control system like that for red cells, a number of chemical substances released from the site of destruction of leucocytes affect the development of the cells. The substances that regulate the development of leucocytes are loosely called **leucopoietins** or **leucocyte-promoting factors**. These substances are various types of interleukins (produced by monocytes, macrophages and endothelial cells), colony-stimulating factors (produced by monocytes and T lymphocytes), prostaglandins (produced by monocytes), other cytokines and lactoferrin.

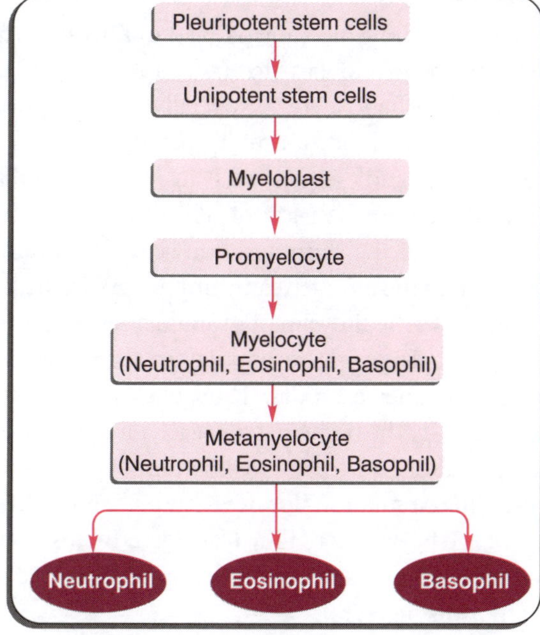


Fig. 9.1 Sequence of development of granulocytes.

## Functions of Leucocytes

The granulocytes act as phagocytic scavengers. They engulf and destroy invading microorganisms, and clear the body of unwanted particulate materials such as dead or injured tissue cells. The neutrophils are said to be the **first line of defence** against acute bacterial invasion. They kill organisms by phagocytosis. The monocytes are also phagocytes and are thought to be the **second line of defence** against microbial invasion. The monocytes enter the tissues where they form tissue macrophages (reticuloendothelial system) and phagocytose microorganisms in the tissues. Lymphocytes and plasma cells act as immunocytes and maintain the body's immunity. Plasma cells are not normally found in blood, but they are formed from B lymphocytes under specific immunologic stimulation. Plasma cells produce antibodies that destroy or inactivate antigens.

## Life History of Leucocytes

Radioactive labelling has shown that the entire maturation process, from myeloblast to neutrophil, takes about three days. The leucocytes, especially the granulocytes that circulate in blood, are marginated on vessel walls (**margination**) and sequestered in closed capillaries. Neutrophils have a half-life of about six hours in the circulation. After their immigration into the tissues, they never return to the bloodstream, and survive in the tissues for a few days. The lifespan of granulocytes is about four to eight days. Their entire population turns over about two and half times each day. Thus, over 100 billion cells are produced by the bone marrow each day. Lymphocytes survive for about 80 to 100 days. Monocytes, after their activities in circulation for few hours, enter different tissues of the body where they transform themselves into tissue macrophages, and stay in the tissues for a long time (a few months or years).

The life history of leucocytes has three phases: marrow phase, circulation phase and tissue phase.

**Marrow phase** This is the phase of development of leucocytes. In this phase there are two pools: *mitosis pool* (development of myeloblast to myelocyte) and *maturation pool* (development of metamyelocytes to matured cells).

**Circulation phase** Many leucocytes, especially neutrophils stick to the endothelial margin of blood vessels (*margination pool*) and remaining circulate in the blood (*active circulation pool*).

**Tissue phase** After activities in circulation, leucocytes enter the tissues (*tissue pool*). Monocytes in the tissue form the *mononuclear phagocyte system* (previously known as reticuloendothelial system)

## Normal Count

| | | |
|---|---|---|
| Adults | : | 4000–11,000/mm$^3$ of blood |
| Newborns | : | 10,000–25,000/mm$^3$ of blood |
| Infants | : | 6000–18,000/mm$^3$ of blood |
| Children | : | 5000–15,000/mm$^3$ of blood |

There is no gender difference.

# METHODS OF COUNTING

White blood cells are counted by two methods: non-automated (manual) and automated. The manual cell count is less accurate, but is still used widely in developing countries, especially in laboratories of medical colleges.

## Manual Method

### Principle

Blood is diluted with an acid solution that removes red cells by hemolysis and accentuates the nuclei of white cells. The counting of the white cells then becomes easy. Counting is done using a microscope under low-power objective, and with knowledge of the volume of fluid examined and the dilution of the blood obtained, the number of white cells per mm$^3$ of undiluted whole blood is calculated.

### Requirements

**I. Apparatus**

1. Microscope
2. Hemocytometer (WBC diluting pipette and counting chamber)
3. Equipment for sterile finger prick
4. Watch glass
5. Coverslip

**II. WBC diluting fluid** Also known as *Türk's fluid.*

*Composition*

1. 1% glacial acetic acid solution
2. Gentian violet stain or aqueous methylene blue (0.3 per cent w/v)

3. Distilled water

*Function of each constituent*

Acetic acid causes destruction of red cells (hemolysis).

Gentian violet stains the nuclei of leucocytes.

Distilled water acts as a solvent.

## Procedure

1. Clean and dry the pipette, watch glass, coverslip and Neubauer's chamber thoroughly.
2. Take enough WBC diluting fluid in a watch glass.
3. Prick the finger under aseptic conditions and wipe off the first drop of blood. Allow a good-sized blood drop to form on the finger tip spontaneously (do not squeeze).
4. Touch the blood drop with the tip of the pipette and suck blood exactly up to the 0.5 mark.
   If blood is drawn above the 0.5 mark, bring the blood column to the 0.5 mark by tapping the tip of the pipette on the palm or finger, or by using non-absorbent material. Do not use gauze or cotton for this adjustment, because the liquid portion of the sample inside the stem will be drawn into the absorbent material, leaving a higher concentration of cells inside the stem.
5. Wipe the tip of the pipette and maintain the blood level at the 0.5 mark by holding the pipette in a horizontal position.
6. Dip the tip of the pipette into the diluting fluid (in the watch glass) well below the surface of the liquid.
7. Suck WBC diluting fluid exactly up to the 11 mark. While the bulb is being filled, you may tap the pipette with a finger to knock the bead down below the surface of the solution in the bulb. This will help prevent the formation of bubbles.
8. While removing the pipette from the diluent, maintain the level of the mixture at the 11 mark by closing the pipette tip with the index finger.
9. Hold the pipette horizontally and close both ends of the WBC pipette, then gently mix the contents of the bulb. For mixing, shake the pipette at right angles to its long axis for a few seconds. The glass bead in the pipette should move from one side to the other.
10. After mixing, place the pipette in a horizontal position to prevent any loss of its contents until the cell count is completed.
11. Discard the first two drops of fluid from the pipette as the fluid in the stem does not contain cells.
12. Charge the Neubauer's chamber as described in Chapter 6 and allow two minutes for the cells to settle down.
13. Place the charged chamber on the stage of the microscope and adjust it for observation under low power.
14. Focus the Neubauer's chamber under the low-power objective and check for uniform distribution of cells in the WBC squares. If the cells are not uniformly distributed, clean the Neubauer's chamber and recharge it.
15. Count the total number of WBCs in the four corner squares under the low-power objective. To avoid counting the same cells again, follow the '**Rules of Counting**'. Using the 'L pattern' counting, count the white cells present in the square and those on its left and lower lines. Ignore those on its right and upper lines. 'Γ (inverted L) pattern' counting may also be followed, i.e., count cells on the left and upper line of the square, in addition to cells in the square. But, 'L pattern' for few squares and 'Γ pattern' for other squares should not be practised. Only one pattern should be followed for the entire counting, and preferably the same should be practised by all the students of the class.

> **Note:** WBCs appear similar to clumped red cell debris or stained particles. They are identified as clear, nucleated and refractile bodies.

16. Draw the WBC squares in your notebook and enter the observation. Calculate the final result.

## Dilution Obtained

The volume of the bulb is 10 (11 – 1 = 10). The stem of the pipette (from the tip of the pipette to mark 1) contains diluting fluid that does not take part in the dilution. Dilution (mixing of blood with diluting fluid) occurs only in the bulb. Thus 10 volumes of diluted blood (in the bulb) contain 0.5 volumes of blood and 9.5 volumes of diluting fluid, giving a dilution of 0.5 in 10. Thus, the dilution obtained is 1 in 20, or 20 times.

## Calculation

Area of 4 WBC squares = $4 \times 1 = 4$ mm$^2$

Volume of 4 WBC squares = $4 \times 1/10 = 4/10\ mm^3$
Dilution factor = 1 : 20
Cells in $4/10\ mm^3$ volume of diluted blood = $n$
Therefore, cells in 1 $mm^3$ volume of diluted blood
= $n \times 10/4$
Therefore, cells in 1 $mm^3$ volume of undiluted blood
= $n \times 10/4 \times 20 = \mathbf{n \times 50}$

### Precautions

(Same as precautions taken for RBC count; for details see Chapter 7.)

1. The pipette, coverslip and Neubauer's chamber should be dry and thoroughly cleaned.
2. The prick should be at least 3 mm deep. Do not squeeze to get blood.
3. Wipe off the first drop of blood.
4. Draw blood exactly up to the 0.5 mark
5. Wipe the tip of the pipette.
6. Suck the WBC diluting fluid exactly up to the 11 mark.
7. Air bubbles should not enter while pipetting the fluid.
8. Before charging the chamber, gently mix the contents of the bulb of the pipette.
9. Discard the first two drops of fluid.
10. Do not overcharge or undercharge.
11. Do not allow air bubbles to enter the chamber.
12. Once the counting chamber is filled (charged), complete the counting as early as possible before the fluid begins to dry.
13. If the distribution of cells is not uniform, discard and recharge.
14. Avoid counting the same cells twice.

### Sources of Error

Fortunately, error in the leucocyte count is not as critical as error in the red cell counts. Even an error of 20 per cent does not affect the result much. The possible sources of error may be the errors inherent in the method or technical errors.

#### *A. Errors Inherent in the Method*

1. **Error of visual count** One potential error is mistaking dirt or clumped red cell debris for leucocytes. This error decreases by making a second count in the Neubauer chamber of the opposite side.
2. **Error due to distribution of cells** Distribution can never be perfectly uniform even with thorough mixing and charging. If there is clumping of leucocytes, recharge the chamber.

#### *B. Technical Errors*

1. **Dilution error** Improper volume measurement of blood and diluent
2. **Pipetting error** Use of defective pipettes
3. **Charging error** Improper charging of the chamber
4. **Counting error** Improper counting
5. **Calculation error** Wrong calculation

### Additional Information

In case of a very high leucocyte count, as seen in leukemia, dilution may have to be increased to 100 times or more. The RBC pipette can be used for this purpose. Blood is sucked up to mark 1 of the RBC pipette and then diluted 100 times. Calculation is done according to the dilution.

## Automated Method

Automated cell counting is done either by impedance counting or by light scattering technology. The principle is the same as that described in Chapter 7.

# DISCUSSION

## Physiological Significance

The total leucocyte count is performed to assess the subject's ability to defend his body against microbial invasions. The leucocytes are a part of the body's defence system that provides protection against infections. The leucocytes constitute the mobile defences of the body. They can pass through the vascular endothelium and enter the tissues by means of *diapedesis*. Leucocytes migrate to the site of injury in response to chemical substances released by the microorganisms, or by the injured or infected cells. The process of migration is called **chemotaxis** and the substances that promote migration are called **chemoattractants**. The white cells, once they reach the site of invasion, engulf and digest the foreign substances (**phagocytosis**). All granulocytes, especially neutrophils, and monocytes kill the organisms by phagocytosis. Lymphocytes are the principal cells of the body's immune system.

## Clinical Significance

Total leucocyte count is a part of the routine hematologic investigation used to assess the nature and severity of an infection, extent of spread of the disease and the body's defence capability. In some diseases, alteration in leucocyte count alone may be diagnostic, but frequently the leucocyte count is ordered with other investigations, especially with the differential leucocyte count, to aid in diagnosis. When the total leucocyte count increases above the normal, the condition is called *leucocytosis*, and when the count decreases below normal, it is called *leucocytopenia*.

## Conditions that Alter Total Leucocyte Count

### Leucocytosis

**I. Physiological**

1. *Newborns and infants* Count is as high as 15,000–20,000/mm$^3$.
2. *Physical exercise* During physical exercise, circulation becomes more dynamic, which causes disruption of margination of the leucocytes along the vascular endothelium. Therefore, leucocytes are shifted from their margination pool into the circulation pool (into general circulation). This is called ***shift leucocytosis***. Leucocytosis does not occur due to increased formation of cells.
3. *After food intake* Following food intake, the body's metabolism increases; this increases the body's temperature. Because of this, circulation improves. This causes disruption of margination of leucocytes and results in leucocytosis.
4. *Exposure to sun* and increased environmental temperature.
5. *Pregnancy* Leucocytosis occurs in spite of hemodilution. The exact cause of leucocytosis in pregnancy is not known, but it may possibly be due to the action of hormones on leucopoiesis.
6. *Parturition* Leucocytosis occurs due to the combined effects of tissue injury, hemorrhage and severe exertion.
7. Pain, nausea and vomiting
8. Menstruation
9. Emotion and anxiety

**II. Pathological**

1. *Acute bacterial infection* Infection with pyogenic bacteria (localised or generalised) is the commonest cause of leucocytosis. Examples of bacterial infections are boils, abscess and pneumonia. But, there are a few bacterial infections in which leucocyte count decreases. One of the typical examples of leucocytopenia in acute bacterial infection is typhoid fever.
2. *Chronic bacterial infection* An example is tuberculosis.
3. Tissue injury
   Infarction
   Burns
   Surgery
4. Hemorrhage
5. Neoplasia
6. Stress states and hyperactivity
   Convulsions
   Severe colic
7. Inflammatory disorders
   Certain collagen diseases
   Rheumatic fever
8. Metabolic disorders such as diabetic ketoacidosis
9. Corticosteroid therapy

### Leucocytopenia

**I. Physiological**

Physiological decrease in leucocyte count is very rare. Exposure to severe cold may sometimes decrease the total WBC count.

**II. Pathological**

1. Infections
   Typhoid fever
   Paratyphoid fever
   Early phases of many viral infections such as infectious hepatitis
2. *Overwhelming sepsis* In severe sepsis, consumption of neutrophils exceeds production.
3. Replacement of hemopoietic tissue in the bone marrow by neoplastic infiltrative cells:
   Acute leukemia
   Lymphoma
   Multiple myeloma
   Myelofibrosis
4. *Aplastic anemia* Hypoplasia of bone marrow decreases all the cell counts.
5. *Cytotoxic therapy* Treatment of malignant diseases by cytotoxic drugs

6. Drugs (especially in sensitive individuals):
   Chloramphenicol
   Sulpha drugs
   Aspirin
7. Hypersplenism
8. Starvation and malnutrition

Leucocytopenia usually occurs due to neutropenia.

## Leukemia

Leukemia is a cancerous disease of the blood-forming tissues. Uncontrolled proliferation of one or more of the various hematopoietic cells occurs, and these progressively displace the normal cellular elements.

### Definition

Leukemia is a malignant neoplasia of hemopoietic cells in which there is abnormal proliferation of leucocytes and their precursors. It results in appearance of abnormal and immature cells with very high leucocytosis in the peripheral blood, and infiltration of tissues by leukemic cells. There is increased infiltration of bone marrow by the proliferating cells. The total leucocyte count is usually very high, except in the subleukemic or aleukemic form of leukemia. Usually, the proliferation involves the leucocytic series; occasionally, erythroid precursors or megakaryocytes may also be involved in the disease process.

### Causes

The exact cause of leukemia is not known. Some of the probable causes are:

1. Heredity and genetic predisposition
2. Environmental factors, especially exposure to gamma radiation producing genetic mutation or chromosomal aberration
3. Various chemicals and drugs
4. Some viral infections

### Classification

Leukemia is broadly classified into two main categories: myeloid (myelocytic) and lymphocytic leukemia. These two types are again classified into acute and chronic forms on the basis of the clinical course and the number of blast cells present.

#### *Acute Lymphoblastic Leukemia (ALL)*

ALL is primarily a disease of children and young adults. This constitutes 80 per cent of childhood acute leukemias. It rarely occurs in adults and the elderly. The most common mode of presentation is with symptoms of anemia or hemorrhage, infective lesions of the mouth and pharynx, fever, prostration, headache and malaise. There is generalised lymphadenopathy, splenomegaly and hepatomegaly. The typical blood picture consists of anemia, thrombocytopenia and moderate or marked increase in leucocytes, the majority of which are blast cells (lymphoblasts; 60–80 per cent).

#### *Acute Myeloblastic Leukemia (AML)*

This primarily affects adults between the ages of 15 and 40 years. It constitutes only 20 per cent of childhood leukemias. The presentation is like that of ALL, but lymphadenopathy and hepatosplenomegaly is not common. Blood picture presents anemia, thrombocytopenia and moderate to high leucocytosis. More than 60 per cent of leucocytes in the peripheral blood are blast (myeloblast) cells.

#### *Chronic Myeloid Leukemia (CML)*

This form of leukemia accounts for about 20 per cent of all cases of leukemia. It is primarily a disease of adults of 30–60 years with peak incidence in the fourth and fifth decades of life. Onset is usually slow with non-specific features like anemia, weight loss, weakness and easy fatigability. *Splenomegaly is the outstanding physical sign*. Hepatomegaly may be present, but lymph node enlargement is rare. Markedly elevated total leucocyte count, usually more than one lakh cells per $mm^3$ of blood, is seen. Neutrophils and metamyelocytes constitute most of the circulating cells. Blast cells are rarely present except in the blastic crises.

#### *Chronic Lymphocytic Leukemia (CLL)*

CLL is the most indolent of all leukemias. It occurs typically in persons over 50 years of age. Men are affected twice as frequently as women. Patients present non-specific symptoms. *Lymphadenopathy is the outstanding physical sign*. Hepatosplenomegaly may be present. Mild to severe increase in leucocyte count is seen. More than 90 per cent of leucocytes are lymphocytes.

## Leukemoid and Leukoerythoblastic Reactions

### Leukemoid Reaction

This is a condition in which the leucocyte count is very high, and may be more than 50,000 per $mm^3$ of blood. This occurs rarely in severe infections, especially in children and may occur in acute hemolysis and malignant diseases such as carcinoma of breast, lungs and kidney. Few immature cells may be seen in peripheral blood. This is not leukemia, but blood picture resembles chronic leukemia. Therefore, it is called leukemoid reaction. This is differentiated from leukemia by demonstrating high leucocyte alkaline phosphatase (LAP) in blood, which is depressed in CML.

## Leukoerythoblastic Reaction

This is similar to that of leukemoid reaction, but in addition, nucleated red cells (erythroblasts) are seen in blood smear, indicating that erythrocytic series is involved in the process. This may occur in severe hypoxia, severe anemia and malignancies infiltrating bone marrow.

## Leukostasis

When leucocyte count is above 100,000 per $mm^3$ of blood, sometimes thrombus consisting mainly of leucocytes are lodged in brain, lung and heart. This is called leukostasis. The risk of leukostasis is high when blood is transfused before TLC is reduced in conditions of high leucocytosis.

# VIVA

1. Which diluting fluid is used for determining total leucocyte count and what is its composition? What is the function of each component?
2. Why are two drops of blood discarded from the pipette before charging the Neubauer's chamber?
3. Why is the dilution obtained 1 in 20, and not 1 in 22?
4. In which condition is the RBC pipette used for white cell counting?
5. What are the precautions for performing total leucocyte count? What are the possible sources of error in total leucocyte count?
6. What are the functions of the white bead present in the WBC pipette?
7. What are the functions of leucocytes?
8. What is the physiological significance of performing a total leucocyte count?
9. What are the causes of physiological leucocytosis?
10. What is the mechanism of leucocytosis in physical exercise?
11. What are the pathological causes of leucocytosis and leucocytopenia?
12. What is leukemia? What are the types of leukemia?
13. What are the most frequently occurring leukemias in children and in adults?
14. What is the principle of bone marrow transplantation (BMT) and what are the indications?

    Ans. BMT is the intravenous transfusion of red bone marrow from a healthy donor to the recipient. Usually, the marrow is taken from ileac crest. However, the donor's marrow should match with the recipient's. The stem cells of the donor settle in recipient's marrow, proliferate and produce cells of different cell lines. This is usually indicated in some form of leukemia, malignancies, severe hemolytic anemia, genetic disorders and severe combined immunodeficiency diseases.
15. What is leukemoid reaction and leucoerythroblastic reaction?
16. How are leucocytes produced (give broad steps of leucopoiesis)?
17. How is leucopoiesis regulated and what are the leucopoietic growth factors (leucopoietins)?
18. What is the lifespan of leucocytes?
19. What is the fate (different phases in the life history) of various leucocytes?
20. What is mononuclear phagocyte system, and what are its components?

    Ans. Monocytes after entering the tissue become tissue macrophages that are combinedly called mononuclear phagocyte system (MPS). They kill microbes by phagocytosis. The cells of MPS in different tissues are:

    A. In blood
       - Monocytes

    B. In bone marrow
       - Monoblasts, Promonocytes

C. In tissues
- Kupffer cell in liver
- Osteoclasts in bone marrow
- Alveolar macrophages in lungs
- Histiocytes in connective tissue
- Microglia in brain
- Red pulp macrophages in spleen
- Macrophages in lymph nodes and thymus
- Mesangial cells in kidney
- Dendritic cells/histiocytes in skin

Chapter 10

# Preparation and Examination of Blood Smear

### Learning Objectives

After completing this practical, you will be able to:

- List the uses of peripheral blood smear.
- Select a spreader for making blood smears.
- Make a good smear using the wedge method.
- Fix and stain the smear.
- List the criteria of an ideal smear.
- Name and explain the functions of each constituent of the Leishman stain.
- List the precautions and sources of error in preparing a smear.
- Identify red cells, platelets, and different leucocytes in a smear.
- List the identifying features of all the cells.
- List the differences between neutrophils and eosinophils, and large lymphocytes and monocytes.

You may also be able to:

- Explain the possible sources and effects of error in making a smear.
- Name the other stains used in staining a smear.
- Explain the principle and advantages of other methods of making smears.
- List the causes of defective staining and the steps to prevent them.

## INTRODUCTION

Microscopic examination of peripheral blood smear is performed as a routine hematologic investigation. It is done by preparing, staining and examining a thin film of blood on a glass slide. The blood film is often called *peripheral blood smear.* The cellular components of blood are noted while examining a blood smear under a microscope.

The unique feature of a blood smear is that it can be retained and preserved as an original record in the laboratory to recheck for errors or to evaluate the progress in the clinical status of the patient, or to assess the response of the patient to treatment. Thus, it can be reused after days, months or years. No other routine hematologic test can be reassessed. Therefore, a peripheral smear is a permanent record. A peripheral smear made for differential count of leucocytes not only provides information regarding them but also about the other cellular elements of blood. It is used to study the morphology of red cells and platelets, and to detect the presence of various parasites like malarial parasites and microfilaria. Peripheral blood smear is also used to verify hemoglobin status, hematocrit and the red cell count of the subject. Because the blood film has many uses, a smear must be carefully prepared and studied.

## METHODS OF PREPARATION OF A SMEAR

The blood smear is prepared in two stages:

1. Making a blood smear
2. Fixing and staining the blood smear

### Making a Blood Smear

A blood smear can be made by three methods:

1. Cover glass method
2. Glass slide (wedge) method
3. Centrifugal method

The glass slide method is commonly practised.

### Wedge or Glass Slide Method

The wedge method is so called because the smear resembles a wedge.

#### Principle

Spreading a drop of blood on the glass slide makes a thin film.

#### Requirements

1. Glass slides
2. *Spreader* These are specially designed glass slides with a smooth edge, the breadth is slightly less than

that of usual glass slides. If spreaders are not available, a glass slide with a smooth edge can be used.
3. Equipment for sterile finger puncture

## Procedure

1. Take four clean and grease-free glass slides and select one as a spreader.
2. Clean the tip of the middle finger with alcohol, allow the finger to air dry and prick the finger tip with a sterile lancet.
3. Discard the first drop of blood.
4. Place a drop of blood on one end (say the right end) of a slide, in the middle, about 1 cm from the end, in such a way that only the top of the blood drop touches the slide. Ensure that the skin of the tip of the finger does not touch the slide.

> **Note:** If the finger touches the slide, moisture or oil from the skin of the finger may spoil the smear.

5. Place the specimen slide on the flat surface of the table, and hold it in position at the left end of the slide (the end opposite the blood drop) with the middle or index finger and thumb of the left hand.
6. Place the smooth clean edge of the spreader slide on the specimen slide just in front of the drop of blood. There should be an approximate angle of 30°– 45° between the two slides (Fig. 10.1A).
7. Using the right hand, draw the spreader back until it touches the drop of blood. Let the blood run along the edge of the spreader (Fig. 10.1B). The spreader can be slightly shaken sideways to facilitate the spread of blood along the edge of the spreader.
8. When the blood has spread evenly across the edge of the spreader slide, push the spreader to the other end of the slide with a smooth, quick and controlled movement.

> **Note:** All the blood should be used up before you reach the other end of the slide.

Keep the angle of the spreader constant throughout the process. As the spreader is moved, a thin film of blood will be deposited behind it. The blood film should cover half to three-fourths of the slide when properly prepared (Fig. 10.1C). It should also be noted that no blood is left at the end of the smear (all blood should be completely used in making the smear), otherwise distribution of cells becomes unequal (for explanation, see Precaution 8).

9. Turn the spreader slide over (this gives another clean edge) and prepare a second blood film using the same procedure.

> **Note:** A third smear can also be prepared. At least two films should be made for the same blood specimen.

10. Dry the blood smears quickly by waving them in the air, or if the moisture is too high, as occurs in the rainy season, dry the films by waving them rapidly about 5 cm above the flame of a spirit lamp. Never bring the smear close to the flame as excess heat may damage it.

> **Note:** If the smears are not dried quickly, the blood cells will shrink and appear distorted.

Never put the slide directly over the flame. However, adequate drying is essential to preserve the quality of the film. Hence, before staining the slide, make sure that the film is completely dry. It is also observed that if the smear is not dry, it washes off when the slide is washed after staining.

## Precautions

1. The glass slides must be scrupulously cleaned. Dirty slides do not give an even smear.
2. Discard the first drop of blood as it contains tissue fluid and is rich in neutrophils.
3. Do not squeeze to make a drop of blood. The puncture should be deep enough to form the blood drop spontaneously.
4. Use a medium-sized blood drop. If the drop is small, the size of the smear decreases, and if it is too large, some blood will be left at the tail end of the smear.
5. Make the smear immediately after placing the drop of blood on the slide. A delay will cause uneven distribution of white cells on the film. Rouleaux formation by the red cells and clumping of platelets occurs if the blood is not spread immediately. The blood may also clot.
6. The spreader slide must be moved steadily and confidently with a single, quick and smooth movement. Loss of contact between the spreader slide and smear slide yields poor smears. Pressing too much on the spreader slide results in accumulation of white cells and platelets at the end of the smear.

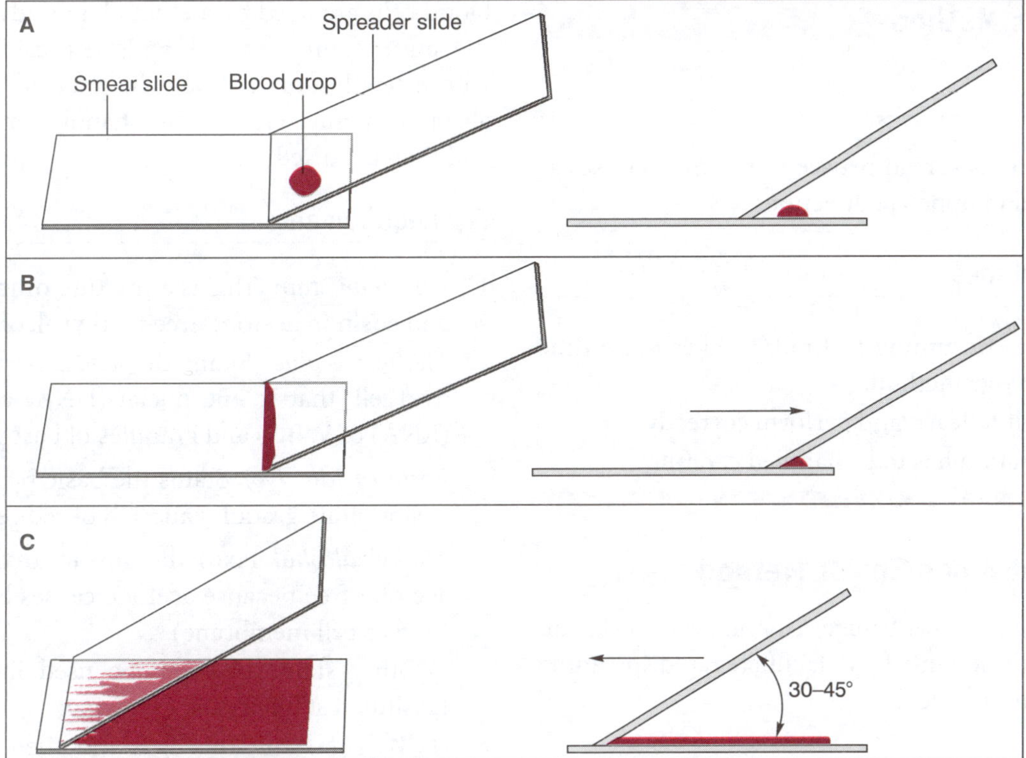


Fig. 10.1 Steps in the preparation of blood smear (arrows indicate the direction of movement of the spreader slide).

Pushing the spreader slide with an uneven movement results in thicker and thinner areas in the body of the smear (Fig. 10.2C). The smear should not be made very fast or slow. The smear *becomes thick if made very fast or thin if made slow*. With practice, the student will learn the optimum speed.

7. Before the smear is made (before the spreader slide is moved), ensure that the blood has spread uniformly along the edge of the spreader; otherwise a thick narrow smear results.
8. The entire amount of blood taken on the slide should be used in making the film. The film should gradually fade away at the feather edge and no blood should be left at the tail end of the smear (Fig. 10.2A). A defined border at the end of the smear indicates that most of the white cells have piled up at the end. When this occurs, the heavier neutrophils accumulate at the end to a greater extent than the other white cells, resulting in uneven distribution of white cells in the body of the smear. Platelets also tend to accumulate at the end of the smear if some blood is left (not used in the smear), decreasing the number in the body of the smear.
9. The angle between the spreader slide and the glass slide should be about 45°. The angle of holding the spreader slide contributes to the thickness of the film.

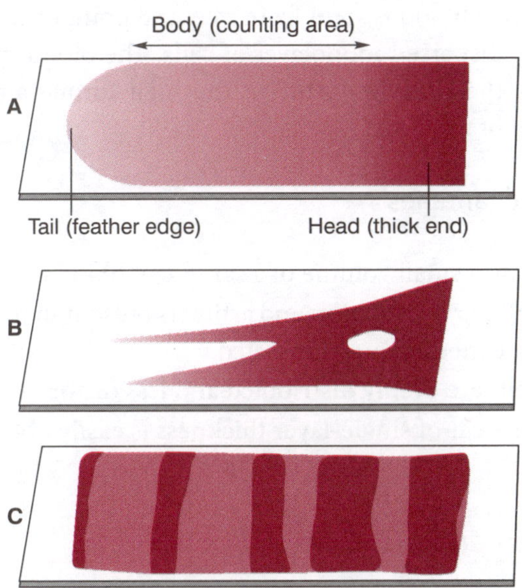


Fig. 10.2 Good (A) and bad (B, C) smears.

Increasing the angle yields a thicker smear, whereas decreasing it gives a thin smear.

10. The smear should be completely dry. A wet smear will not stick to the slide when staining. The cells are distorted if the smear takes a long time to dry.

### Cover Glass Method

#### Principle

A drop of blood is spread between two cover glasses as they are pulled in opposite directions.

#### Disadvantages

1. It is a time-consuming method. It takes more time than the wedge method.
2. It is difficult to learn and perform correctly.
3. The preparation has to be handled carefully.

### Centrifugal Blood Smear Method

With the use of a cytocentrifuge, a monolayer of cells can be prepared. These centrifuges facilitate rapid spreading of the cells across a slide.

#### Principle

A drop of blood is spun from a central point creating an evenly dispersed monolayer of cells. The blood spreads across the slide by virtue of the high torque and low inertia of motion.

#### Advantages

1. Only a small volume of a sample of blood is used.
2. Cellular destruction and artifacts present in the glass slide method are eliminated.
3. Cells are evenly distributed and less distorted.
4. A smear of single-layer thickness is easily obtained.

## Fixing and Staining a Smear

### Method of Fixing and Staining a Smear

#### Principle

The staining method for blood films fixes dead cells, as opposed to supravital staining which is used with living cells. *Fixation* is the process by which blood cells are made to adhere to the slide, and *staining* is the process by which the cells (cytoplasm and nuclei) are stained. The blood cells are fixed by methanol. It is advisable to stain the smear soon after making it. If it cannot be stained within few hours, it should be fixed by immersion in absolute methyl alcohol (methanol) for 2–3 seconds, and then air-dried.

#### Requirements

1. *Leishman stain* This is a mixture of methylene blue and eosin in acetone-free methyl alcohol.
   *Methylene blue* Stains the acidic part of the (basic dye) cell, that is, the nuclei (DNA) and cytoplasm (RNA) of WBCs and granules of basophils.
   *Eosin (acidic dye)* Stains the basic part of the cell—eosinophilic granules and Hb of red cells.
   *Methyl alcohol* Fixes the smear to the slide. It is acetone-free because acetone causes lysis of the cell (breaks cell membrane).
   Other stains that can be used in place of the Leishman stain are the following:
   i) *Wright stain* This is a modified Romanowsky stain, very similar to the Leishman stain. It produces the same colour reaction with the cellular components of blood as the Leishman stain.
   ii) *May–Grunwald and Giemsa stain* The slide is first stained with the May–Grunwald stain for 5 minutes, and then replaced by the Giemsa stain for 10 minutes. Staining of the cells is similar to that of the Leishman stain.
   iii) *Field stain* It was originally introduced for thick films for malarial parasites in field study. Staining is rapid and convenient. It is used for rapid screening of blood smears.
2. *Staining rack* This consists of two glass rods placed in parallel, about 5 cm apart, on a tray. The glass rods hold the slides and the tray holds the stain and water poured on the slides.
3. Distilled water
4. Pasteur pipette
5. Blood smears

#### Procedure

1. Place the slides on the staining rack with the blood smear (dull side of the slide) facing up. If the staining rack is not available, place two glass rods over a tray to hold the slide.

2. Pour 8–12 drops of Leishman stain on the slide. The stain should just cover the smear.
3. Note the time and leave it for 1½ to 2 minutes.

> Note: During this period, the alcohol in the stain fixes the cells (fixation time).

4. Add double the amount of distilled water on the smear, with the help of a dropper, taking care that the water does not spill.
5. Mix the stain and the water evenly by blowing gently or by blowing air through a Pasteur pipette.

> Note: A metallic shiny layer (greenish scum) should form on the top of this mixture.

6. Note the time and leave it for 7–10 minutes.

> Note: This is the time when staining occurs (staining time). Staining time may have to be adjusted according to the reaction of the stain. Reduce the time if it is overstained, and increase the time if it is poorly stained.

7. Pour off the stain, and wash the slide gently and thoroughly under tap water.

> Note: Make sure that the stream of water does not fall directly on the smear. While pouring off the stain, it should be ensured that the greenish scum does not stick to the surface of the smear.

8. Shake off all water adhering to the slide and set the slide in an upright position in a drying rack.

> Note: Keep the smeared surface of the slide face down. This prevents dust from settling on the smear.

### Precautions

1. The smear should dry completely before staining. Unless completely dry, the smear will not stick to the slide and is removed while washing.
2. Adequate quantity (8–10 drops) of stain should be poured on the smear and the stain should cover the entire smear. Do not pour excess stain (it should just cover the smear).
3. Allow adequate fixing time (check the recommended time of fixation for the given sample of stain).
4. The distilled water should just cover the slide. Care should be taken to prevent spill-over of the mixture of water and stain.
5. It is important that the staining rack be kept on a level surface so that the stain is uniform throughout the film and the mixture does not spill over.
6. Water and stain should be mixed by gentle blowing. Mixing should be done immediately after pouring the distilled water.
7. Exact timing for staining should be followed (check the recommended time).
8. When the mixture of stained water is poured off the slide, take care to prevent deposition of scum on the smear.
9. While washing, ensure that the smear is not directly under the stream of water.

## EXAMINATION OF A STAINED BLOOD SMEAR

After the initial preparation of the smear, it is examined under the low-power and high-power objectives, and then under the oil-immersion objective. Examination under the low-power and high-power objectives includes:

- Evaluation of the quality of the smear
- Rough estimation of the red cell and leucocyte numbers
- Distribution of the cells in the smear
- A scan of the film

Examination under the oil-immersion objective includes:

- Examination of the erythrocytes for alterations and variations in morphology
- Evaluation of platelet numbers and morphology
- Differential count of leucocytes

## Steps of Examination

Examination of a smear takes place in three steps: general scanning, selection of the site for examination, and identification and count of cells.

### General Scanning

First, examine the stained blood smear under low-power objective for screening. This allows you to scan the entire slide of blood smear quickly. Note the background colour and distribution of white cells. In an ideal stained smear, three zones can be identified (Fig. 10.2A):

i) the thick area or the 'head' of the smear
ii) the 'body' of the smear
iii) the thin end or 'tail' of the smear

Towards the tail end, the red cells lie singly, and neutrophils and monocytes predominate, while in the body, the red cells overlap each other to a certain extent and the lymphocytes predominate. Towards the head end, the red cells considerably overlap and eosinophils predominate. This non-uniform distribution of various types of leucocytes is inherent to the smear prepared by the glass slide method. Therefore, the smear should be examined in a zigzag fashion (Fig. 11.1) across the length of the smear but not along the breadth of the smear, to get an accurate differential count. If the scanning indicates very irregular distribution of leucocytes (neutrophils and monocytes are fully concentrated in the tail), the smear will give an inaccurate differential count. In this case, make a new smear. The scanning of the entire slide also gives an opportunity to detect the presence of large abnormal cells like megakaryoblasts, and parasites like microfilariae.

## Selection of Site for Examination

If the smear is an ideal one (one-cell thickness), it should be examined throughout its length excluding the extreme, thin portion of the tail and the very thick portion of the head. But, if the smear is not an ideal one (which often happens in practice) select the portion of the blood smear where the red cells just touch each other or slightly overlap but are not piled on top of one another. This area is usually found near the feather edge (between the body and tail) of the film. Place a drop of immersion oil on the slide (do not place on a coverslip) directly on the smear. Now switch to the oil-immersion objective. Ensure that the objective makes contact with the oil. Look through the microscope and increase the light by opening the iris as needed.

## Identification of Cells

Identify various types of cells on the basis of the following characteristics as a result of staining with the Leishman stain. Even if the smear is not properly stained, the shape and size of the cells provide sufficient clues for their identification (Fig. 10.3).

### a) Red Blood Cells

*Appearance* Red cells appear as round bodies containing no nucleus, granules or discrete materials.

*Staining* Stain orange-red. The red colour is darker at the edge of the cell than in the centre (giving the appearance of a central halo). This variation is caused by the biconcave shape of the cells which contains less hemoglobin in its (thinner) centre.

*Size* The diameter of the cells is about 7.2 μm.

### b) Platelets

*Appearance* Under high power, they look like dirt and stain deposits. Under oil-immersion, they look like pin heads. They contain no nuclei. On fine adjustment, platelets look refractile; this is a characteristic feature that distinguishes them from deposited stained particles.

*Staining* : Stain mauve-pink.

*Distribution* : Usually they are present in groups or aggregates (many platelets lying close to each other), but presence of a single (isolated) platelet is not unusual.

*Size* : They are the smallest cells in the peripheral smear. The diameter of the platelets is 2–4 μm.

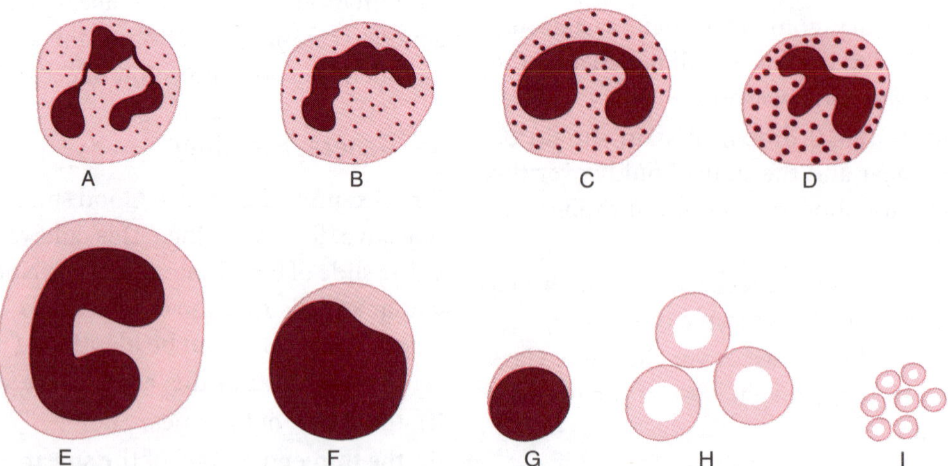


Fig. 10.3 Cells observed in a normal peripheral smear. A. Segmented neutrophil; B. Band neutrophil; C. Eosinophil; D. Basophil; E. Monocyte; F. Large lymphocyte; G. Small lymphocyte; H. Red cells; I. Platelets.

*c) Leucocytes*

i) Neutrophils (Fig. 10.4)

*Size* : 10–14 µm

*Nucleus* : Multilobed (2–6 lobes), lobes are connected by thin strands. In band-form, the nucleus is sausage-shaped (also called stab form).

*Cytoplasm* : Looks pale pink, contains fine pink granules.

ii) Eosinophils (Fig. 10.5)

*Size* : 10–14 µm

*Nucleus* : Usually bilobed, lobes are connected by a thick strand, giving the appearance of spectacles (spectacle-shaped nucleus).

*Cytoplasm* : Stains faint pink containing coarse brick-red or red-orange granules. The cytoplasm is usually not visible as it is obscured by granules.

iii) Basophils

*Size* : 10–14 µm

*Nucleus* : Usually bilobed or trilobed, but lobes are usually not distinctly visible because the cell is studded with granules.

*Cytoplasm* : Contains numerous coarse granules. Granules are blue-black and fill the cells and obscure the nucleus.

iv) Large lymphocytes (Fig. 10.6)

Size : 10–14 µm

*Nucleus* : Occupies 80–90 per cent of the cell. It is eccentrically placed and oval or round with or without a dent. It is homogeneous (compact) and violet in colour.

*Cytoplasm* : Clear blue cytoplasm; usually contains no granules.

v) Small lymphocytes (Fig. 10.7)

*Size* : 6–9 µm (same as or slightly larger than red cells)

*Nucleus* : Occupies almost the whole cell. It is homogeneous (compact) and deep violet in colour.

*Cytoplasm* : May not be present or sometimes there may be a thin rim of clear blue cytoplasm present at the periphery. There are no granules.

vi) Monocytes (Fig. 10.8)

*Size* : 12–24 µm, the largest leucocytes

*Nucleus* : Occupies 50 per cent of the cell, centrally or slightly eccentrically placed. It is usually kidney-shaped or horseshoe-shaped, but may be round, oval, dumb-bell shaped, or irregular. Non-homogeneous (spongy) in appearance and pinkish violet in colour

*Cytoplasm* : Ground-glass (hazy, turbid) appearance
- grey-blue in colour
- usually contains no granules, but sometimes (15–30 per cent of monocytes) fine granules may be present.

The differences in structure and function of leucocytes are summarised in Table 10.1.

Table 10.1 Structure and functions of various leucocytes.

| Leucocytes | % in DLC | Structure | Functions |
|---|---|---|---|
| Neutrophils | 50–70% | 10–14 µm diameter; nucleus is multilobed, connected by thin strands of chromatin; cytoplasm has fine, pink granules. | Phagocytosis of organisms (first line of defence) |
| Eosinophils | 1–4% | 10–14 µm diameter; nucleus is bilobed; coarse brick-red granules in cytoplasm | Combat the effects of histamine in allergic reactions, kill parasitic worms |
| Basophils | 0–1% | 10–14 µm diameter; nucleus is bilobed or irregular in shape; Large cytoplasmic granules are deep blue-purple | Release heparin, histamine, and serotonin in allergic reactions that promote overall inflammatory response |
| Lymphocytes | 20–40% | Small lymphocytes are 6–9 µm in diameter; large lymphocytes are 10–14 µm in diameter; nucleus is round or slightly indented; cytoplasm forms a clear rim around the nucleus | Mediate immune responses |
| Monocytes | 2–8% | 12–25 µm diameter; nucleus is oval or kidney-shaped or horseshoe-shaped; cytoplasm turbid in appearance | Phagocytosis (after transforming into tissue macrophages) |

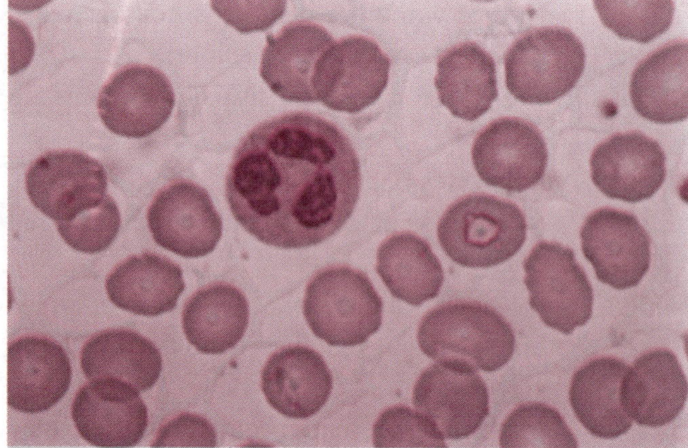

Fig. 10.4 Neutrophil.

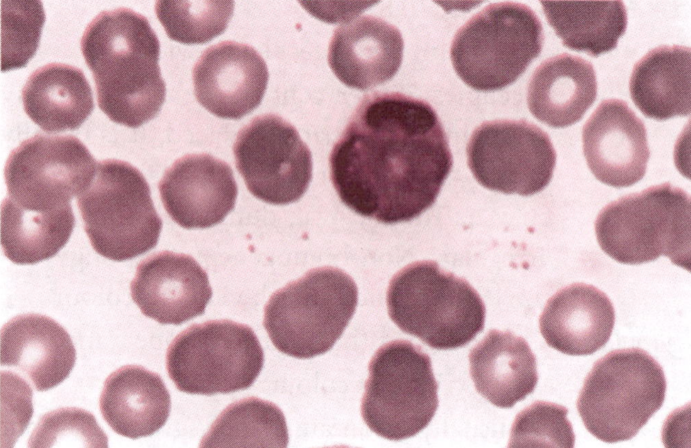

Fig. 10.5 Eosinophil.

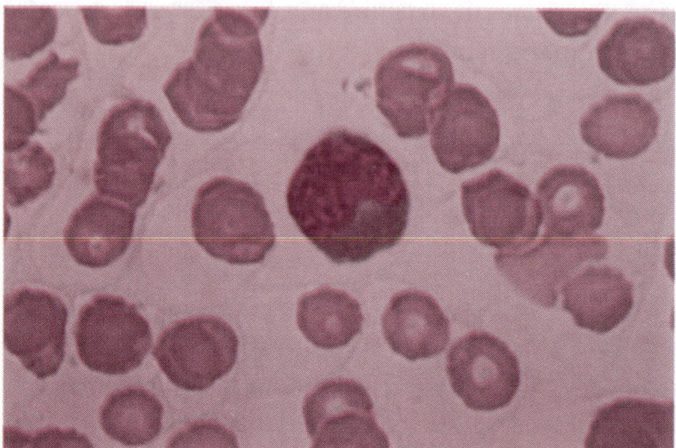

Fig. 10.6 Large lymphocyte.

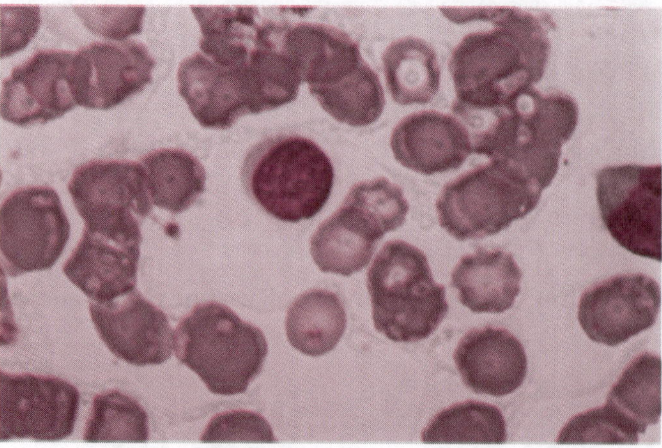

Fig. 10.7 Small lymphocyte.

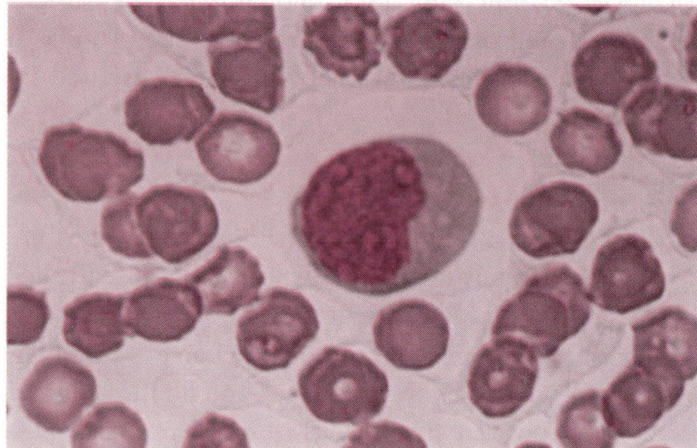

Fig. 10.8 Monocyte.

## DISCUSSION

A bad smear results from lack of sincerity and interest in making the smear. If all the steps for preparing and staining the smear are properly followed, the smear will definitely be a good one. The smear may be prepared well but improper staining may spoil it completely.

## Staining Defects

The following staining defects are frequently observed.

1. *Presence of more precipitated stained particles* This occurs due to either improper washing or using an old stain that has not been properly filtered. Improper washing means inadequate washing of metallic scum. It can be corrected by using a freshly prepared or adequately filtered stain or by correcting the washing procedure. The smear should be washed for about one minute.
2. *Excessively red appearance* This occurs due to understaining, overwashing or use of a highly acidic stain or water (for staining). It can be rectified by increasing the fixing and staining time, and properly washing the smear. Buffered water (pH 6.8) or distilled water should be used for staining.

Table 10.2 Differences between neutrophils and eosinophils, and large lymphocytes and monocytes.

| | Neutrophils | Eosinophils |
|---|---|---|
| 1. Size | Double the size of red cells | Double the size of red cells |
| 2. Nucleus | Multilobed (2–6 lobes), obes connected by thin strands | Usually bilobed,lobes connected by a thick strand (gives spectacular appearance) |
| 3. Cytoplasm | Contains fine pink granules | Contains coarse brick-red granules |
| | **Large lymphocyte** | **Monocyte** |
| 1. Size | About double the size of red cells | Triple the size of red cells, or more |
| 2. Nucleus | i) Oval or round, usually with a dent | Kidney or horse-shoe shaped nucleus. But may be round, oval or dumb-bell shaped |
| | ii) Compact (homogeneous) | Spongy (non-homogeneous) |
| | iii) Eccentric | Centrally placed |
| | iv) Occupies 80–90 per cent of the cell | Occupies 50 per cent of the cell |
| 3. Cytoplasm | Clear, sky blue, contains no granules | Hazy, ground glass in appearance, sometimes (15–20% monocytes) may contain fine granules |
| 4. Nuclear-Cytoplasmic ratio | 20 : 80 to 90 | 50 : 50 |

3. *Excessively blue appearance* This results from overfixing, overstaining, inadequate washing or use of a highly alkaline stain or water (for staining). It can be rectified by decreasing the fixing and staining time, proper washing of the smear and using proper stain and water.
4. *Faded appearance of the cells* This results from overwashing, understaining, underfixing or from an improperly made stain.

## Morphological Differences in Leucocytes

Usually, students confuse neutrophils with eosinophils, and large lymphocytes with monocytes. The important points that help to differentiate between these cells are given in Table 10.2.

## Criteria of an Ideal Smear

1. A good blood smear should cover one-half to three-quarters of the length of the slide.
2. It should be thickest at the origin and gradually thin out rather than having alternate thick and thin areas. The thin end of the smear should have a good feather edge, that is, the film should fade away without a defined border at the end. It should be tongue-shaped.
3. There should be no streaks or gaps in the smear.
4. It should be one-cell thick (of red cells), that is, the red cells should not overlap each other nor should they remain far away from each other. If a film is thick, the cells pile up.

   Thickness of the film is determined by:
   i) Size of the drop of blood used—a thick film results when the drop of blood is large and a thin film from a small drop of blood.
   ii) The speed of the stroke used to move the spreader slide—a thick film results from fast spreader movement and a thin film from slow movement.
   iii) The angle at which the spreader slide is moved—a thick film results when the angle is greater than 45° and a thin film results when the angle is less than 30°.
5. It appears salmon pink to the naked eye if stained properly.
6. It should not contain precipitated stained particles.
7. When examined microscopically, the background or space between the cells should be clear, the red cells should appear light red-orange, the platelets should look pink, and the leucocytes should have the proper colour for the nucleus, cytoplasm and granules.

## Preparation of Thick and Thin Smears

Thick smears are mainly prepared for detection of microfilariae in the peripheral blood. A drop of blood is placed at the centre of the slide and spread with the corner of another slide. The film is allowed to dry for 30 min at 37°C and then stained. The entire film is scanned using a low-power objective.

## VIVA

1. What are the methods of making a blood smear?
2 Why is the glass slide method called the wedge method?
3. What are the advantages of making a smear by the centrifugal method?
4. How is a spreader selected for making a smear?
5. Why should the angle between the spreader and the specimen slide be between 30° and 45°?
6. Why should the smear be dried quickly after preparing it?
7. What is the method of drying the blood smear?
8. What are the precautions to be taken while preparing a blood smear?
9. Why is the smear immediately made after placing the drop of blood on the slide?
10. Why is the smear made by a steady and smooth movement of the spreader?
11. Why should the initial drop of blood be fully used in making a smear?
12. Name the factors that determine the thickness of a smear.
13. Why is the fixing done immediately after making a smear?
14. What is the method of fixing a smear if staining is to be delayed?
15. Which is the stain usually used in staining the blood smear? What are its constituents and what are the functions of each constituent?
16. Why is the alcohol present in the Leishman stain acetone-free?
17. Why is distilled water added to the stain after fixation?

    Ans. In the first two minutes, methanol in the stain causes fixation of cells. Distilled water is added after that to cause ionisation of the stain (ionisation of methylene blue and eosin). Stains work only in their ionised form. Therefore, distilled water is added to the stain after fixation has taken place.
18. Why is water not used as a solvent for the Leishman stain?

    Ans. Staining of cells is done only after they are fixed, by adding distilled water. Water opposes fixation of cells.

    If water is present in the stain, the cells will stain but will not fix to the smear. Therefore, stain is water-free. Water also enhances rouleaux formation of red cells, but this rarely happens after the smear is made.
19. Why is buffer water preferred to distilled water for staining?

    Ans. Ionisation of stain particles occurs maximally at pH 6.8. The pH of buffer water is 6.8. Tap water is not used as it contains impurities.
20. Name the other stains that can also be used for staining the smear.
21. In which special circumstances is the Field stain used?
22. What are the precautions for staining a smear?
23. Why is the stain diluted with distilled water after 1½ to 2 minutes and not earlier?
24. What is the significance of the appearance of scum on the staining fluid after addition of distilled water?

    Ans. It indicates that the staining has been done properly. If the greenish scum does not float on the diluted stained surface, this indicates that the scum is deposited on the surface of the smear. In that case, the cells look hazy when examined under a microscope.
25. Why is the smear examined under low-power objective before being examined under an oil-immersion objective?
26. What is the purpose of general scanning of the smear prior to DLC?
27. Which is the most ideal area of the smear for DLC and why?
28. What are the uses of a blood smear?

    Ans. A blood smear is used for:

    i) DLC and detection of abnormalities of leucocytes if present, for example, immature and abnormal leucocytes as seen in different leukemias.
    ii) Study of red cell morphology (size, shape, hemoglobin content).
    iii) Rough estimation of red cells and PCV.
    iv) Determination of indirect platelet count and morphology of platelets.
    v) Detection of the presence of parasites, for example, malarial parasite, microfilariae and so on.

vi) Sex can be differentiated by identifying the presence of Barr body in the nucleus of neutrophils (it needs special staining).

29. How do you identify red blood cells and platelets in a smear?
30. How will you differentiate neutrophils from eosinophils and large lymphocytes from monocytes?
31. What are the criteria of an ideal smear?
32. What are the causes of deposition of precipitated stains in the smear and how do you prevent it?
33. What are the causes of excessive red or blue appearance of the smear and how do you prevent it?
34. What are the causes of the faded appearance of the cells in the smear and how do you prevent it?
35. What is punctate basophilia (basophilic stippling) and what does it indicate?

    Ans. Punctate basophilia or basophilic stippling is the presence of numerous basophilic granules in red cells. It indicates disturbed rather than increased erythropoiesis. It occurs in thalassemia, megaloblastic anemia, infections, liver disease, poisoning by lead and heavy metals, unstable hemoglobins and pyrimidine 5'-nucleotidase deficiency.

36. What are Dhol bodies, and what do they indicate?

    Ans. Dhol bodies are small, round or oval, pale blue-grey bodies usually found in the periphery of neutrophils. They consist of ribosomes and endoplasmic reticulum. Their presence indicates bacterial infections. But they are also seen in tissue damage, inflammation and pregnancy.

Chapter 11

# Differential Leucocyte Count

### Learning Objectives

After completing this practical, you will be able to:

- Describe the importance of performing DLC in practical physiology.
- select a good spreader slide.
- prepare a good smear for making DLC.
- identify the leucocytes.
- perform a differential count within the stipulated time.
- Describe the structure and functions of various leucocytes.
- list the common causes of increase or decrease in different leucocytes.

You may also be able to:

- explain the functions of different leucocytes.
- State the physiological basis of alteration in cell counts in different clinical conditions.

## INTRODUCTION

The types and numbers of each type of leucocyte counted are traditionally reported as percentages. Determination of percentage distribution of leucocytes in peripheral blood is known as differential leucocyte count (DLC). Increase or decrease in individual cell lines are reported separately and give more meaningful information to the physician regarding the status of the leucocytes in the blood. Five types of leucocytes are encountered in normal peripheral blood. They are divided into granulocytes and agranulocytes. Neutrophils, eosinophils and basophils are granulocytes, and lymphocytes and monocytes are agranulocytes. In 15–30 per cent of monocytes, fine granules are seen. However, since this is not a constant feature, monocytes are classified under agranulocytes.

The size of the cells, whether small, medium or large, cannot be directly measured in the smear in the microscopic field but can easily be compared with the size of the surrounding normal red blood cells in the same field, which are approximately 7.5 m in diameter. The various characteristics of the nucleus and the cytoplasm of the cells are considered for identifying leucocytes. The features of the nucleus include the shape and size compared to the rest of the cell, and the pattern of chromatins in the nucleus. The features of the cytoplasm include the presence or absence of granules, the nature of granules and their staining characteristics and colour, and the relative amount of cytoplasm.

## STRUCTURE AND FUNCTIONS OF LEUCOCYTES

### Neutrophils

Neutrophils are the commonest leucocytes. They constitute 50–70 per cent of the total leucocytes. Typically, there are two types: segmented and band neutrophils.

#### Segmented Neutrophils

*Structure*

The diameter of neutrophils (Fig. 10.4, Chapter 10) varies from 10 to 14 μm, and the nucleus forms a relatively small part of the cell. The nucleus can assume various shapes, but its usual configuration is lobular (a series of lobes connected by narrow strands of chromatin filaments). It usually contains 2–5 lobes, but sometimes may contain more. No nucleoli are visible in the nucleus. The cytoplasm has a faint pink colour and contains a large number of fine pink granules. About two-thirds of the granules are specific neutrophilic granules, while the remaining one-third are azurophilic granules.

*Functions*

Neutrophils are actively phagocytic (Table 10.1, Chapter 10). The granules have many hydrolytic enzymes and appear to be lysosomal in character. Phagocytosis occurs through a series of events, which include opsonisation, chemotaxis, ingestion and degranulation. During phagocytosis, a number of chemicals are released, such as hydrogen peroxide, and hypochlorite and hydroxyl radicals, all of which are strongly bactericidal. Neutrophils form the *first line of defence* against acute bacterial infections.

### Band Neutrophils

These neutrophils are younger neutrophils. The relative band neutrophil count in adults is 2–5 per cent (of the total neutrophils).

#### Structure

Band neutrophils resemble segmented neutrophils except for the shape of their nucleus. The nucleus may be rod- or band-shaped. There may be slight indentations, but without definite lobes. The number of granules in band neutrophils is more than in segmented neutrophils.

#### Functions

The functions are the same as that of segmented neutrophils except that the cells are more active (phagocytic).

## Eosinophils

#### Structure

Eosinophils (Fig. 10.5) are slightly larger than neutrophils. Their diameter is 10–14 μm. The nucleus usually has 2 lobes (sometimes 3). The lobes are plumper. No nucleoli are visible. The cytoplasm is packed with brick-red coarse granules. The cytoplasm is pale blue, but is usually obscured by granules. The granules are hard, firm bodies that are not easily damaged. Eosinophilic granules are also highly refractile, a feature that is often valuable in distinguishing them from neutrophilic granules.

#### Functions

Eosinophils are involved in defending the body from allergic reactions (Table 10.1, Chapter 10). Eosinophil granules contain a number of chemicals like MBP (major basic proteins), protein X, ECF-A (eosinophil chemotactic factor of anaphylaxis) and lysozymes that neutralise allergens and are also larvicidal and parasiticidal.

## Basophils

Basophils are the rarest leucocytes, constituting 0.5 per cent of the total leucocyte population in peripheral blood.

#### Structure

They are about the same size as neutrophils. The nucleus occupies a relatively greater portion of the cell. The nucleus is often irregular in shape. The cytoplasm is colourless and contains coarse granules. The nucleus and cytoplasm are very often totally obscured by granules which are large, deeply stained and blue-black or deep brown in colour.

#### Functions

The exact function of basophils is not known. Basophil granules contain heparin, histamine and a slow-reacting substance (SRS). The cells are phagocytic. After their activities in the blood, they enter the tissue.

## Monocytes

Monocytes constitute 2–8 per cent of the total leucocytes.

#### Structure

Monocytes (Fig. 10.8, Chapter 10) are the largest leucocytes, 12–25 μm in diameter. The nucleus is large and occupies 50 per cent of the cell. The nucleus is frequently kidney-shaped or horseshoe-shaped, but it may be oval, lobular, notched or polymorphic. It never undergoes segmentation. Nuclear chromatins are sharply segregated and distributed in a linear arrangement of delicate strands which gives the nucleus a stringy appearance. The cytoplasm is abundant and is ground-glass or muddy blue in appearance. Sometimes, it contains extremely fine pink granules. The granules are azurophilic.

#### Functions

Monocytes are actively phagocytic (Table 10.1, Chapter 10). They remain in circulation for a few hours and then migrate into the tissues and transform themselves into tissue macrophages. They are the **second line of defence** of the body. They protect the body against bacteria, viruses, fungi and parasites. They also participate in immunity. They act as the antigen-presenting cells, and also secrete a number of cytokines that mediate various immunologic responses.

## Lymphocytes

Lymphocytes constitute 20–40 per cent of leucocytes in adults. But the count is slightly higher in infants and children, who have more lymphocytes and less neutrophils.

*Structure*

Structurally, lymphocytes are of two types—small and large. The majority (80 per cent) of the circulating lymphocytes are small. Only 20 per cent of lymphocytes are large.

### Small lymphocytes

The size of small lymphocytes (Fig. 10.7) is the same as or slightly bigger than the red cells. Their diameter ranges from 7 to 10 μm. The cells are mainly occupied by the nucleus. The nucleus is round or slightly notched. Almost the entire nucleus stains deep purple. The cytoplasm may not be present, but there may be a thin rim of cytoplasm to one side at the periphery.

### Large Lymphocytes

Large lymphocytes (Fig. 10.6) are of the same size as or slightly larger than neutrophils. Their diameter varies from 10 to 16 μm, but may be as much as 20 mm. A large lymphocyte is confused with monocytes. The nucleus is large and occupies about 90 per cent of the cell. The nucleus contains homogeneous chromatin with some clumping at the nuclear periphery. This gives the nucleus of lymphocytes a compact appearance in contrast to the spongy appearance of the nucleus of monocytes. The cytoplasm is clear and navy blue in colour, in contrast to the hazy or turbid cytoplasm of monocytes. The cytoplasm contains no granules, but on very rare occasions, a few fine azurophil granules may be seen.

*Functions*

Lymphocytes mediate the immunologic responses of the body (Table 10.1, Chapter 10). Functionally, lymphocytes are divided broadly into two categories: T lymphocytes and B lymphocytes. The majority (80 per cent) of the circulating lymphocytes are T lymphocytes. T lymphocytes mediate cellular immunity, which is concerned with viral and fungal infections, parasitic infestation, cancer cells, transplant rejection and rejection of tumour cells. B lymphocytes mediate humoral immunity by producing antibodies concerned with protecting the body against bacterial and other infections. B lymphocytes do not directly synthesise antibodies, which are produced by *plasma cells*. B cells, on specific immunologic stimulation, transform themselves into plasma cells. Therefore, plasma cells are not normally found in the blood.

## Normal Count

For a differential leucoctye count, a minimum of 100 cells should be counted, though ideally, 200 or more cells should be counted to find out the more accurate percentage of each type of leucocyte. The percentage distribution of cells in a normal leucocyte count in adults is:

| | |
|---|---|
| Neutrophil | : 50–70 per cent |
| Eosinophil | : 1–4 per cent |
| Basophil | : 0–1 per cent |
| Lymphocyte | : 20–40 per cent |
| Monocyte | : 2–8 per cent |

Infants and children have fewer neutrophils (40–60 per cent) and more lymphocytes (25–55 per cent).

# METHODS

## Method of Counting Leucocytes

### Principle

A blood film stained with the Leishman stain is examined under an oil-immersion objective and the different types of white blood cells are identified. The percentage distribution of these cells is then determined.

### Requirements

1. Glass slides
2. Leishman stain
3. Microscope
4. Distilled water
5. Pasteur pipette

### Procedure

1. Prepare blood smears and stain the smears with Leishman stain as described in Chapter 10.
2. First, examine the smear under a low-power objective for general scanning and assessing the quality of the smear, and for studying the distribution pattern of the cells.
3. Place a drop of cedar wood oil on the smear at the feather edge. Bring the oil-immersion objective into position and make the lower end of the objective touch the drop of oil. Using the fine adjustment screw, adjust the objective and focus the cells.

4. For counting cells, start from one end of the smear and move the slide in a zigzag manner (Fig. 11.1). Count individual white cells that you come across and enter your observation in a table (as described below) in your rough notebook. Continue counting until 100 cells are counted.
5. Calculate the percentage of each leucocyte and report your observation.

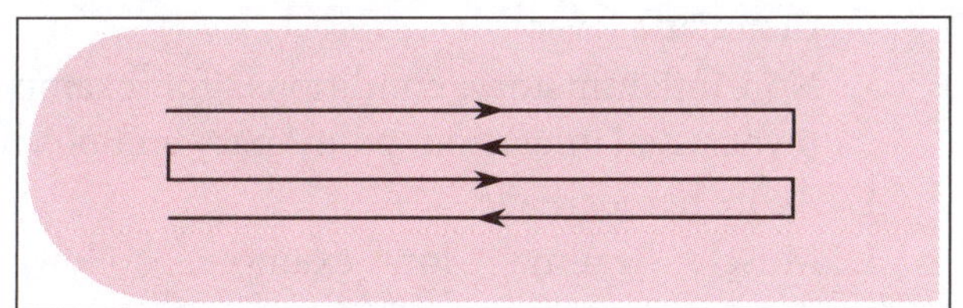

Fig. 11.1 Zigzag way of counting leucocytes for differential count. Arrows indicate the direction of counting.

## Precautions

All the precautions described in the previous chapter are applicable to this practical. In addition, the following precautions should be observed:

1. The quality of the smear should be assessed before starting the count. The smear should be discarded if it is not good and a fresh smear should be prepared.
2. Count cells throughout the length of the smear, except the extreme ends of head and tail.
3. Counting should be done in a zigzag pattern to prevent double counting of a cell.
4. A minimum of 100 cells should be counted.
5. The slide should be preserved for future rechecking of the result.

## Observation and Result

Different leucocytes are placed in groups of 5, five lines indicating five cells (four vertical lines and one oblique line placed over the four lines indicates the fifth cell). In this way, 100 cells are counted. An example of such type of counting is shown below.

| | | |
|---|---|---|
| Neutrophils | 卌 卌 卌 卌 卌 卌 卌 卌 卌 卌 卌 | = 55 cells |
| Eosinophils | 卌 卌 卌 | = 15 cells |
| Basophils | | = nil |
| Lymphocyte | 卌 卌 卌 卌 卌 | = 25 cells |
| Monocytes | 卌 | = 5 cells |
| | Total | = 100 cells |

| | | |
|---|---|---|
| Neutrophils | : | 55 per cent |
| Eosinophils | : | 15 per cent |
| Basophils | : | 0 per cent |
| Lymphocytes | : | 25 per cent |
| Monocytes | : | 5 per cent |

Alternatively, a table of 100 small squares can be drawn and each cell counted can be entered in the small squares of the table, till 100 cells are filled. On the right side of the table, against each row, the number of different leucocytes present in that row can be entered in separate columns and finally, the percentage can be taken as shown below.

| N | N | N | L | L | N | N | N | E | M |
|---|---|---|---|---|---|---|---|---|---|
| N | L | L | N | L | E | E | N | N | N |
| N | N | N | L | E | N | E | M | N | N |
| N | L | L | E | N | N | N | L | N | N |
| N | N | N | L | L | L | N | E | N | E |
| N | N | N | L | L | N | N | N | N | M |
| N | L | L | N | E | E | N | L | E | N |
| N | N | N | L | L | N | E | M | N | N |
| N | L | L | E | E | N | M | L | N | N |
| N | N | N | L | L | L | N | E | N | N |

| N | E | B | L | M |
|---|---|---|---|---|
| 6 | 1 | 0 | 2 | 1 |
| 5 | 2 | 0 | 3 | 0 |
| 6 | 2 | 0 | 1 | 1 |
| 6 | 1 | 0 | 3 | 0 |
| 5 | 2 | 0 | 3 | 0 |
| 7 | 0 | 0 | 2 | 1 |
| 4 | 3 | 0 | 3 | 0 |
| 6 | 1 | 0 | 2 | 1 |
| 4 | 2 | 0 | 3 | 1 |
| 6 | 1 | 0 | 3 | 0 |
| **55** | **15** | **0** | **25** | **5** |

Neutrophils : 55 per cent
Eosinophils : 15 per cent
Basophils : 0 per cent
Lymphocytes : 25 per cent
Monocytes : 5 per cent

### Inference

There is moderate eosinophilia of 15 per cent. Other leucocytes are in the normal range.

## DISCUSSION

Differential count is a frequently ordered investigation in clinical medicine. Usually it is done along with other hematologic tests, like total leucocyte count, to assess the ability of the subject to defend the body from microbial invasion, and also to assist in diagnosing the disease.

## Clinical Significance

Differential count is vital for the diagnosis of a number of blood-related diseases involving leucocytes or red cells. Its primary use is to identify changes in the distribution of white cells, which may be related to a particular disease like a specific infection (for example, typhoid) or a malignant condition (like leukemia). Clinical terms like increase in specific white cells (neutrophilia, eosinophilia, lymphocytosis and monocytosis) or their decrease (neutropenia, eosinopenia, lymphocytopenia and monocytopenia) are based on the result of the differential count. In addition, a study of the blood smear reveals morphological abnormalities of blood cells, the presence of abnormal cells, and the presence of blood parasites. Differential count also helps in the approximate estimation of other cells (RBCs and platelets). Morphological studies of red cells enable a physician to recognise the hemoglobin status and types of anemia, and also help to check reports on blood indices.

### Conditions that Alter Different Cell Counts

*I. Neutrophilia*

**A. Physiological**

1. Exercise
2. Pregnancy
3. Parturition
4. Food intake
5. Emotional stress
6. Exposure to cold

**B. Pathological**

1. Acute pyogenic infections, for example, tonsillitis, pneumonia
2. Non-infective inflammations, for example, rheumatic fever
3. Non-inflammatory conditions, for example, myocardial infarction, pulmonary embolism
4. Acute hemorrhage
5. Muscle trauma, for example, following surgery
6. Leukemia, for example, chronic myeloid leukemia
7. Toxic conditions, for example, uremia, hepatic coma
8. Corticosteroid therapy

*II. Neutropenia*

**A. Physiological** Physiological neutropenia is very rare. Sometimes, it occurs after chronic exposure to severe cold.

**B. Pathological**

1. Starvation and debility
2. Typhoid and paratyphoid fever
3. Aplastic anemia (bone marrow failure)
4. Parasitic infections, like malaria, kala azar
5. Viral infections like measles, influenza, viral hepatitis
6. Hypersplenism
7. Drug-induced neutropenia

*III. Eosinophilia*

1. Allergic conditions
   Bronchial asthma
   Urticaria
   Food allergy
   Hay fever
2. Parasitic infestations
   Hookworm
   Filariasis
   Hydatid disease
3. Skin diseases
   Psoriasis
   Pemphigus

4. Collagen diseases
   Periarteritis nodosa
5. Hodgkin's disease
6. Addison's disease
7. Certain leukemias

*IV. Eosinopenia*

1. ACTH therapy
2. Cushing's disease
3. Acute pyogenic infections
4. Aplastic anemia

*V. Basophilia*

1. Chronic myeloid leukemia
2. Polycythemia

*VI. Basophilopenia*

It occurs rarely, as seen in severe septicemia or aplastic anemia.

*VII. Lymphocytosis*

1. Chronic infections
   Tuberculosis
   Pertussis (whooping cough)
   Syphilis
   Brucellosis
2. Infectious mononucleosis
3. Lymphocytic leukemia
4. Lymphomas
5. Viral infections

*VIII. Lymphocytopenia*

1. Immunosuppressive therapy
2. ACTH therapy
3. Hodgkin's disease
4. Bone marrow failure

*IX. Monocytosis*

1. Protozoan diseases
   Malaria
   Kala azar
2. Hodgkin's disease
3. Monocytic or myelomonocytic leukemia
4. ACTH therapy

*X. Monocytopenia (rare)*

1. Bone marrow failure
2. Aplastic anemia
3. Septicemia

## VIVA

All the 36 questions listed in the previous chapter are suitable for this chapter also. The following are some additional questions:

37. What are the functions of neutrophils, eosinophils and basophils?
38. What are the functions of lymphocytes and monocytes?
39. What is the normal percentage distribution of different leucocytes in peripheral blood?
40. What is the clinical significance of performing DLC?
41. What are the conditions that increase or decrease the different types of leucocytes?
42. How do you calculate the absolute count of each type of leucocyte by using the value of TLC and DLC?

    Ans. Absolute count of a cell is equal to the number of that cell counted in DLC divided by 100 × TLC

    For example, if TLC = 7000/ $mm^3$ of blood, DLC is as follows:

    | | | | |
    |---|---|---|---|
    | Neutrophils | : 55 per cent | Lymphocytes | : 25 per cent |
    | Eosinophils | : 15 per cent | Monocytes | : 5 per cent |
    | Basophils | : 0 per cent | | |

    Absolute count of the various leucocytes is as follows:

    Neutrophils = (55/100) × 7000 = 3850/$mm^3$ of blood
    Eosinophils = (15/100) × 7000 = 1050/$mm^3$ of blood
    Lymphocytes = (25/100) × 7000 = 1750/$mm^3$ of blood
    Monocytes = (5/100) × 7000 = 350/$mm^3$ of blood

Chapter 12

# Arneth Count

## Learning Objectives

After completing this practical, you will be able to:

- Identify neutrophils of various stages.
- State the percentage distribution of neutrophils in various stages.
- Perform the Arneth count.
- List the precautions taken while doing the Arneth count.
- List the functions of neutrophils.
- Explain the meaning and causes of 'shift to right' and 'shift to left'.

You may also be able to:

- Explain the clinical significance of the Arneth count.
- Explain the mechanism of 'shift to right' and shift to left' that occur in various conditions.

## INTRODUCTION

Arneth count (also called Cooke–Arneth count) is the determination of the percentage distribution of different types of neutrophils on the basis of the number of their nuclear lobes. Joseph Arneth, a German physiologist classified neutrophils into five types (stages) according to the number of lobes of their nuclei (Fig. 12.1).

$N_1$ (Stage 1): The nucleus is unilobed. This is called *band neutrophil* because the nucleus is rod- or band-shaped. There may be slight indentations, but distinct lobes (clearly separated lobes by thin strands) are not found. In some of the neutrophils, the nucleus may be U-shaped (these are called *stab neutrophils.*)

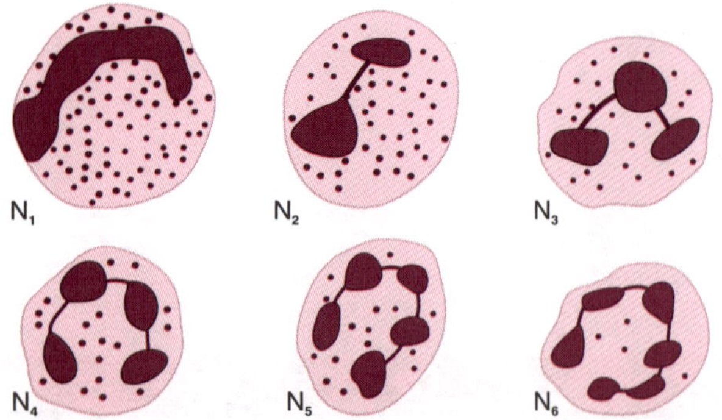


Fig. 12.1 Stages of neutrophils. Note that with maturation, the number of nuclear lobes increases but the number of granules and cell size decrease.

$N_2$ (Stage 2): The nucleus is bilobed (two lobes, separated by a thin strand).

$N_3$ (Stage 3): The nucleus is trilobed (three lobes, separated by thin strands).

$N_4$ (Stage 4): The nucleus is tetralobed (four lobes, separated by thin strands).

$N_5$ (Stage 5): The nucleus is pentalobed (five lobes, separated by thin strands).

Rarely, $N_6$ (six lobes) and $N_7$ (seven lobes) may be encountered.

This staging of neutrophils is based on the degree of maturity. The younger neutrophils contain fewer nuclear lobes than the older ones.

Sometimes it is difficult to stage neutrophils, especially when the lobes of the nucleus are folded. In such situations, two other parameters may be considered: (1) the number of granules and (2) the cell size. The younger cells contain more granules. As the cells participate in physiologic activities, they lose their granules (degranulation), and therefore, the older cells contain less granules. The neutrophils of Stage 6 or 7 contain very few or no granules. The size of the cell also decreases as the age advances. In older cells ($N_5$, $N_6$ and $N_7$), the nucleus may also exhibit the features of degeneration in the form of fragmentation (of lobes) and pyknosis.

**Normal count**

$N_1$ : 2–10 per cent
$N_2$ : 20–30 per cent
$N_3$ : 40–50 per cent
$N_4$ : 10–15 per cent
$N_5$ : 2–5 per cent

# METHODS

## Method for Arneth Count

### Principle

Neutrophils are grouped into different stages based on their nuclear lobes. The percentage distribution of different stages of neutrophils is determined by examining a stained smear under an oil-immersion objective.

### Requirements

Same as for differential leucocyte count (Chapter 11).

### Procedure

1. Prepare blood smears and stain with Leishman stain as described under DLC.
2. Examine the smear under a low-power objective to assess the distribution of cells.
3. Count neutrophils under an oil-immersion objective as $N_1$, $N_2$, $N_3$, $N_4$ and $N_5$ for neutrophils of Stage 1, 2, 3, 4 and 5, respectively.

> Note: For counting the cells, start from one end of the smear and proceed in a zigzag manner as described under DLC.

4. Count at least 100 neutrophils and enter your observation in a tabular format (in 100 small squares).

### Observation

Note the percentage distribution of various stages of neutrophils and plot a graph (Fig. 12.2).

### Precautions

1. The smear should be one-cell thick.
2. Staining should be proper.
3. Lobes of the neutrophil should be counted accurately. If there is confusion in staging a neutrophil, the number of granules and the size of the cell should be considered.
4. At least 100 neutrophils should be counted.

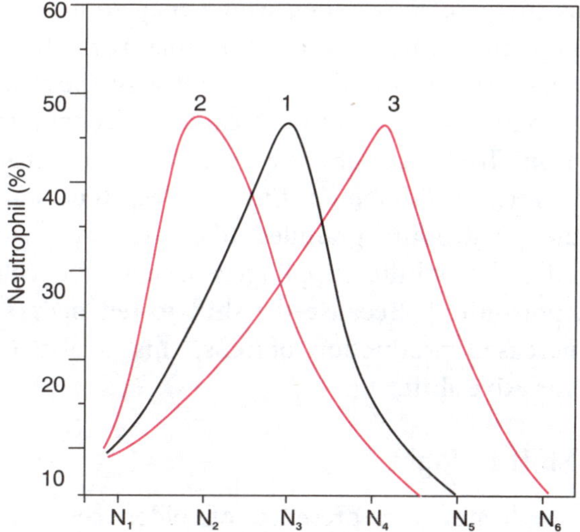


Fig. 12.2 Arneth curve. Normal count (1), shift to left (2) and shift to right (3).

# DISCUSSION

Neutrophils are active phagocytic cells in the blood. They are the first line of defence against acute bacterial infections. They are actively mobile; therefore, they migrate immediately to the site of infection and kill the organisms. In acute infections, the neutrophil count increases in the blood proportionate to the degree of assault.

## Clinical Significance

Arneth count is not usually ordered in clinical practice, but in some clinical conditions, it is used to determine the number of younger or older neutrophils in circulation. When there are more younger cells, the change is called **shift to left**; and when there are more older cells, the change is called **shift to right**. In shift to left, the total cells counted in $N_1$ and $N_2$ are more than 50 per cent, and in shift to right, the total cells counted in $N_4$ and $N_5$ are more then 20 per cent. As Arneth count reveals the production of neutrophils, it indirectly reflects the activity of the bone marrow.

### Shift to Left

This indicates that the bone marrow is hyperactive, therefore the circulating neutrophils are mainly $N_1$ and $N_2$. This occurs due to the active response of the bone marrow to different stimuli to form and release more neutrophils into the circulation. The band forms increase in number, which may sometimes be accompanied by the presence of immature neutrophils. If immature neutrophils are present with the younger neutrophils, the condition is called a **leucoblastotic reaction**. Toxic changes may manifest in neutrophils in the form of *basophilic stippling*, deep blue staining of the neutrophil granules like that of basophil granules (basophilic stippling is seen in red cells in lead poisoning). Because the shift to left occurs due to increased production of cells, this is also called **regenerative shift**.

### Shift to Right

This indicates the presence of older cells in the circulation. It occurs due to decreased production of cells by the bone marrow (inadequate hematopoiesis) as occurs in aplastic anemia. Sometimes, neutrophils of Stage 6 or 7 may also appear in the blood. Neutrophils may undergo toxic changes in the form of presence of basophilic granules (dark blue granules that resemble basophilic granules), vacuolisation of cytoplasm, hypersegmentation (more than five lobes) of nucleus, and degeneration and pyknosis of the nucleus. As shift to right occurs due to hypofunction of the bone marrow, this is also called **degenerative shift**.

## Conditions that Affect Arneth Count

### Shift to Left

1. Acute pyogenic infections
2. Tuberculosis (In tuberculosis, lymphocytosis occurs. However, in Arneth count, a shift to left is observed. This may be due to increased destruction of older neutrophils)
3. Hemorrhage
4. Irradiation (exposure to radiation): Low-dose irradiation stimulates the bone marrow and increases production of cells. However, exposure of bone marrow to a high dose of irradiation causes shift to right as the bone marrow is suppressed.

### Shift to Right

1. Megaloblastic anemia
2. Aplastic anemia
3. Septicemia
4. Uremia

## VIVA

All questions of Chapters 10 and 11 are suitable for this chapter also.

1. What are the functions of neutrophils?
2. What is the half-life of neutrophils in circulation and how long do they survive in tissues?
3. What is the normal percentage distribution of neutrophils in different stages of Arneth count?
4. What is the relationship between the lobes and age of the neutrophils?
5. What is 'shift to left' and what is its clinical significance?
6. What is 'shift to right' and what is its clinical significance?

Chapter 13

# Absolute Eosinophil Count

## Learning Objectives

After completing this practical, you will be able to:

- Describe the importance of performing absolute eosinophil count (AEC) in practical physiology.
- Describe the structure and functions of eosinophils.
- State the normal value of AEC.
- Count eosinophils by using the principle of hemocytometry.
- List the precautions taken for AEC.
- Explain the composition and function of each constituent of the Pilot solution.
- List the common causes of eosinophilia and eosinopenia.

You may also be able to:

- Explain the principle of indirect absolute eosinophil count.
- Describe other diluting fluids used for eosinophil count.
- Name the chemicals present in the granules of eosinophils and list their functions.
- State the physiologic basis of alteration of eosinophil count in different conditions.

## INTRODUCTION

Differential count of leucocytes yields the relative number of eosinophils in the leucocyte population. It is possible to find the absolute number of eosinophils in circulation by performing direct and indirect absolute counts. The direct method of absolute eosinophil count (AEC) is done by using the principle of hemocytometry. Indirect AEC is done by calculating the number of eosinophils as a percentage of the total leucocytes present in the circulation. Therefore, for indirect count, two tests should be performed: the differential count and the total count of leucocytes. The sources of error are greater in the indirect count as it multiplies the error of both the methods. The direct count on the other hand is more accurate. The staining properties of eosinophils make the direct count possible.

### Structure and Development of Eosinophils

Eosinophils usually have bilobed nuclei. In a stained preparation, the granules take on a deep red or brick-red colour. Eosinophils are distinguished from neutrophils primarily on the basis of granules rather than the number of lobes in the nuclei. In absolute count, other leucocytes and red cells are destroyed, making it easy to distinguish eosinophils.

Development of eosinophils occurs along the same lines as that of other granulocytes (as described in Chapter 9). Production of eosinophils is regulated by GM-CSF and interleukins $IL_3$ and $IL_5$.

### Life History

Once released into the bloodstream, most eosinophils migrate within 30–60 minutes into extravascular tissues where they survive for 8–12 days. Like neutrophils, eosinophils are mobile cells whose movement is directed by chemotactic factors derived from a variety of sources including mast cells and lymphocytes.

### Functions

1. Eosinophils are present in large numbers in parasitic infestations in which they appear to serve an important defence function. The granules of eosinophils contain a number of chemicals. Some of these chemicals directly kill the larvae of the parasites (larvicidal) and also the adult parasites (parasiticidal).

   **Granular contents** The granules of the eosinophils contain the following chemicals.

   *Major basic protein (MBP)* The MBP makes 50 per cent of the mass of the granules. It is a potent tissue toxin that kills larvae and adult parasites.

   *Eosinophilic cationic proteins (ECP)* The ECP is a bactericidal and larvicidal agent.

   *Eosinophil peroxidase* This enzyme participates in inflammatory activities.

*Aryl sulphatase B* This enzyme inactivates leukotrienes that are involved in hypersensitivity reactions. It also inactivates the slow-releasing substance A.

*Lysophospholipase* This is a membrane-bound enzyme that causes hydrolysis of intracellular lipoproteins.

*Histaminase* It causes degradation of histamine.

2. Eosinophil count also increases in patients suffering from allergic diseases in which exposure to abnormal exogenous or endogenous antigens leads to an immunologic reaction. In these allergic conditions, eosinophils dampen the host's response by limiting the antigen-induced release of mediators of inflammation.
3. Eosinophils are also phagocytic and destroy organisms through oxidative mechanisms similar but not identical to those of neutrophils. Eosinophils can phagocytose bacteria, fungi and inert particles, but are less efficient than neutrophils.

## Normal Count

The normal range is 40 to 440 per l of blood. There is no sex and age variation.

# METHODS OF COUNTING

Absolute count of eosinophils is done by two methods: (1) directly by using the principle of hemocytometry and (2) indirectly by studying the smear and total leucocyte count.

## Direct Method

### Principle

Blood is diluted 10 times in a WBC pipette with a special diluting fluid, which removes red cells and stains the eosinophils. The diluted blood specimen is then charged in a counting chamber and the cells are counted under a high-power objective. The population of eosinophils is then calculated for the undiluted blood.

### Requirements

*I. Equipment*

1. Microscope
2. Hemocytometer (WBC pipette and counting chamber). Three counting chambers are commonly used.
   i) Fuchs–Rosenthal counting chamber
   ii) Neubauer counting chamber
   iii) Speir counting chamber

   *Fuchs–Rosenthal counting chamber* is preferred because it is specially designed for the eosinophil count. It has a depth of 0.2 mm to accommodate more diluting fluid.

   The Speir chamber is very similar to the Fuchs–Rosenthal counting chamber.

   However, as these chambers are not usually available, the Neubauer chamber is commonly used in our laboratories.
3. Materials for sterile finger puncture
4. Watch glass
5. Filter paper
6. Petri dish

*II. Reagent (diluting fluid)*

There are three diluting fluids available for eosinophil count: Pilot solution, Randolph solution and Dunger solution.

**Pilot solution** This is the most frequently used diluting fluid.

*Composition*

| | | |
|---|---|---|
| i) | Phloxine B (1% solution in water) | : 10 ml |
| ii) | Propylene glycol | : 50 ml |
| iii) | Sodium carbonate solution (10% solution in water) | : 1 ml |
| iv) | Heparin | : 100 units |
| v) | Distilled water | : 40 ml |

*Function of each constituent*

| | |
|---|---|
| Phloxine | : Stains eosinophil granules |
| Propylene glycol | : Lyses the red cells |
| Sodium carbonate (with water) | : Lyses all white cells except eosinophils |
| Heparin | : Prevents coagulation |

Heparin is usually not added to the solution as red cells are lysed by propylene glycol. However, to prevent clumping of red cell fragments, heparin should be added to the solution.

**Randolph solution** This is very similar to the Pilot solution except that methylene blue is added to help in differentiating other leucocytes (blue) from eosinophils (orange-red).

**Dunger solution**

*Composition*

i) Aqueous eosin (1%) : Stains eosinophil.
ii) Acetone : Fixes white cells
iii) Distilled water : Lyses red cells

This solution does not remove other white cells, which appear as grey bodies.

### *III. Specimen*

Capillary blood or EDTA-anticoagulated venous blood is used.

## Procedure

1. Clean the watch glass, coverslip, WBC pipette and Neubauer's chamber thoroughly and ensure that these are dry.
2. Take adequate Pilot fluid in a watch glass.
3. Prick the finger tip under aseptic conditions.
4. Suck blood exactly up to the 0.5 mark and clean the tip of the pipette.
5. Suck Pilot fluid up to the 11 mark.
6. Shake the pipette for at least 2 minutes to mix the blood thoroughly with the diluting fluid.
7. Keep the pipette for 15 minutes under the cover of a petri dish lined with moist filter paper.
8. After 15 minutes, take out the pipette, mix the solution by gently shaking the pipette and discard 2–3 drops of the solution from the pipette.
9. Charge the Neubauer's chamber (as described in Chapter 6).
10. Count eosinophils in four WBC squares under the high-power objective of the microscope.
11. Enter the observations in your rough notebook in similarly drawn squares.

## Calculation

Dilution is 1 in 20. Therefore, the number of eosinophils counted per $mm^3$ of blood will be $n \times 50$ (for details see Chapter 9) where $n$ represents the total number of cells counted.

## Precautions and Sources of Error

All the precautions observed for pipetting and charging the chamber (described in Chapter 6) should be followed for this experiment too. In addition, the following precautions should also be observed.

1. Counting with capillary blood gives a higher result (about 10–20 per cent more) than with venous blood.
2. Counting should be done within 30 minutes of charging the chamber because eosinophils slowly disintegrate in the diluting fluid.
3. For mixing the contents of the pipette, shake gently to avoid undue rupture of the eosinophil membranes.
4. After diluting the blood, the pipette should be kept under the cover of a petri dish lined with moist filter paper, for 15 minutes (staining time) to prevent evaporation.
5. Use the indirect counting method simultaneously to check the result of direct counting.

## Indirect Method

This is one of the ways to check the result of the absolute eosinophil count. It should tally with the value obtained in the differential leucocyte count (relative count). In the indirect method, the value of the total leucocyte count is required in addition to the value of the eosinophil percentage of the differential count.

$$\text{AEC} = \frac{\text{Differential count}}{100} \times \text{Total leucocyte count}$$

For example, if the eosinophil percentage in DLC is 4 and the TLC is $7000/mm^3$ of blood, then the AEC = $(4/100) \times 7000 = 280/mm^3$ of blood.

> Note: If the results of the direct and indirect methods differ significantly, the absolute count of eosinophils by the direct method should be repeated.

# DISCUSSION

Absolute count of eosinophils by the direct method is not a routine hematologic test. In clinical practice, the absolute count of eosinophils is usually done using the indirect method. However, sometimes, it becomes mandatory to determine the number of eosinophils in a particular volume of blood because this gives an accurate result.

## Clinical Significance

The number of eosinophils in the blood is altered significantly in different allergic diseases and parasitic infestations. The eosinophil count is also taken as an index of ACTH activity in the blood. If ACTH is injected intramuscularly in a subject with normal adrenocortical function, it results in the reduction of the total number of circulating eosinophils. This effect has been used as a test of adrenocortical function. This is called the **Thorn test**. It is not a specific test and the value of the test is limited. Therefore, with the availability of superior methods, the Thorn test is not usually used for assessment of adrenocortical function.

The condition in which the eosinophil count increases is called *eosinophilia* and the condition in which the count decreases is called *eosinopenia*.

## Conditions that Alter Eosinophil Count

### Eosinophilia

1. Allergic diseases
   Bronchial asthma
   Hay fever
   Food allergy
2. Parasitic infestations
   Hookworm
   Roundworm
   Tapeworm
   Filaria
3. Skin diseases
   Eczema
   Pemphigus
   Dermatitis herpetiformis
4. Tropical pulmonary eosinophilia and Loeffler's syndrome
5. Malignant neoplasia
   Eosinophilic leukemia
   Lymphoproliferative disorders, for example, Hodgkin's disease
   Secondary carcinomas
6. Addison's disease

### Eosinopenia

1. Cushing syndrome
2. Aplastic anemia
3. ACTH therapy

## VIVA

1. What are the methods of absolute eosinophil count?
2. What are the other counting chambers used for absolute eosinophil count in addition to Neubauer's chamber, and what are their advantages?
3. What are the different diluting fluids used for absolute eosinophil count?
4. What is the composition of Pilot solution and what are the functions of each constituent?
5. After diluting the blood, why is the pipette kept under the cover of a petri dish lined with moistened filter paper?
6. Why should the counting be performed within half an hour of diluting the blood?
7. Why is the blood with the diluting fluid in the pipette mixed gently?
8. What are the precautions for absolute eosinophil count?
9. How are eosinophils counted by the indirect method?
10. Why is the direct count preferred to the indirect count for obtaining the absolute value of eosinophils?
11. What is the structure of an eosinophil and what are the chemicals present in the eosinophil granules?
12. What is the half-life and fate of eosinophils?
13. What are the functions of eosinophils?
14. What is the normal eosinophil count?
15. What is the clinical significance of this investigation?
16. Name the conditions that alter eosinophil count.
17. What is the Thorn test? What is its significance?

# Chapter 14

# Determination of Erythrocyte Sedimentation Rate

## Learning Objectives

After completing this practical, you will be able to:

- Explain the importance of determining ESR in practical physiology.
- Explain what ESR is and how it differs from PCV.
- List the factors that affect ESR.
- List the methods of determination of ESR.
- Identify the Westergren pipette and Wintrobe tube.
- Load the ESR tubes with blood.
- List the precautions and sources of error in determination of ESR.
- State the normal value of ESR in males and females with each method.
- Name the common conditions in which there is alteration of ESR.

You may also be able to:

- Explain the role of fibrinogen and other factors in determining ESR.
- Explain the physiological basis of variation in ESR in different physiological and pathological conditions.

## INTRODUCTION

Sedimentation of the red cells occurs when anti-coagulated blood is allowed to settle. The rate at which the red cells fall is known as the **erythrocyte sedimentation rate** (ESR). Students should not confuse ESR with PCV. In the case of hematocrit, the packing of red cells is accomplished by centrifugation, while in ESR, the column of red cells settles by gravity. Sedimentation of red cells occurs due to rouleau (singular rouleaux) formation. Rouleaux is the piling up of red cells, so they look like a stack of coins. When the red cells form rouleau, the cells (together) become heavier as they sit on one another. Sedimentation is faster when the size and number of rouleau are large. Therefore, any factor that facilitates rouleaux formation increases ESR and any factor that inhibits it decreases ESR.

### Factors Affecting ESR

ESR mainly depends on four factors: (1) the size of the rouleau, (2) plasma factors, (3) the shape and number of red cells and (4) technical and mechanical factors.

#### Size of the Rouleau

The ESR primarily depends on the size or mass of the falling particles, that is, the rouleaux. The larger the particle, the faster is the fall. The size of the falling particles depends on the formation of red cell aggregates, that is, rouleaux formation.

#### Plasma Factors

1. **Plasma proteins** The size of the rouleaux depends on the presence of certain factors in the plasma, especially its fibrinogen and globulin content. Normally, red cells tend to repel each other, as they are negatively charged (zeta potential) due to the negative electrostatic charges imparted by sialic acid moieties on the cell membrane. Fibrinogen neutralises the charges on the red cells and makes them sticky. Therefore, when the fibrinogen concentration increases in the plasma, the repelling force on the red cells is removed; this facilitates rouleaux formation. In some pathological conditions, in addition to fibrinogen, other plasma factors called acute-phase reactants increase in the blood. These phase reactants also neutralise the charges on the red cell surface and facilitate rouleaux formation. A rise in C-reactive protein in the plasma in acute rheumatic fever is an example of such acute phase reactants.

2. **Viscosity** When the medium in which red cells settle becomes thick (more viscous), the rate of sedimentation decreases and conversely when the medium becomes thin (less viscous), the rate of sedimentation increases. Thus, in the conditions in which the viscosity of blood increases, the ESR decreases, and in which viscosity decreases, ESR increases. Viscosity of blood increases in polycythemia and decreases in anemia. Therefore, ESR is low in polycythemia and high in anemia.

### Shape and Number of Red Cells

Red cells are biconcave discs. This shape favours rouleaux formation. A change in the shape of red cells opposes rouleaux formation. Therefore, in sickle cell disease and hereditary spherocytosis, the ESR is low in spite of anemia. Polycythemia lowers ESR and anemia raises ESR.

### Technical and Mechanical Factors

Some technical and mechanical factors also affect ESR:

1. **Temperature** The rate of sedimentation increases with temperature. Increase in temperature increases ESR by decreasing the viscosity of blood.
2. **Position of the pipette** ESR pipettes are kept vertical in the rack. Slanting of the tubes in the rack facilitates ESR.

## Normal Values

Wintrobe method

Males : 0–9 mm/h

Females : 0–20 mm/h

Westergren method

Males : 3–5 mm/h

Females : 5–12 mm/h

## METHODS OF DETERMINATION

There are two traditional methods for determining ESR: the Westergren method and the Wintrobe method. The Westergren method is more sensitive and provides more accurate values than the Wintrobe method, because the former uses longer and narrower tubes for ESR measurement.

## Westergren Method

### Principle

Anticoagulated blood is taken in a pipette and left undisturbed in a vertical position. The level of the column of red cells is noted in the beginning (0 h) and after 1 and 2 hours. The distance (mm) the column moves is noted as the ESR (mm/h).

### Requirements

**I. Apparatus required**

1. *Westergren pipette* The Westergren pipette is an open-ended tube. It is 300 mm in length with an internal bore of 2.5 mm. It is graduated from 0–200 mm along the lower two-thirds of its length. The graduated volume of the pipette is 1.0 ml. The pipettes are held vertically in the Westergren rack after filling with blood, and the rack is provided with rubber pads at the lower end and metal clips at the upper end (Fig. 14.1).
2. *Westergren rack* This is a special rack designed to hold Westergren pipettes in a vertical position. It is constructed in such a way that the rubber stoppers attached to springs close the open ends of the tubes when they are placed in the rack (Fig. 14.1).

**II. Blood sample** Anticoagulated blood is taken for the study. Sodium citrate solution (3.8%) is the preferred anticoagulant. The ratio of blood to the anticoagulant is 4 : 1, that is, 4 parts blood (say 2.0 ml) is mixed with 1 part anticoagulant (0.5 ml). EDTA can also be used.

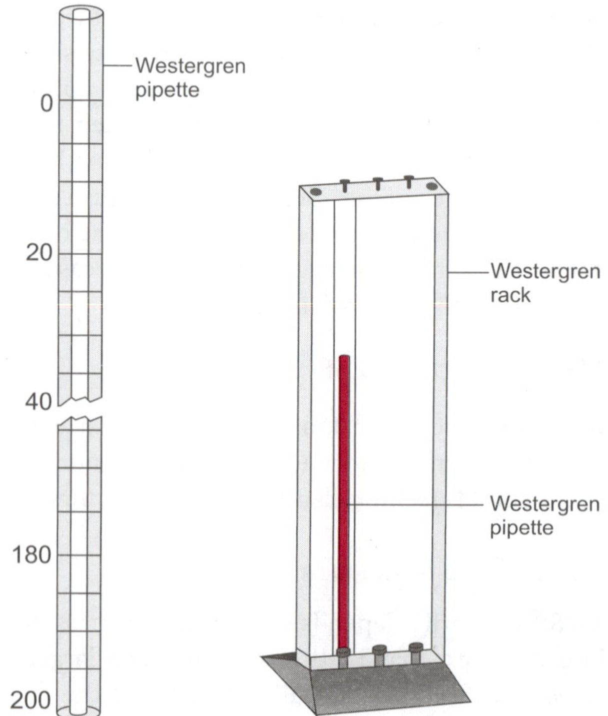


Fig. 14.1 Westergren pipette and rack.

## Procedure

1. Mix the blood thoroughly by inversion or swirling.
2. Fill the citrated blood into the Westergren pipette up to the 0 mark, making sure that there is no air bubble in the blood column drawn through the tube. The Westergren pipette can either be filled by mouth suction (not usually recommended) or by means of a rubber bulb if available.
3. Immediately close the upper end of the Westergren tube to prevent the blood from running down.

> Note: The upper level of the blood column should coincide with the 0 mark of the pipette. If a difference exists, it should be noted and adjusted accordingly with the final result.

4. Place the Westergren tube in the rubber pad of the Westergren rack and fix it vertically with the metal clips provided on the rack.
5. Note the time and allow the tube to stand for 1 hour.
6. Record your observations (note the level to which the red cell column has fallen) after 1 hour.

> Note: Ideally, observations should also be recorded at the end of the second hour.

## Precautions

1. Concentration of anticoagulant should be appropriate.
2. Blood should be properly mixed before pipetting.
3. The pipette should be clean and dry.
4. Blood should be filled exactly up to the 0 mark and should not contain air bubbles. If the upper level of the blood is above the 0 mark (say 2 mm), care must be taken to add the additional distance travelled by the blood column (2 mm) in the final report. This means that if the reading is 12 mm after 1 hour, report it as 14 mm/1$^{st}$ h.
5. The tube should be kept vertically in the rack.
6. The reading should be taken at the end of 1 hour and 2 hours.

## Sources of Error

1. The concentration of anticoagulant affects the ESR value. A false low value is reported in case of higher concentration of anticoagulant.
2. Be accurate about timing. Do not take a reading after 30 minutes and report it as a one-hour reading by multiplying by two. The rate of sedimentation is slow in the beginning and fast after about 45 minutes. A one-hour reading gives the final picture. Therefore, the reading should be taken only after one hour.
3. Temperature directly affects ESR. High temperatures lead to false high values; conversely, low temperatures give false low values. Therefore the specimen must be brought to room temperature before setting up the test.
4. Tilting of the tube increases the ESR.

## Wintrobe Method

This method is not usually followed for the determination of ESR in clinical practice. It is used in some laboratories, because it provides two results simultaneously from the same sample, that is, ESR and hematocrit. The ESR reading is taken in the first hour, then the tube is centrifuged for hematocrit value. The Wintrobe tube is made in such a way that both the readings are available on two different graduations marked on the tube. However, the ESR result by this method is not as accurate as that of the Westergren method.

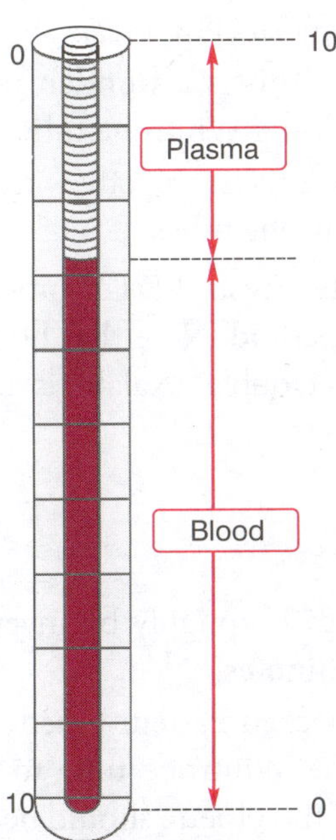


Fig. 14.2 Wintrobe tube filled with blood.

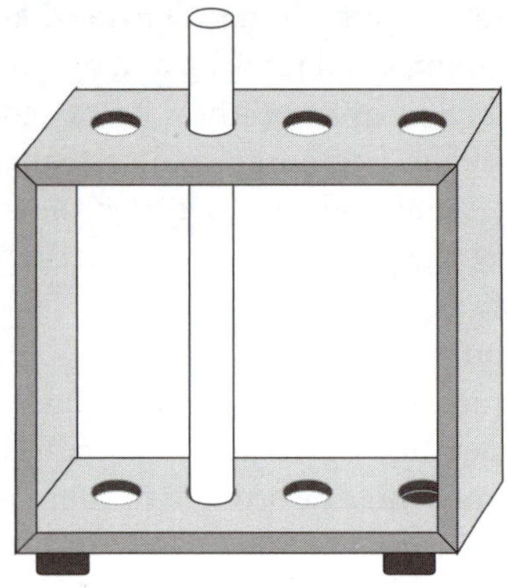

Fig. 14.3 Wintrobe rack.

## Principle

The principle is the same as that of the Westergren method.

## Requirements

**I. Apparatus required**

1. *Wintrobe tube* The Wintrobe tube is a thick-walled cylindrical tube, 11 cm in length with an internal bore of 3 mm. The tube is graduated in mm in both directions from 0 to 10 cm. The marking 0–10 from above downwards is used for reading ESR. The marking 0–10 from below upwards is used for reading hematocrit (Fig. 14.2).
2. *Wintrobe rack* This is a wooden rack with holes at the top for holding Wintrobe tubes (Fig. 14.3).
3. *Pasteur pipette* This is a pipette with a long neck used for filling Wintrobe tubes.

**II. Blood sample** Fresh EDTA-anticoagulated blood is used for this method. Note that blood is not diluted in this method. Double oxalate is also preferred as anticoagulant.

## Procedure

1. Mix the blood thoroughly by inversion or swirling for at least 2 minutes.
2. With a long-necked Pasteur pipette or with a special syringe, fill the Wintrobe tube to the 0 mark. For this, the tip of the pipette should be introduced right down to the bottom of the Wintrobe tube and the blood slowly forced out of the pipette into the tube from below upwards. While filling, draw out the pipette tip as the tube is filled with blood. This will prevent air bubble formation.
3. Place the Wintrobe tube in an exactly vertical position in the rack. Note the time.
4. Note the reading of the erythrocyte column at the end of one hour and report ESR as mm/1st hr.

## Precautions

1. The Wintrobe tube should be very clean and dry.
2. Do not use hemolysed blood.
3. Blood should be mixed properly before pipetting.
4. Blood should be filled exactly up to the 0 mark. If blood is drawn above the mark, do not use absorbent material to adjust the level. Use a dropper for this purpose.
5. The blood column should not contain air bubbles or blood clots.
6. The tube should be kept vertical in the rack.
7. The reading should be taken after an hour.
8. While filling the pipette, the tip of the pipette should be kept below the level of blood.

## Sources of Error

1. Be accurate about timing. Do not take a reading after 30 minutes and report it as a one-hour reading by multiplying by two. The rate of sedimentation is slow in the beginning and fast after about 45 minutes. A one-hour reading gives the final picture. Therefore the reading should be taken only after one hour.
2. Temperature directly affects ESR. High temperatures lead to false high values; conversely, low temperatures give false low values. Therefore, the specimen must be brought to room temperature before setting up the test.
3. Tilting of the tube increases the ESR rate.

# DISCUSSION

## Clinical Significance

ESR is a non-specific test to detect inflammation. ESR increases in inflammatory conditions, be it infective or non-infective. A rise in plasma fibrinogen as occurs in acute infections (pneumonia), a rise in plasma globulin as seen in chronic infections (like tuberculosis), and a rise in phase reactant as seen in non-infective inflammations (like rheumatoid arthritis)—all these conditions increase ESR. ESR also increases in malignant diseases like carcinoma and leukemia. ESR is the index of inflammatory activity in the body. It increases with an increase in the rate of inflammation and decreases with a decline in inflammatory activity. Thus, ESR gives a clue to the physician regarding the progress of the disease and the response of the disease to treatment. Sometimes ESR remains elevated long after the clinical manifestations have disappeared, indicating that the defence mechanism of the body continues to be more active than normal.

## Conditions that alter ESR

*I. Increased ESR*

**A. Physiological**

1. Pregnancy (due to increased fibrinogen and globulin)
2. After a meal (therefore, blood for ESR measurement is collected early in the morning on an empty stomach).

**B. Pathological**

1. Acute infection (e.g., pneumonia)
2. Chronic infection (e.g., tuberculosis)
3. Acute non-infective inflammation (e.g., gout)
4. Collagen vascular disease (e.g., rheumatoid arthritis, systemic lupus erythematosus, etc.)
5. Malignant disease (e.g., carcinoma of breast, leukemia)
6. Anemia

*II. Decreased ESR*

1. Polycythemia
2. Afibrinogenemia
3. Sickle cell anemia
4. Hereditary spherocytosis

## Zeta Sedimentation Ratio (ZSR)

Blood in special capillary tubes is spun in the vertical position for four 45-second cycles in a centrifugal device, called the Zetafuge. This leads to rapid compaction of red cells, allowing rouleaux to form and sediment in just three minutes. The capillary tube is then read like a microhematocrit. The value obtained is referred to as **zetacrit**. The true hematocrit is divided by zetacrit giving a value in percentage, which is known as ZSR. The interpretation is easier as ZSR is not affected by anemia. It is an equally sensitive test like that of recording ESR. The advantages of ZSR are that it requires only 100 microlitres of blood and its measurement is considerably faster. The normal value in adults is 40% to 50% for both genders. As zetafuge is not available now, recording ZSR is impossible, though it is a satisfactory alternative to ESR.

## VIVA

1. What is ESR? How does it differ from hematocrit?
2. What are the factors that affect ESR?
3. What is the role of plasma fibrinogen in ESR?
4. What are the methods of determining ESR?
5. Why should the anticoagulant concentration be appropriate for ESR estimation?
6. What are the precautions and sources of error in the Wintrobe method?
7. What are the precautions and sources of error in the Westergren method?
8. Why is the Westergren method more accurate than the Wintrobe method?
9. What is the clinical significance of determining ESR?
10. Why is the blood collected on an empty stomach for determining ESR?
11. What are the physiological conditions of increased ESR?
12. What are the diseases in which ESR increases? What are the diseases in which ESR decreases?
13. What is ZSR?

CHAPTER 15

# Determination of Blood Group

## LEARNING OBJECTIVES

After completing this practical, you will be able to:

- Describe the clinical significance of determination of blood group.
- Name the blood groups of the ABO and Rh systems.
- State the physiological significance of the ABO and Rh systems.
- Define Landsteiner's law.
- State the principle of determination of blood groups.
- Determine blood groups by using anti-A and anti-B antisera.
- List the precautions taken while determining the blood group.
- List the common indications of blood transfusion.
- List the common hazards of transfusion.
- Name the diseases transmitted by blood transfusion.
- Explain universal donor and universal recipient.
- Explain the importance of cross-matching.

You may also be able to:

- Name and explain the importance of other blood group systems.
- State the physiological basis of development of blood groups.
- Explain the physiological basis of major and minor cross-matching.
- List and explain all the effects of mismatched transfusion.
- Explain the procedure of storage of blood in the blood bank.
- Explain the physiological changes in red cells during storage and after transfusion.
- List the cause, features, treatment and prevention of erythroblastosis fetalis.
- Name the diseases associated with different blood groups.

## INTRODUCTION

There are more than 30 blood group systems containing about 400 antigens. Fortunately, most of these antigens are not significant immunologically. Moreover, many of them have cold antibodies that do not react at body temperature. The antigens that are involved in blood groups are called **agglutinogens** and the antibodies that are produced against these antigens are called **agglutinins**. Clinically, the important blood group systems are: (1) the ABO system and (2) the Rh system. The MN system is important from the medico-legal point of view.

### The ABO System

The ABO blood group system is the most important of all blood group systems because of the presence of natural A and B antibodies in individuals, from birth, who lack corresponding antigen on their red cells. In addition, transfusion of incompatible ABO blood groups immediately leads to serious consequences.

In this system, there are two antigens, antigen A and antigen B. Based on the presence or absence of these antigens, blood groups are classified as:

Group A : Antigen A is present
Group B : Antigen B is present
Group AB : Both antigens A and B are present
Group O : Neither antigen A nor B is present

The A antigen is of two types, A and $A_1$. Therefore, Group A is further divided into two subgroups:

Group $A_1$ : Containing A and $A_1$ antigens.
Group $A_2$ : Containing the A antigen only.

Similarly, the AB blood group is subdivided into the $A_1B$ and $A_2B$ blood groups.

The antibodies in the ABO system are of two types, anti-A ($\alpha$) and anti-B ($\beta$). These antibodies are naturally occurring and are present in the blood of individuals in whom the respective antigens are absent. Thus, Group A (having A agglutinogen on the red cell membrane) will have anti-B and Group B (having B agglutinogen on the red cell membrane) will have anti-A agglutinins in their plasma. The AB group will have no antibody and Group O will possess both the antibodies.

A and B agglutinogens are complex oligosaccharides that differ in their terminal sugars. On the RBC membrane, they are glycolipids, and in tissues and body fluids, they are soluble glycoproteins. **H antigen** is the fucose-containing antigen, which is found in all individuals. Usually, H antigen has no antigenic activity.

Therefore, an individual with blood group O having no antigens of the ABO system, has no antigenic activity at all, and hence, identified as 'O'.

### Distribution

In the Indian population, the distribution of the ABO blood group is as follows:

A : 28 per cent
B : 22 per cent
AB : 5 per cent
O : 45 per cent

In the A blood groups, the distribution of $A_1$ group is 75 per cent and that of $A_2$ is 25 per cent.

### Landsteiner's Law (Karl Landsteiner, 1900)

This law states that if an agglutinogen is present on the red cell membrane, the corresponding agglutinin must be absent in the plasma. If the agglutinogen is absent in the red cells, the corresponding agglutinin must be present in the plasma. The second half of the definition may not be applicable to all blood group systems. For example, in Rh-negative individuals, absence of Rh agglutinogen in the red cells is not accompanied by the presence of anti-Rh agglutinin in the serum.

## The Rh (Rhesus) System

This system was first discovered in Rhesus monkeys; hence it is called the Rh system. In this system, there are six antigens, but there are no naturally occurring antibodies. The antigens are C, D, E, c, d and e. Of these six antigens, immunologically, D is the most significant. Therefore, the Rh system has two blood groups:

Rh-positive : D antigen present
Rh-negative : D antigen absent

The antibody in this system is called anti-D antibody and is produced only when an Rh-negative individual receives the Rh-positive blood. These antibodies develop slowly in the first encounter, but rapidly in subsequent encounters.

In the Indian population, 95–98 per cent are Rh-positive and 2–5 per cent are Rh-negative.

## The MN System

In this system, there are three blood groups: M, N and MN. This system is usually required for paternity tests. It can only determine who is not the father of a baby but cannot confirm who is. For example, if the baby's blood group is M and the suspected father's is N, then it can definitely be said that N is not the father of M. But, it can never specifically be said who the father of the baby is. Determination of other blood groups assists in establishing paternity.

MN groups are also useful for anthropological and genetic studies.

## The Lewis System

The antigens of the Lewis system are Lea and Leb. These are not really red cell antigens because they are produced in the plasma and are then absorbed into the red cells. The antibodies are of the IgM type. They do not cross the placental barrier and, therefore, do not cause hemolytic disease of the newborn.

## The Ii System

There are two antigens in the Ii system, I and i. This system differs from other blood groups in several ways:

1. At birth, the I antigen is poorly developed, but red cells of the fetus and neonates are rich in i antigens.
2. There occurs a gradual changeover from i to I in the first two years of life.
3. In conditions like hemoglobinopathies, red cells show increased i antigen without any decrease in the I antigen.

## The Duffy System

There are two blood group antigens in this system, the Fya and the Fyb antigens. This system has three blood groups: Fya, Fyb and Fyab. A close relationship between the Duffy blood group and malaria has been well established. The Fyab blood groups are resistant to *Plasmodium vivax*, whereas Fya and Fyb are susceptible to vivax malaria. This is because the Fya and Fyb antigens, if present separately on the red cell membrane, increase the entry of the malarial parasite into the red cells.

## The Kell System

In this system there is only one antigen called the K antigen. People with K-positive blood group (containing K antigen on the red cell membrane) are susceptible to chronic granulomatous diseases.

# METHODS

## Determination of Blood Group

### Principle

Red cells contain different types of agglutinogens while plasma contains agglutinins. The red cells of the subject are allowed to react with commercially made agglutinins. The presence or absence of the clumping of red cells in different agglutinins determines the blood groups.

### Requirements

1. Anti-A serum (containing anti-A agglutinin)
2. Anti-B serum (containing anti-B agglutinin)
3. Test tubes
4. Slides
5. 0.9 per cent saline
6. Microscope
7. Equipment for sterile finger prick
8. Capillary pipette
9. Glass-marking pencil
10. Glass rods

### Procedure

1. Take 2 ml of 0.9 per cent saline solution in a test tube.
2. Make a sterile finger prick and collect a large drop of blood into the test tube containing the saline solution.
3. Mix the solution to obtain red cell suspension.
4. On one of the slides, place a drop of anti-A serum on its left half and label it 'anti-A' with the help of the glass-marking pencil. On the left half of another slide, place a drop of anti-B serum and label it 'anti-B'.
5. Place a drop of saline on the right half of each slide and mark it as control (C).
6. To each of these drops, add a drop of red cell suspension by using a capillary pipette.
7. Mix the red cell suspension with the sera using separate glass rods or by gently shaking the slides. Wait for 5–10 minutes.
8. Observe the serum-cell mixtures for agglutination (clumping). Compare it with the cells in the saline controls (Fig. 15.1).

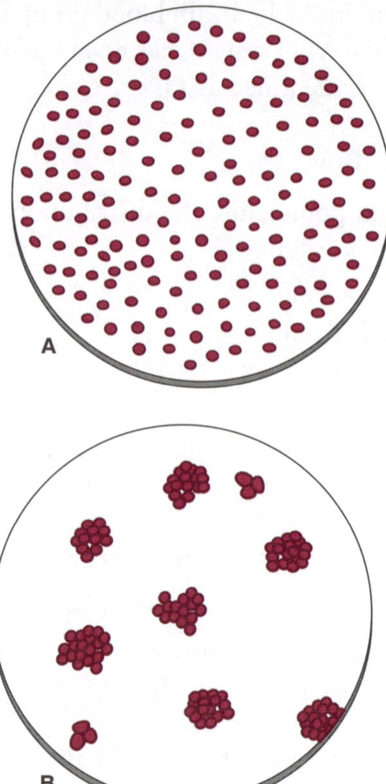


Fig. 15.1 Confirmation of blood grouping under low-power microscope. A: No agglutination (cells are uniformly distributed); B: Agglutination present.

9. Confirm your findings under the low-power objective.

> **Note:** The serum–cell mixture should be examined before it dries up to differentiate clumping (actual agglutination) from rouleaux formation of red cells.

10. Record the presence or absence of agglutination in each slide and interpret the result as follows.

> **Note:** A false-positive result if present should be excluded by comparing with the control (control will also show clumping of cells). False-negative results may occur because of decreased immmunocompetence of antisera which may occur due to use of improperly stored antisera.

### Precautions

1. The slides must be labelled correctly.
2. While mixing the red cell suspension with antisera, care must be taken not to mix anti-A and anti-B sera with the same glass rod.

| Anti-A serum | Anti-B serum | Agglutinogens (on RBC) | Blood group |
|---|---|---|---|
| + | – | A | A |
| – | + | B | B |
| + | + | AB | AB |
| – | – | Nil | O |
| +: agglutination | | – : no agglutination | |

3. If there is no clumping in either of the slides, wait for at least 15 minutes.
4. The observations should finally be checked under the microscope.
5. A control should always be used to exclude false-positive results.
6. Blood should always be diluted for blood grouping test. Use of undiluted blood may give false-positive results (rouleaux formation may be confused with clumping). Dilution of blood decreases rouleaux formation.
7. Cell-sera suspension should be examined for clumping before the preparation dries up.

## DISCUSSION

To be able to donate or receive blood, an individual should know his or her blood group. This may be required in many medical emergencies. Therefore, the blood group is always noted on the identity card of a person. The blood group is always determined prior to any surgical intervention.

## Physiological and Clinical Significance

### Uses of Blood Grouping

The uses of blood groups are to:
1. Ensure compatible blood transfusion
2. Eliminate hemolytic disease of the newborn due to Rh incompatibility
3. Solve paternity disputes
4. Detect susceptibility to various diseases
5. Detect personality

## Blood Transfusion

### Indications

1. *Acute blood loss* Whole blood is preferred.
2. *Chronic anemia* Packed red cells are preferred.
3. Bone marrow failure
   Leukemia
   Aplastic anemia
   Bone marrow infiltration by neoplastic cells
   In bone marrow failure, fresh blood and specific blood components are required. Red cells are administered along with granulocytes to fight infections.
4. *Purpura* Platelet transfusion is preferred (so blood grouping may not be necessary).
5. *Clotting factor deficiencies* Fresh frozen plasma is preferred. In hemophilia, cryoprecipitate (rich in factor VIII and fibrinogen) is given.

### Procedure

Blood grouping and cross-matching are always done before blood transfusion to ensure a safe and compatible transfusion. A satisfactory compatibility procedure should include:
i) ABO and Rh typing
ii) Cross-matching
iii) Antibody screening of the patient (to detect the presence of clinically significant antibodies)

### Cross-Matching

There are two types of cross-matching (i) major cross-matching and (ii) minor cross-matching.

**Major cross-matching** The cells of the donor are directly matched against the plasma of the recipient. It is important to ensure that antibodies present in the recipient's plasma do not harm the donor's red cells.

**Minor cross-matching** The donor's plasma is checked against the red cells of the recipient. It is called minor cross-matching because it is not very important, as the small volume of the donor's plasma is diluted in a large volume of the recipient's plasma. Therefore, the titre of antibodies present in the donor's plasma falls to such a low level after transfusion that they are quite unlikely to damage the red cells of the recipient.

## Universal Donor and Recipient

### Universal Donor

Persons with blood group O-negative are considered to be universal donors because the red cells contain no antigens. Therefore, their blood can be given safely to anyone.

### Universal Recipient

Persons with blood group AB-positive are considered to be universal recipients because their plasma contains no antibodies. Therefore, they can receive blood from anyone.

Though technically this concept is true, its use sometimes may lead to mismatched transfusion due to the presence of various other minor blood groups. Therefore, prior to transfusion, blood should always be cross-matched to eliminate the possibilities of mismatch. However, in emergency conditions, this concept may be used in selecting the donor.

## Hazards of Blood Transfusion

### I. Due to Mismatched Transfusion

When an incompatible blood group is transfused, reactions occur primarily due to agglutination of the donor's red cells. This results in hemolysis. The severity of the reaction depends on the degree of hemolysis. The complications of mismatched transfusion are:

1. Shivering and fever
2. Hemoglobinemia and hemoglobinuria
3. Jaundice
4. Acute renal failure, which occurs due to:
   - Hemoglobin casts blocking the renal tubules and damaging the tubes
   - Release of toxic substances from the lysed red cells causing renal vasoconstriction
   - Circulatory shock
5. Hyperkalemia (due to release of potassium ions from red cells) that causes cardiac problems

### II. Due to Faulty Techniques of Giving Blood

1. **Thrombophlebitis** This is a common complication in those who receive repeated transfusions.
2. **Air embolism** Air enters the venous circulation and lodges at the outlet of the right ventricle and blocks the flow of blood to the lungs. Death may occur in severe cases. The use of plastic bags has reduced this complication.

### III. Due to Massive Transfusion

This occurs when more than 10 units of blood are given within 24 hours or when the total blood volume is exchanged within 24 hours. *Cardiac arrhythmias* or *cardiac arrest* may occur due to high potassium levels in the stored blood.

### IV. Febrile Reaction

The patient feels cold and may develop rigour due to raised body temperature. This occurs mainly due to the presence of pyrogens in the transfusion apparatus.

### V. Allergic Reactions

This is less frequent and is characterised by itching, erythema, nausea, vomiting and, in severe cases, anaphylactic reactions.

### VI. Transmission of Diseases

1. Hepatitis
2. Malaria
3. AIDS
4. Syphilis

## Rh Incompatibility

If an Rh-negative individual receives Rh-positive blood, there will be no immediate reaction because Rh-negative individuals do not normally have anti-Rh antibodies. However, the donor's red cells induce an immune response in the recipient to synthesise anti-Rh antibodies. These take about 2–4 months to reach a significant titre, but by that time the donor's red cells die a natural death. The anti-Rh antibody cannot cause any harm to the recipient's red cells because the recipient's red cells contain no Rh antigens. But, if the same Rh-negative person receives a subsequent Rh-positive transfusion, the anti-Rh antibodies are synthesised in large amounts immediately by the memory cells, causing a mismatch reaction.

### Erythroblastosis Fetalis

#### *Etiopathogenesis*

This is a hemolytic disease of the newborn which occurs due to Rh incompatibility, when an Rh-negative mother carries an Rh-positive fetus. Usually, no reaction occurs in the first pregnancy. However, if the mother has received transfusion of Rh-positive blood earlier, reaction may occur in the first pregnancy. A small amount of blood leaking into maternal circulation at the time of delivery induces formation of anti-Rh agglutinins in the mother. In subsequent pregnancies, the mother's agglutinin crosses the placenta to the fetus and causes hemolysis in the fetus.

#### *Clinical Features*

If the hemolysis is severe, the fetus may die *in utero* or if the fetus is born alive, he may have the following features.

1. Anemia
2. Jaundice
3. Edema (hydrops fetalis)
4. Kernicterus: This is a neurologic syndrome that occurs due to the deposition of bile pigments in the basal ganglia. Bile pigments cannot cross the blood-brain barrier (BBB) in adults but can do so in fetuses and infants because the BBB is not fully developed.
5. Presence of erythroblasts (nucleated red cells) in the blood.

#### *Treatment*

The best treatment is to carry out an exchange transfusion soon after birth.

#### *Prevention*

The disease is prevented by administering a single dose of anti-Rh antibodies in the form of Rh immunoglobulin during the postpartum period following the first delivery. The disease can also be prevented by passive immunisation of the mother with a small dose of Rh immunoglobulins during pregnancy.

## Storage of Blood for Transfusion

### Procedure

Blood is stored in the blood bank at 4°C. Disodium hydrogen citrate is used instead of trisodium citrate as anticoagulant, because this favours the fall of pH, which is required for survival of red cells. Stored blood should ideally be used within two weeks of storage. Blood should not be used if it is stored for more than four weeks, because gross hemolysis occurs after this period.

### Red Cell Changes During Storage

Red cells undergo rapid changes during storage in simple citrate solutions even at 4°C. During cold storage, the changes that occur are mainly due to reduction of metabolism of cells. They are:

1. Increase in sodium and decrease in potassium concentration in the red cells. This occurs due to decreased active transport of ions across the cell membrane. There is mainly a decrease in $Na^+$–$K^+$ pump activity. This results in net increase in the total base and water of the cell.
2. Cells swell and become more spherocytic. This results in spontaneous hemolysis.
3. The ATP content in the cell decreases and inorganic phosphate concentration increases. This is due to an imbalance between the phosphorylation and dephosphorylation processes in the cells.

### Changes in Stored Blood after Transfusion

Within 24 hours of transfusion, the cell metabolism greatly increases; consequently, the sodium is extruded from the cells and the potassium is drawn back into the cells. The volume, shape and fragility of the red cells revert to normal within 24–48 hours. Red cells show 80 per cent survival 24 hours after transfusion if the transfusion is given within 14 days of storage of the blood. But the survival rate greatly decreases if the blood is stored for more than two weeks. Therefore, it is ideal to use blood within 14 days of storage.

## Diseases Associated with Blood Groups

Different blood groups are prone to different diseases.

| | |
|---|---|
| Group A | : Carcinoma of stomach |
| O | : Duodenal ulcer |
| Fya & Fyb | : Vivax malaria |
| K | : Chronic granulomatous diseases |
| Rh-negative | : Autoimmune hemolytic anemia |
| Li | : Hemoglobinopathies |

## VIVA

1. What is the physiological basis of determination of blood groups?
2. What are the precautions taken for determination of ABO blood groups?
3. How will you confirm the clumping (agglutination) of red cells?
4. What is the mode of inheritance of blood groups?

Ans. Blood groups are genetically determined. In general, the presence of a blood group antigen is a codominant characteristic. Therefore, the antigen is present in the phenotype regardless of the genotype (whether homozygous or heterozygous). However, the homozygous or heterozygous state determines the type of contributions the individual can make to the progeny. This is why the blood group of a child may be different from that of both parents.

5. What is Landsteiner's law and what are the exceptions to this law?
6. What is a 'universal donor' and a 'universal recipient'?
7. What is cross-matching of blood and what is its clinical significance?
8. Why is minor cross-matching usually not done for blood transfusion?
9. What is Rh incompatibility and how does it differ from ABO incompatibility?

   Ans. When an Rh-negative person receives blood from an Rh-positive person, there is a reaction. This is called Rh incompatibility. This differs from ABO incompatibility in terms of the speed with which the transfusion reactions develop. In ABO incompatibility, the reaction develops immediately, but Rh incompatibility reaction may not occur at all in the first exposure. Though the reaction does not occur in the first transfusion, the donor's red cells induce an immune response in the recipient as a result of which anti-Rh agglutinins are slowly formed in the recipient's plasma. When the same individual receives a second transfusion of Rh-positive blood, the transfusion reaction occurs immediately.

10. What is erythroblastosis fetalis and how can it be prevented?
11. How is blood stored in the blood bank?

    Ans. Blood is collected from the donor in a labelled plastic bag or glass bottle. Disodium hydrogen citrate is used as anticoagulant because it favours survival of red cells by decreasing the pH.

    Blood is stored in the blood bank at 4°C.

12. What are the physiological changes that occur in the red cells during storage?
13. What is the cause of hemolysis of stored blood?
14. What are cold and warm antibodies for blood group antigens? What are the differences among them?

    Ans. The terms 'cold' and 'warm' antibodies are applied to the antibodies of the ABO system and Rh systems of blood group, respectively. Their important features and differences among them are:

| | Antibodies of ABO system | Antibodies of Rh system |
|---|---|---|
| i) | These are larger molecules, of the IgM type; cannot cross the placenta. | They are of the IgG type; can easily cross the placenta. |
| ii) | React with the antigens best at low temp. between 5–20°C. Hence called 'cold' antibodies. | React with antigens best at body temperature. Hence called 'warm' antibodies. |
| iii) | ABO incompatibility between a mother and fetus does not occur. | Rh incompatibility occurs. |

15. What is the importance of using a control on each side of the 3 test sides? What are false-positive and false-negative results?

    Ans. The control sample for blood group testing in each case is only a suspension of red cells in normal saline. Its purpose is to avoid 'false-positive' and 'false-negative' results?

    False-Positive Reaction: It means that though there is no actual agglutination, the reaction appears to be so. Formation of large rouleaux (this may happen if undiluted blood is used) may give a false impression of agglutination, but the cells will quickly disperse on tilting the slide a few times. Bacterial contamination of an antiserum, or of normal saline, may show agglutination in all tests or in all controls.

    False-Negative Reaction: It may occur due to loss of potency of the antisera because of faulty storage. All tests will come out negative with such an antiserum.

16. What is zone phenomenon?

    Ans. For agglutination to occur, the concentration of agglutinogens and agglutinin should be approximately the same. This is called zone phenomenon. With a gross difference in these concentrations, the agglutination may not be significant.

17. What is autologus transfusion and pre-donation?

    Ans. In addition to receiving blood from a donor, an individual may also receive one's own stored blood, i.e. during elective surgery on him in the future. The blood is collected much before surgery and the same blood is transfused during surgery. This is called autologous transfusion. This is also called predonation. The benefit of this procedure is that it avoids transmission of diseases such as AIIDS, hepatitis, etc. as well as risk of transfusion reaction.

Predonation (Predeposit) is a form of autologous transfusion in which a course of iron tablets is given and after that two units of blood are collected (first unit 16 days before and second unit 8 days before surgery). An important technical innovation is the cell-saver machine which sucks up blood from the wound during the operation, recycles it, and returns it to the patient's body.

18. What is blood doping and what is its advantage?

    Ans. Blood 'doping' is the athletic mispractice, in which one or two units of an athelete's blood (or red cells) is removed and stored 2 weeks before the athletic event. The blood is re-injected in 2 sessions just few days before the event. Since oxygen delivery to active muscles is the limiting factor, increased red cell count enhances their performance in marathon events. This practice is banned by the International Athletic and Olympic Committees.

19. Which blood substitute is preferred if suitable blood donor is not available?

    Ans. Whole blood is ideal to replace lost blood as occurs in hemorrhage as it replaces cells and plasma in physiological ratio. But in a situation where it may not be available, an intravenous drip of a crystalloid or colloid solution is immediately started.

    Crystalloid solutions: In clinical practice, the commonly used one is intravenous fluid of glucose saline, i.e., 6% glucose in 0.9% sodium chloride. As crystalloids leave the circulation in a short time, the restoration of the volume is temporary.

    Colloid solutions: The colloid substitutes are plasma expanders, such as human albumin, dextrose and dextrose with NaCl, and a polymer from degraded gelatin. Plasma separated from donated blood can be stored in a liquid form (fresh frozen plasma) for many months. It can be dried and kept still longer, which is reconstituted with distilled water just before use.

    Blood Substitutes: Sometimes, especially if there is a chance of volume overload, instead of whole blood or plasma, a blood component is used to avoid circulatory overload and lower the risk of transfusion. The blood substitutes include packed red cells, WBC concentrates, immunoglobulins, and clotting factor concentrate.

20. What is the speciality of Bombay blood group?

    Ans. The Bombay blood type is a rare variety in which the H antigen is absent. Since there is no H antigen, there is no antigen A or antigen B on the red cells. However, the plasma contains anti-A, anti-B and anti-H antibodies. Therefore, such a person can receive blood only from a person having Bombay blood group.

21. What are forward and reverse blood typing?

    Ans. In blood grouping or typing, the red cells of a donor or a person whose blood type is to be determined are tested against anti-A and anti-B sera. This is called blood typing or forward blood typing.

    In **reverse blood typing**, (also called **serum typing** or **backward blood typing**), the serum of the recipient is tested against red cells containing known antigens, i.e., red cells from persons with blood types A, B, AB, and O. If agglutination occurs with A and AB red cells, the blood type is B; if agglutination occurs with B and AB red cells, the blood type is A; if agglutination occurs with A, B, and AB red cells, the blood type is O and if there is no agglutination in any RBCs, the blood type is AB.

    For blood transfusion in leukemic patients, serum typing is done along with blood typing as an extra precaution, because in leukemias, the RBC antigens may become considerably weak. This is also performed in pseudomonas infection, since in these infections, RBCs become agglutinated by all antisera due to unmasking of hidden antigens.

22. What is the MN system and what is its clinical use?
23. Why does mismatching of blood of the Lewis system not cause hemolysis?
24. What is the clinical significance of the Ii system?
25. Which disease is closely associated with the Duffy system and why?
26. What is the clinical use of the Kell system?
27. What are the different diseases associated with different blood groups?
28. What is Bombay blood group and what is its significance?

    Ans. Bombay blood group is a rare occurrence, in which H antigen is not expressed. Due to absence of H antigen, agglutinogens A and B are absent on the membrane of red cells. However, in spite of absence of these three blood group agglutinogens, anti-A, anti-B and anti-H agglutinins are present in the plasma. Therefore, a person having Bombay blood group can receive blood only from a person having Bombay blood group, and not from others.

CHAPTER 16

# Osmotic Fragility of Red Cells

## LEARNING OBJECTIVES

After completing this practical, you will be able to:

- Describe the utility of this practical in clinical physiology.
- Prepare saline solutions of different percentage.
- Perform the osmotic fragility test.
- Explain the mechanism of hemolysis when red cells are exposed to hypotonic solutions.
- List the precautions taken for the osmotic fragility test.
- Define and explain osmotic fragility.
- List the conditions that alter the osmotic fragility of red cells.

You may also be able to:

- Correlate the applicability of this practical in different clinical conditions.
- Explain the physiological basis of alteration in osmotic fragility in different diseases of red cells.

## INTRODUCTION

Osmotic fragility of red cells is defined as the ease with which the RBCs are ruptured (hemolysed) when they are exposed to hypotonic solutions. It assesses the integrity of the membrane of red cells.

The osmotic fragility test helps in the diagnosis of anemia in which the physical properties of the red cells are altered. This test detects whether or not the red cells can be easily hemolysed. The red cell membrane allows water to pass through while restricting solutes. This is called osmosis. Red cells shrink due to exosmosis when they are placed in a solution that is more concentrated than the concentration of the solute inside. On the other hand, red cells absorb water by endosmosis, when kept in a hypotonic solution like water which results in hemolysis due to swelling and rupture of the cells. In an isotonic solution, that is, solution of equal concentration as the red cell content (for example, 0.85% NaCl), the red cells stay intact.

The test of osmotic fragility attempts to determine the concentration of solute inside the red cells by placing the cell in different concentrations of sodium chloride and observing hemolysis in a hypotonic solution. When red cells are introduced into a hypotonic solution of sodium chloride, they take up water and swell until a critical volume is reached and then rupture. When the critical volume is reached, the cells become spherical. As the cells take up water, they become more fragile. The red cells that are already spherical, as seen in hereditary spherocytosis, have increased osmotic fragility in hypotonic solutions because they can swell only a little before they burst. Conversely, the cells that are biconcave or flat have decreased osmotic fragility in hypotonic solutions because they can swell considerably before they reach the spherical shape and burst. The osmotic fragility is thus a measure of the rate of hemolysis of the red cells when exposed to hypotonic solutions of sodium chloride.

## METHODS

### Osmotic Fragility Test

#### Principle

When the red cells are suspended in a hypotonic solution of sodium chloride, they take up water and swell until a critical volume is reached and hemolysis occurs. As the cells take up water, they become increasingly fragile. Thus, the intracellular solute concentration, as reflected by red cell fragility, can be helpful in establishing the functional state of the red cells.

#### Requirements

**I. Apparatus**

1. Clean test tubes
2. Test tube rack
3. Distilled water
4. 1% NaCl solution
5. Dropper

**II. Specimen** Freshly drawn heparinised or defibrinated venous blood is prepared for this test. The test should be carried out within two hours of blood collection. Heparin is frequently used as an anticoagulant because it causes less distortion of the red cells.

## Procedure

1. Arrange the test tubes in the rack and number them serially from 1 to 12.
2. Prepare solutions of increasing hypotonicity by mixing the required number of drops of 1 per cent sodium chloride solution and distilled water in the test tubes serially from 1 to 12, as given in Table 16.1. Use one dropper for all saline solutions and another for distilled water.

   Note that the first tube contains saline, which is nearly isotonic and the last tube is filled with only distilled water (tonicity nil).
3. Shake the tubes thoroughly and add a drop of blood in each tube.
4. Invert each tube gently once to mix the blood with saline, and then place them in a rack.
5. After 30 minutes, observe the tubes against a white background without disturbing the tubes. Note the number of the first tube that shows partial hemolysis and the number of the tube in which hemolysis is complete. A tube with partial hemolysis shows an upward supernatant fluid with pink colour proportionate to the degree of hemolysis and a lower layer of sedimented red cells at the bottom of the tube. A tube with complete hemolysis shows a clear, uniformly pink solution in the absence of red cells at the bottom. A tube with no hemolysis shows a clear, straw-coloured supernatant fluid with few red cells settled at the bottom (Fig. 16.1).

## Observation

Beginning of hemolysis: in per cent saline.

Completion of hemolysis: in per cent saline.

Express the result, giving the range from the beginning of hemolysis to its completion.

## Normal Value

Normally, osmotic fragility begins at 0.45 to 0.50 and completes at 0.30 to 0.33 per cent saline.

Table 16.1

| Test tube no. | 1 | 2 | 3 | 4 | 5 | 6 | 7 | 8 | 9 | 10 | 11 | 12 |
|---|---|---|---|---|---|---|---|---|---|---|---|---|
| Distilled water drops | 3 | 9 | 10 | 11 | 12 | 13 | 14 | 15 | 16 | 17 | 18 | 25 |
| 1 per cent saline drops | 22 | 16 | 15 | 14 | 13 | 12 | 11 | 10 | 9 | 8 | 7 | 0 |
| % saline soln. obtained | 0.88 | 0.64 | 0.60 | 0.56 | 0.52 | 0.48 | 0.44 | 0.40 | 0.36 | 0.32 | 0.28 | 0 |

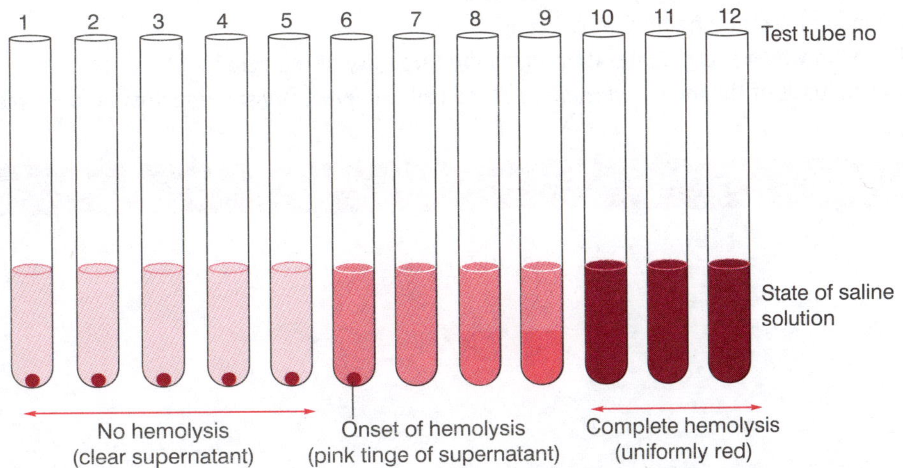


Fig. 16.1 Osmotic fragility test. Note that hemolysis starts in the sixth tube (slight pink tinge of the supernatant) and is completed in the tenth tube (solution is uniformly red). No hemolysis is observed in test tubes 1 to 5 (clear supernatant with red cell clumps at the bottom).

### Precautions

1. Separate droppers should be used for pouring the drops of distilled water and 1% saline into the test tubes.
2. Drops should be counted exactly as recommended in the table.
3. A minimum time of 30 minutes should be allowed for hemolysis to occur.
4. Hemolysis should be checked against a white background by placing a white paper behind the tubes.
5. The tubes should not be disturbed while recording the observation.

## DISCUSSION

When the rate of hemolysis of the red cell is increased, the osmotic fragility is increased, and when the rate of hemolysis is decreased, the osmotic fragility is decreased. Increased osmotic fragility of red cells denotes decreased resistance of these cells to rupture. Osmotic fragility is related to the shape of red cells. The shape of red cells is dependent on the volume, surface area and functional state of the red cell membrane. As the resistance of the red cell membrane to rupture is related to its geometric configuration, red cells which are spherical (spherocytes) demonstrate increased hemolysis, while the cells that are flat (sickle cell or target cells) demonstrate decreased hemolysis. Hypochromic red cells (as seen in iron deficiency anemia) are very thin and contain less hemoglobin; therefore, they can swell to a greater extent before they rupture.

## Conditions that Alter Fragility of RBC

### Diminished Fragility

1. Iron deficiency anemia
2. Thalassemia
3. Sickle cell anemia
4. Obstructive jaundice
5. After splenectomy
6. Variety of anemias where target cells are seen in the peripheral blood

### Increased Fragility

1. Hereditary spherocytosis
2. Congenital hemolytic anemia
3. Other conditions in which spherocytes are found in the blood

## VIVA

1. What do you mean by osmotic fragility of red cells? What are the factors that determine this?
2. What is the principle of the osmotic fragility test of red cells?
3. What is the normal range of osmotic fragility of red cells?
4. What are the conditions in which there is alteration in osmotic fragility of red cells?
5. What is the physiological basis of the increased fragility of red cells in hereditary spherocytosis and decreased fragility in sickle cell disease?

CHAPTER 17

# Determination of Bleeding Time and Coagulation Time

## LEARNING OBJECTIVES

After completing this practical, you will be able to:

- Describe the importance of determining BT and CT in clinical physiology.
- List the steps of blood coagulation.
- Determine BT by the Duke method.
- Determine CT by capillary tube method.
- Give the normal values of BT and CT.
- List the precautions taken for determination of BT and CT.
- Name the diseases in which BT and CT are prolonged.
- List the tests to determine platelet function and to assess the efficiency of intrinsic and extrinsic pathway of blood coagulation.

You may also be able to:

- Explain the mechanism of intrinsic and extrinsic pathway of blood coagulation.
- Describe the role of platelets in blood coagulation.
- Explain the principle and clinical significance of different tests for investigation of bleeding disorders.

## INTRODUCTION

Bleeding and clotting times are determined to assess the integrity of hemostatic mechanisms. Hemostasis is the stoppage of bleeding. It is a complex process that involves three major steps in sequence: (1) vasoconstriction, (2) platelet plug formation and (3) coagulation or clot formation. Bleeding time (BT) depends on the effectiveness of vasoconstriction and platelet plug formation whereas clotting time (CT) mainly depends on the effectiveness of the clotting mechanism. *BT is the time from onset of bleeding till the stoppage of bleeding* and *CT is the time from onset of bleeding till clot formation.*

### Vasoconstriction

Vascular response is the immediate response of blood vessels to injury. The response is vasoconstriction. This decreases the loss of blood and assists in the process of platelet plug formation. The contraction of the smooth muscles of the blood vessels in response to injury is the immediate cause of vasoconstriction. It is potentiated by the release of chemicals like serotonin from the platelets aggregated at the site of injury.

The effectiveness of vascular response is detected by the capillary fragility test, but vascular response cannot be clearly separated from platelet response. Therefore, determination of **bleeding time** and **capillary fragility test** is necessary to measure the integrity of both the responses.

### Platelet Plug Formation

Platelet plug (*temporary hemostatic plug*) formation occurs due to three properties of platelets: adhesion, aggregation and release reaction. BT is the time from onset of bleeding to temporary hemostatic plug formation that stops bleeding. The response of platelets in hemostasis includes change in shape, increase in surface adhesiveness and the tendency to aggregate with other platelets to form a plug. Platelets adhere to the injured vessel wall. Adhesion is followed by aggregation of platelets, which are activated to release a number of chemicals (*release reaction*) that cause vasoconstriction and temporary hemostatic plug formation (*see* Chapter 18).

The effectiveness of platelets in hemostasis can be assessed by:

- Bleeding time
- Platelet count
- Platelet aggregation studies
- Platelet adhesiveness test
- Clot retraction test
- Prothrombin consumption test

### Coagulation or Clot Formation

Blood coagulation occurs in three stages: (1) activation of Stuart–Prower factor, (2) formation of thrombin from prothrombin and (3) formation of fibrin from fibrinogen (Fig. 17.1). CT is the time from the onset of bleeding to the clot (*definitive hemostatic plug*) formation.

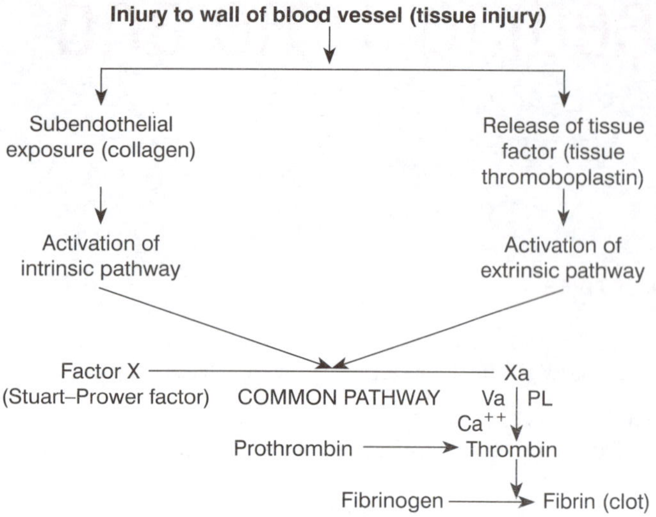


Fig. 17.1 Stages of blood coagulation.

**Activation of Stuart–Prower factor** The tissue extract (tissue thromboplastin or factor III) enters the blood through the site of injury and combines with factor VII and calcium (factor IV). This is called the *extrinsic system*. It originates outside the blood vessels and includes factor III, IV and VII. In the meantime, there is activation of the *intrinsic system* when factor XII is activated by its contact with the negatively charged surface of the collagen fibres of the injured vessel walls. The intrinsic system originates inside the blood vessels and includes factors XII, XI, IX, VIII, and calcium (IV). Finally, both extrinsic and intrinsic systems follow a common pathway, which results in the formation of active Stuart–Prower factor (Xa).

Any defect in the intrinsic system of stage 1 is recognised by the activated partial thromboplastin time (PTT).

**Formation of thrombin from prothrombin** In stage 2, prothrombin (factor II) is activated by Xa in the presence of Va, calcium and platelet phospholipid, the end product of stage 1. This results in the formation of thrombin. Any defect in this stage results in prolongation of prothrombin time.

**Formation of fibrin from fibrinogen** This is the final stage of the coagulation process. Fibrin is formed from fibrinogen by thrombin, the end product of stage 2. First, fibrin monomers are formed, then polymerisation of fibrin takes place with the help of activated factor XIII, to form the fibrin clot.

Thrombin time is prolonged if there is a defect in the formation of fibrin from fibrinogen.

## METHODS OF DETERMINATION OF BLEEDING TIME

Bleeding time (BT) is usually determined by two methods: (1) Duke method and (2) Ivy method.

### Duke Method

The Duke method is the more frequently used method to determine BT in clinical laboratories as it is easy to perform and requires minimal equipment and laboratory skill.

#### Principle

A deep skin puncture is made and the length of time required for bleeding to stop is recorded. It determines the function of the platelets and the integrity of the capillaries.

#### Requirements

1. Equipment for sterile finger puncture
2. Blotting paper or filter paper
3. Stopwatch

#### Procedure

1. Assemble all necessary material and supply proper instructions to the subjects (this can be done by the student).
2. Clean the finger tip or the ear lobe of the subject with alcohol, and allow the skin to dry completely.

> Note: Though the ear lobe is a good site for this test, the finger tip is more convenient.

3. Make a deep puncture (blood should flow freely without squeezing) with the help of a sterile lancet.
4. Immediately start the stopwatch.
5. Blot the drop of blood coming out of the incision every 30 seconds by using the blotting paper or circular filter paper. Place each subsequent drop a little further along the side of the filter paper.

> Note: Do not allow the filter paper to press on the bleeding spot. Note that the drops become progressively smaller.

6. Stop the stopwatch as soon as bleeding ceases.
7. Count the number of drops on the filter paper and multiply it by 30 seconds.

**Note:** If the bleeding does not stop in 10 minutes, discontinue the test and apply pressure to the spot to stop bleeding.

## Precautions

1. Gather all the necessary materials before starting the test.
2. Do not rub too much while cleaning the skin as rubbing increases blood flow and alters BT.
3. The skin should dry completely before pricking.
4. The puncture should be deep (about 4 mm).
5. Do not squeeze. Blood should flow freely.
6. Blot the blood exactly every 30 seconds.
7. Do not allow the filter paper to press on the bleeding spot as it may interfere with bleeding.
8. If bleeding continues for more than 10 minutes, discontinue the test and ask the subject to apply pressure to the wound.

## Normal Value

The normal range of BT by the Duke method varies from 1 to 5 minutes.

## Clinical Significance

Prolongation of BT is found in *thrombocytopenia, thrombasthenia* and *von Willebrand disease.* It occurs when platelet count is less than 50,000/μl of blood. Thrombasthenia is the condition of platelet dysfunction in which platelet count remains normal, but the platelets are functionally abnormal. In von Willebrand disease, platelet defect is combined with factor VIII deficiency.

# Ivy Method

The Ivy method is more reliable than the Duke method, but it is more painful to the subject. Skill is required for using a sphygmomanometer. Therefore, the Duke method is commonly preferred in clinical laboratories.

## Principle

A standard incision is made on the forearm under a standardised condition, and the length of time required for bleeding to cease is recorded.

## Requirements

1. Sphygmomanometer
2. Sterile lancet, capable of making an incision 1 mm wide and 3 mm deep
3. Blotting paper
4. Alcohol
5. Cotton wool

## Procedure

1. Explain the procedure to the subject.
2. Tie the sphygmomanometer cuff on the patient's arm above the elbow.
3. Raise the cuff pressure to 40 mm Hg, and maintain it for the entire period.
4. Select an area approximately 5 cm below the cubital fossa on the anterior aspect of the forearm and clean with alcohol.
5. Hold the skin tightly by grasping the underside of the forearm firmly and make two separate punctures 5 cm apart in quick succession using the sterile lancet. Start the stopwatch.
6. Blot the blood from each incision site on a separate piece of blotting paper, every 30 seconds.
7. When the bleeding stops, stop the watch and release the pressure from the sphygmomanometer cuff.
8. Record the bleeding time of both the punctures. The longer of the two bleeding times is more accurate than the average of the two.
9. If the bleeding continues for more than 15 minutes, discontinue the test and apply pressure to the puncture to stop bleeding, and report as BT more than 15 minutes.

## Precautions

1. Explain the procedure to the subject.
2. The area selected for puncture should be properly cleaned.
3. Two incisions should ideally be made for determination of BT by this method.
4. A constant pressure of 40 mmHg should be maintained throughout the procedure.
5. The incision should be made deep into the skin.
6. The longer of the two bleeding times (rather than the average) should be taken for the result.

### Normal Value

The normal range of BT by the Ivy method varies from 5 to 11 minutes.

### Clinical Significance

The clinical significance is the same as that of the Duke method. Though the Duke method is commonly followed, the Ivy method should be the method of choice, as it is more reliable.

# METHODS OF DETERMINATION OF CLOTTING TIME

Clotting time (CT) is usually determined by two methods: (1) capillary tube method and (2) Lee–White (venipuncture) method. The capillary tube method is routinely used in clinical laboratories to determine CT.

## Capillary Tube Method

### Principle

A standard incision is made in the skin of the patient and blood is taken into a capillary glass tube. The length of time that it takes for the blood to clot (as detected by the appearance of fibrin string) is reported as CT.

### Requirements

1. Materials for sterile finger prick
2. Capillary tubing (10–15 cm in length and 1.5 mm in diameter) without anticoagulant

### Procedure

1. Explain the procedure to the subject.
2. Make a sterile finger puncture by using the lancet to a depth of 3 mm.
3. As soon as blood is visible, start the stopwatch.
4. Wipe off the first drop of blood and allow the next drop of blood to flow into the capillary tube by introducing one end of the tube into the drop and holding the other end at a lower level.
5. Hold the capillary tube filled with blood between the palms so as to maintain it at body temperature.
6. After 2 minutes, break off the capillary tubing 1–2 cm from one end every 30 seconds and look for appearance of a thread of fibrin.
7. When a thin string of fibrin is seen between the broken ends, stop the watch and note the time.
8. In the report, mention the use of the capillary method.

### Precautions

1. Explain the procedure to the subject.
2. The fingertip should be cleaned with alcohol before pricking.
3. The puncture should be deep and blood should flow spontaneously.
4. Immediately after filling, the capillary tube should be held between the palms to maintain its temperature. Temperature affects clotting.
5. With each break of the capillary tube, appearance of the fibrin string should be looked for.

### Normal Value

The normal range of CT by capillary glass tube method is 2–8 minutes.

### Clinical Significance

CT is prolonged in diseases in which clotting factors are deficient. If the CT is more than 10 minutes, the patient should be subjected to detailed investigations to identify the missing coagulation factors.

## Lee–White Method

This is more reliable and sensitive than the capillary method, but it needs special arrangements for venipuncture and a temperature-controlled water-bath.

### Principle

Venous blood is collected in a clean glass tube without any anticoagulant. The time taken by blood to clot at 37°C is noted as clotting time.

### Requirements

1. Materials for drawing blood by venipuncture

2. Test tubes
3. Water bath at 37°C
4. Stopwatch

### Procedure

1. Explain the procedure to the subject.
2. Collect over 2 ml of venous blood by making a sterile venipuncture. Start the stopwatch as soon as the blood enters the syringe.
3. Remove the needle from the syringe and fill each of the two tubes to the 1 ml mark.
4. Plug the tubes with non-absorbent cotton wool and place them in the water bath at 37°C.
5. After 3 minutes, remove the first tube from the water bath and tilt the tube gently to 45° to check whether the blood has clotted. If not, return the tube to the water-bath and examine every 30 seconds to check the appearance of a clot.
6. When blood clots, the tube can be tilted through an angle of 90° without spilling the contents. As soon as the blood is clotted, examine the second tube. The blood in the second tube usually clots as soon as blood clots in the first tube.
7. Stop the stopwatch and note the time.
8. The CT is the clotting time of the second tube.

### Precautions and Sources of Error

1. One important source of error is inappropriate volume of blood taken for the test (less than 1 ml gives a shorter CT).
2. The temperature of the tubes should be maintained at 37°C.
3. While collecting blood, air bubbles should not enter the syringe. Presence of air bubbles shortens the CT.

### Normal Value

The normal range of CT by the Lee–White method is 5–12 minutes.

### Clinical Significance

This method is more reliable than the capillary tube method. The clinical significance of this method is the same as that of the capillary tube method.

## OTHER TESTS FOR BLEEDING DISORDERS

There are many other tests that are performed to detect the nature and degree of various bleeding disorders. As these tests are not routinely carried out in physiology laboratories but asked in viva, the basic principle and clinical significance of each test are described.

## Capillary Fragility Test

### Principle

This is also called Capillary Fragility Test of Hess or Tourniquet test. This test measures the ability of the capillaries to withstand increased stress. Petechiae appear in the forearm of the subject when the blood pressure cuff in the arm is inflated to a maximum pressure of 100 mm Hg for about 5 minutes.

### Clinical Significance

Normally, 0–10 petechiae appear. More than 10 petechiae indicates capillary weakness, thrombo-cytopenia or both.

## Platelet Aggregation Test

### Principle

An aggregating agent is added to a suspension of platelets in plasma and the response is measured turbidometrically as a change in the transmission of light by an instrument called the *aggregometer*.

### Clinical Significance

Measurement of platelet aggregation is an essential part of the investigation of any patient with suspected platelet dysfunction.

## Platelet Adhesiveness Test

### Principle

This test measures the ability of platelets to adhere to a glass surface. When anticoagulated blood is allowed to pass at a constant rate through a plastic tube containing glass beads, some platelets adhere to the glass beads. The percentage difference of the platelet count prior to and after passing through the glass bead column indicates the functional status of platelets.

### Clinical Significance

The normal range is 75–95 per cent of platelet retention. The platelet adhesiveness test is non-specific. The results are abnormal in several platelet functional disorders.

## Clot Retraction Time

### Principle

Blood clots when collected in a glass tube without any anticoagulant. The clot begins to retract (after blood has clotted) within 30 seconds, and is about 50 per cent at the end of 1 hour. At the end of 18–24 hours the clot should have retracted completely.

### Clinical Significance

Abnormal clot retraction is reported when less than 50 per cent retraction occurs at 1 hour. Clot retraction is primarily dependent on platelet function. Hematocrit and fibrinogen levels also affect it. Poor clot retractability is usually seen when platelet count is less than 1,00,000.

## Clot Lysis Time

### Principle

The clot is lysed due to fibrinolysis, which is a natural process. Due to lysis, the clot becomes fluid and red cells sink to the bottom of the test tube.

### Clinical Significance

The lysis time for the normal clot is about 72 hours. If lysis is seen within 24 hours, fibrinolysis is considered to be abnormal.

## Prothrombin Consumption Test

### Principle

This test determines the amount of prothrombin present in the serum after clot formation.

### Clinical Significance

Normally, in the coagulation process, more than 95 per cent of prothrombin is used up as it is converted to thrombin. The presence of more than 5 per cent of prothrombin in the serum indicates a quantitative or qualitative platelet deficiency.

## Prothrombin Time (PT)

### Principle

A preparation of rabbit brain emulsion (which contains tissue thromboplastin) is added to plasma in the presence of calcium. This, in the presence of factor VII, triggers stage 2 of the coagulation mechanism, and the clotting time is recorded after the addition of calcified thromboplastin to the plasma.

### Normal Value

The normal value is 12–16 seconds.

### Clinical Significance

Prolonged PT suggests the possibility of deficiency of factors II, V, VII and X. In stage 2, prothrombin is converted to thrombin which triggers the transformation of fibrinogen to fibrin. Abnormal prothrombin time suggests a stage 2 defect.

## Partial Thromboplastin Time (PTT)

### Principle

The platelet substitute, in the form of partial thromboplastin, is prepared from rabbit brain as chloroform extract. When mixed with test plasma containing excess of calcium, it leads to clot formation.

### Normal Value

The normal value is 60–80 seconds.

### Clinical Significance

PTT is prolonged when there is a deficiency of one or more clotting factors XII, XI, IX, VIII, X, V, II and I. Abnormal PTT indicates a stage 1 defect and the absence of one or more of the intrinsic factors.

## Activated Partial Thromboplastin Time (APTT)

### Principle

The platelet substitute, in the form of partial thromboplastin, is prepared from rabbit brain. This is incubated with a contacting agent (kaolin) to provide optimal activation of the intrinsic coagulation factors. The clotting time is determined after the addition of excess of calcium.

### Normal Value

The normal value is 25–40 seconds.

### Clinical Significance

APTT is prolonged in deficiencies of factors XII, XI, X, IX and VIII. APTT is a more reliable test than PTT. When used in conjunction with PT, it provides a simple method for differentiating between stage 1 intrinsic defects and other factor deficiencies. APTT is mainly determined in hemophilias that involve the deficiency of factors VIII, IX or XI.

## Thrombin Time (TT)

### Principle

Thrombin (commercially available) is added to the plasma along with calcium and the clotting time is determined.

### Normal Value

The normal value is 15–20 seconds.

### Clinical Significance

Thrombin time detects the effectiveness of stage 3 of coagulation in which fibrinogen is converted to fibrin. Prolonged TT is considered to be due to either a decrease in fibrinogen concentration or the presence of dysfunctional fibrinogen.

## Plasma Recalcification Time (PRT)

### Principle

When excess of calcium is added to the citrated plasma, clotting occurs. Because platelet factor III is also involved in clotting through the intrinsic pathway of coagulation, the clotting occurs in a shorter time in platelet-rich plasma than in platelet-poor plasma.

### Normal Value

Platelet-rich plasma : 100–150 seconds
Platelet-poor plasma : 135–240 seconds

### Clinical Significance

This is an easy screening test that detects deficiency of the factors of the intrinsic pathway, that is, factors XII, XI, IX, VIII, X, V and II (all coagulation factors except VII and XIII).

## DISCUSSION

Bleeding occurs when a blood vessel is injured and stops by a process called hemostasis. Abnormal bleeding occurs spontaneously or following trauma, due to the derangement of hemostasis which warrants investigation. Patients prepared for surgery must be routinely checked for bleeding disorders to ensure normal hemostasis during the procedure.

## Clinical Significance

Laboratory investigations for bleeding disorders are required for patients who have a history of spontaneous bleeding or excessive bleeding following injury or surgery. Hemorrhagic disorders are broadly classified into *inherited* and *acquired defects*. Acquired defects are more common than inherited defects. The platelet defects are more common than the coagulation defects. Deficiencies of factor VIII (hemophilia) and factor IX (Christmas disease) are more common inherited coagulation defects. The common acquired defects are thrombocytopenia, vitamin K deficiency, disseminated intravascular coagulation and liver failure.

Bleeding time is prolonged in conditions in which platelets are defective or less in number, and the vascular response to injury is impaired. Clotting time is prolonged in conditions in which clotting factors are defective or deficient.

***Conditions in which BT is prolonged, but CT is normal***

- Thrombocytopenia due to any cause
- Thrombasthenia

- Idiopathic thrombocytopenic purpura

***Conditions in which CT is prolonged, but BT is normal***

- Hemophilia
- Christmas disease
- Any bleeding disorder in which clotting factors are deficient.

## Hemophilia

Hemophilia occurs due to the deficiency of factor VIII. It is an X-linked recessive bleeding disorder. The abnormality is located on the X chromosome. Women are carriers and usually do not suffer from the disease because they are protected by the second X chromosome, which is usually normal. The disease manifests with a bleeding tendency that usually appears in infancy, but, which in mild cases may appear in adult life. Bleeding from wounds is a characteristic symptom, which is usually slow and persists from days to weeks in spite of the presence of large clots. Bleeding may also occur spontaneously into the tissues, joints and cavities of the body. The patient is treated with fresh blood transfusions because factor VIII is lost rapidly on storage. The better alternative is to administer a factor VIII concentrate.

## Christmas Disease

Christmas disease occurs due to deficiency of factor IX. It is clinically indistinguishable from hemophilia. Therefore, it is also called hemophilia B.

## Purpura

Purpura is a group of diseases that occur due to thrombocytopenia. The two commonest forms of purpura are *idiopathic thrombocytopenic purpura* (ITP) and *drug-induced purpura* (which is also commonly seen in *von Willebrand disease*). Purpura induced by a vascular defect may be seen in vitamin C deficiency.

# VIVA

1. What are the methods of determination of BT, and what are their normal values?
2. What are the precautions taken for determining BT by the Duke and Ivy methods?
3. Which method is more reliable for determining BT, and why?
4. What is the clinical significance of determining BT by the Duke and Ivy methods?
5. What are the methods of determination of CT, and what are their normal values?
6. What are the precautions to be taken while determining CT by the capillary tube and Lee-White methods? Which method is more reliable, and why?
7. What is the clinical significance of determination of CT by the capillary tube and Lee-White methods?
8. Why is CT normally more than BT?
   Ans. BT is the time from onset of bleeding to stoppage of bleeding. Bleeding stops due to the formation of a temporary hemostatic plug. CT is the time taken from onset of bleeding to formation of the definitive hemostatic plug (clot). Temporary hemostatic plug formation occurs earlier than the definitive hemostatic plug. Therefore, normally, CT is more than BT.
9. What are hemostasis and homeostasis?
   Ans. Hemostasis means arrest of bleeding. Homeostasis is defined as maintenance of constancy of the internal environment of the body, that is, milieu interior. As hemostasis tries to maintain constancy of blood volume, it is part of the total homeostatic mechanism.
10. What are the mechanisms of hemostasis?
11. What are the steps of blood coagulation, and how do you detect the defects in these steps?
12. What are the tests to detect defects in the vascular response of hemostasis?
13. What are the tests to detect defects in platelets?
    Ans. Defects in platelets can be detected by:
    - bleeding time
    - platelet count
    - platelet aggregation studies
    - platelet adhesiveness test
    - clot retraction test
    - prothrombin consumption test
14. What is normal prothrombin time and what is its clinical significance?

15. What is the normal partial thromboplastin time and what is its clinical significance?
16. What is the normal value of activated partial thromboplastin time (APTT), and what is its clinical significance?
17. What is normal thrombin time (TT), and what is its clinical significance?
18. What is plasma recalcification time (PRT), and what is its clinical significance?
19. What is hemophilia?
20. What is 'Simplate Method' of BT determination, and what is its advantage?
    Ans. In Duke and Ivy bleeding time methods, there is no full control on the depth of the wound made by a lancet or a needle. The widely practised technique is to use an automated scalpel to control the depth and length of the wound, which is usually 1 mm deep and 9 mm long. The blood pressure cuff is inflated to 40 mm of Hg to distend the capillary bed of the forearm. The normal bleeding time in this method is < 7 minutes.
21. What are the factors that influence BT and CT?
    Ans.
    *Factors influencing BT*
    a) Size (breadth and depth) of the wound
    b) Degree of hyperemia of skin puncture site
    c) Number of platelets and their functional status
    d) Functional status of the blood vessels
    e) Body temperature or temperature of the part to be pricked: If the part is cold, bleeding is less due to vasoconstrictions. Rubbing the part (hyperemia) promotes bleeding.
    f) Environmental temperature: In cold weather, due to low temperature, BT becomes less (due to vasoconstriction)

    *Factors influencing CT*
    a) Nature of contact surface. Siliconised surface may prolong the CT.
    b) Blood level of clotting factors.
    c) Skin temperature: Low temperature may prolong the CT.
22. Name the conditions in which bleeding time is prolonged, but CT is normal.
    Ans. Prolongation of BT with normal CT is seen in:
    i) Thrombocytopenia (Decreased production of platelets or increased destruction of platelets).
    ii) Thrombasthenia (functional platelet defects).
    iii) Drugs—aspirin, large doses of penicillin, corticosteroids, sulfa drugs.
    iv) von Willebrand disease
    v) Other diseases—uremia, cirrhosis, leukemia, etc.
    vi) Vessel wall defects (acquired, but may be inherited).
    vii) Allergic purpura—there is damage to capillary wall by antibodies.
    viii) Infections—typhus, bacterial endocarditis, hemolytic streptococci, etc.
    ix) Vitamin C deficiency—Petechia, and bleeding from gums occur due to decreased intracellular substance and less stable capillary basement membrane.
    x) Senile purpura—in the elderly, small vessels rupture due to increased mobility of skin resulting from loss of elastic and connective tissues around blood vessels.
    xi) Connective tissue diseases
23. How is the severity of bleeding linked to the level of platelet count?
    Ans. The level of platelet deficiency is the main factor that contributes to severity of bleeding.

| | |
|---|---|
| Above 100,000/mm$^3$ | No clinical symptoms, bleeding is rare. |
| 50,000–100,000/mm$^3$ | Bleeding may occur after major surgeries |
| 20,000–50,000/mm$^3$ | Bleeding occurs with minor trauma |
| Below 20,000/mm$^3$ | Spontaneous hemorrhages in urinary and GI tract, nose bleeds, etc. |
| At < 20,000/mm$^3$ | Cerebral hemorrhages may occur |

24. Give the causes of thrombocytopenia.
    Ans.
    A. Decreased production
       - Bone marrow suppression: Drugs (sulphas, chloramphenicol, cytotoxic drugs); irradiation, toxemic conditions, and aplastic anemia.

- Bone marrow infiltration: Leukemias and secondary deposits of malignant disease.
- Periodic thrombocytopenic purpura (purpura hemorrhagica)

B. Increased destruction
- Drugs: Thiazides, quinine, ethanol, estrogens, methyl dopa, quinidine
- Hypersplenism (Sequestration and destruction in spleen)
- Hemorrhage with severe transfusion.
- Idiopathic thrombocytopenic purpura
- Disseminated intravascular coagulation

25. Give the causes of thrombocytosis

A. Primary thrombocytosis (thrombocythemia): – It is a myeloproliferative disease involving megakaryocytes.

B. Secondary (or reactive) thrombocytosis: – Often occurs after removal of spleen or after severe hemorrhage.

26. What is the mechanism of clotting in the glass capillary tube in your experiment?

Ans. When blood comes in contact with the glass surface of the capillary tube (similar to the injury of blood vessel), it initiates intrinsic blood coagulation. Activation of platelets causes release of phospholipids (PPL). The PPL, along with high molecular weight kininogens and kallikrein, converts factor XII to XIIa that facilitates the intrinsic mechanism of clotting.

27. Give the causes of prolongation of clotting time

Ans.

A. Hereditary Coagulation Disorders
- Hemophilias A, B, C, D
- Afibrinogenemia and dysfibrinogenemia
- von Willebrand disease
- Deficiency of factor XIII

B. Acquired Coagulation Disorders
- Vitamin K deficiency
- Liver diseases: There is a decrease of all clotting factors except VIII. There is also a reduced uptake of vitamin K, and abnormalities of platelet function.
- Intravascular clotting: Clotting factors are used up and bleeding may occur.
- Anticoagulant therapy: Patients receiving heparin or wafarin show an increased CT.
- Newborns: Premature babies have a tendency to bleed due to low levels of certain clotting factors in the plasma, especially prothrombin. Usually, normal levels of the clotting factors are reached by the 2nd or 3rd week after birth.

28. How is the fluid state of blood maintained in the body?

Ans. A balance between clotting and anticlotting mechanisms prevents intravascular clotting. In addition, continuous nature of blood flow and endothelial factors contribute to fluidity of blood.

1. Continuous flow of blood (dynamic circulation)
2. Endothelial factors:
   - Smoothness of endothelial surface (damage to endothelium causes this activation).
   - The glycocalyx layer on the endothelium repels clotting factors and platelets.
   - Thrombomodulin removes thrombin as soon as it is formed.
   - Prostacyclin secreted by endothelium counteracts platelet aggregation.
3. Antithrombin action of antithrombin III – Heparin complex and fibrin.
4. Fibrinolytic (Plasmin System).

29. Define thrombosis and embolism and give the causes for each.

Ans. Thrombosis is an intravascular clot. Generally, thrombosis develops due to two mechanisms:
- Local damage or roughness of endothelial surface of blood vessel: This usually occurs at the site of atheromatous plaques (sites more prone are coronaries, carotid arteries, cerebral arteries), on damaged cardiac valves, or in veins of the lower limbs. At the site of atheromatous plaque, platelets aggregate, adhere and are activated, and slowly initiate the intrinsic system of clotting.
- Slowing of blood flow (stasis): Decreased flow of blood in the pelvic and leg veins causes accumulation of clotting factors. This usually occurs in prolonged confinement to bed (fractures, major surgery, severe burns), during long flights in aeroplanes, as a complication of pregnancy, etc.

Emboli are small fragments of a thrombus that after getting dislodged from thrombus enter the downstream blood and block smaller vessels. This process is called embolism. Also, an embolus can be a blood clot, an air bubble, fat globules from broken bones, and a piece of tissue debris. Lodgment of emboli (embolism) in smaller arteries of any vital organ such as heart, lung or brain could be life-threatening and should be treated with fibrinolytics and anticoagulant agents.

Chapter 18

# Platelet Count

## Learning Objectives

After completing this practical, you will be able to:

- Describe the importance of performing platelet count in practical physiology.
- List the methods of performing platelet count.
- Perform platelet count by the Rees–Ecker method and peripheral blood smear method.
- List the precautions and possible sources of error in the Rees–Ecker method.
- State the normal value of platelet count.
- List the functions of platelets.
- Name the conditions that alter platelet count.

You may also be able to:

- Explain the role of platelets in hemostasis (temporary hemostatic plug formation and blood coagulation).
- Name the granules of platelets and list the chemicals present in these granules.
- Describe the regulation of thrombopoiesis.
- List the principle and advantages of platelet count by the Brecher–Cronkite method.
- Explain the causes of thrombocytopenia and thrombocytosis.

## INTRODUCTION

Platelets are anuclear cytoplasmic fragments of megakaryocytes. They play an important role in hemostasis (the control of bleeding) and the formation of clots within the blood vessels.

### Development

Platelets are developed from megakaryocytes, the giant cells in the bone marrow. The development of platelets is known as *thrombopoiesis*. The steps of thrombopoiesis are:

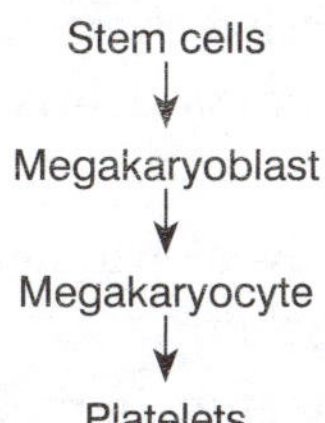


Megakaryocytes form platelets by pinching off bits of cytoplasm and extruding them into the circulation. The production and release of platelets from the bone marrow normally remains constant. Production is depressed by transfusion of platelets, and is enhanced by removal of platelets from the blood (thrombocytopheresis). This indicates that there is a feedback regulatory mechanism for platelet production. Thrombopoietin, a hormone, is probably involved in this process. Platelet production is also regulated by the colony stimulating factors (GM-CSF), $IL_1$, $IL_3$ and $IL_6$.

### Life History

Platelets normally have a half-life of about 4 days. Their survival time in circulation is about 8–12 days. Aged platelets are removed from the circulation by the reticuloendothelial system. The spleen is an important site of destruction of platelets. Therefore, platelet count increases after splenectomy and decreases in hypersplenism.

### Normal Count

In adults: 1.5–4 lakhs/mm$^3$ of blood

### Structure

Platelets are small, anucleated, granulated, spherical or oval bodies, 2–4 μm in diameter. They contain microtubules and microfilaments. The cytoplasm contains two types of granules: alpha and dense. The *alpha granules* contain PDGF (platelet-derived growth factor), platelet factor 3 (a phospholipid), fibronectin, plasminogen, platelet fibrinogen, proaccelerin (factor 5), thrombospondin, alpha-2 plasmin inhibitor and hydrolases. The *dense granules* contain serotonin, ADP and calcium ions.

## Functions

Platelets perform four main functions in the body: (1) temporary hemostasis (arrest of bleeding), (2) clotting of blood, (3) phagocytosis of small particles and organisms and (4) storage and transport of chemicals.

### Temporary Hemostasis

The most important function of platelets is the arrest of bleeding. The initial events following damage to the blood vessels are vasoconstriction and temporary hemostatic plug formation. This is followed by conversion of the temporary plug into the definitive clot. The formation of a hemostatic plug at the site of injury immediately stops bleeding. This hemostatic plug is formed by platelets and is their primary function. The hemostatic plug is known as the **platelet plug**. The temporary hemostatic plug is formed by three properties of platelets: adhesion, aggregation and release reaction.

**Platelet adhesion** Platelets adhere to the exposed collagen of the lining of the damaged blood vessels. The von Willebrand factor facilitates platelet adhesion.

**Platelet aggregation** Platelets have the tendency to stick to each other and to the damaged vessel wall. This phenomenon is called platelet aggregation. Fibrinogen, thrombin and PAF (platelet activating factors) foster platelet aggregation.

**Platelet activation and release reaction** The binding of platelets to collagen initiates platelet activation. Activation is also produced by ADP and thrombin. The activated platelets change their shape, put out pseudopodia, and discharge the contents of their granules. This is known as **release reaction** of platelets. When platelets adhere to the collagen in the damaged vessel wall, ATP in the adhered platelets is converted to ADP. ADP and collagen activate phospholipase $A_2$, which causes hydrolysis of membrane phospholipids to form arachidonic acid. Arachidonic acid is then converted to endoperoxides by cyclo-oxygenase. Endoperoxides, when acted upon by thromboxane synthase, form thromboxane $A_2$. Thromboxane $A_2$ causes vasoconstriction and platelet aggregation, and also increases calcium influx into the platelets. Increased intracellular calcium brings about contraction of microfilaments that cause movement of granules to the canaliculi of the cells. Granules fuse with the canalicular membrane and finally discharge their contents to the exterior through the open canaliculi (release reaction).

### Blood Clotting

Platelets participate in the clotting process because platelet factor 3 (platelet phospholipids) is needed for formation of $X_a$ (activation of the Stuart–Prower factor) and for the conversion of prothrombin to thrombin by factor $X_a$ and $V_a$. Another important function of platelets is to promote clot retraction. This is the shrinkage of the clot, which depends on metabolically active platelets. This is produced by contraction of attached platelet pseudopodia in the polymerised fibrin, which contains actin–myosin-like proteins. If the clot does not retract, it may not be stable and may disintegrate.

### Phagocytosis

Carbon particles, immune complexes and viruses undergo phagocytosis by platelets in the circulation.

### Storage and Transport

Platelets take up 5 HT and synthesise, store and transport serotonin. They also store and transport heparin.

## METHODS OF COUNTING

Several problems are encountered in the counting of platelets because:

1. They are small and difficult to discern.
2. They have an adhesive character and attach readily to glassware, particles or debris in the diluting fluid.
3. They clump easily.
4. They are not evenly distributed in the mixture of blood and diluting fluid.
5. They readily disintegrate in blood diluted with fluid making it difficult to distinguish them from debris.

Therefore, unless carefully done, accurate counting of platelets becomes impossible.

Three methods are frequently used for platelet count. These are:

1. Hemocytometry (direct count)
2. Study of blood smear (indirect count)
3. Automated counting

## Platelet Count by Hemocytometry

Two methods of platelet count by hemocytometry are frequently used: (1) the Rees–Ecker method and (2) the Brecher–Cronkite method. The details of the Rees–Ecker method will be discussed, as this is the method usually followed in our laboratories.

## The Rees–Ecker Method for Manual Platelet Count

### Principle

Whole blood is diluted with a solution of brilliant cresyl blue which stains the platelets light blue. The diluent also prevents coagulation. No attempt is made to lyse the red cells. Platelets are then counted by hemocytometry.

### Requirements

**I. Equipment**

1. Microscope
2. Hemocytometer (RBC pipette and counting chamber)
3. Materials for sterile finger prick
4. Petri dish
5. Filter papers

Instead of Neubauer's hemocytometer, a specially designed *Spencer–Brightline hemocytometer* is used for platelet counts. This uses the Spencer–Brightline counting chamber. The metallic surface of this chamber makes it easier to see the platelets. The cell distribution also appears better, since the chamber's surface is smoother. If the Spencer–Brightline hemocytometer is not available, Neubauer's hemocytometer may be used.

**II. Reagent** The diluent used for counting platelets must meet certain requirements. It must:

1. Provide fixation to reduce the adhesiveness of the platelets
2. Prevent coagulation
3. Prevent hemolysis
4. Provide a low specific gravity so that the platelets settle in one plane.

The Rees–Ecker fluid meets all these requirements. 1% ammonium oxalate can be used, but it is not as good as the Rees–Ecker fluid.

*Composition of the Rees–Ecker fluid*

1. Sodium citrate—prevents coagulation, preserves RBC and provides the necessary low specific gravity.
2. Formalin—acts as a fixative
3. Brilliant cresyl blue—identifies the diluent.
   Note Brilliant cresyl blue does not stain the platelets, as it is not essential for counting. Dye is used only for identification of the diluent.
4. Deionised water—acts as a solvent.

> Note: The Rees–Ecker fluid must be stored in the refrigerator and filtered before each use.

**III. Specimen** Capillary blood (from a finger puncture) can be used. Generally, venous blood gives more satisfactory results, as platelet count in capillary blood is usually less than that of venous blood. This difference is due to clumping of platelets at the site of puncture in finger prick blood collection. The venous blood that is collected should be anticoagulated with EDTA because EDTA reduces the tendency of platelet clumping. If venous blood is used, the test should be performed within 2 hours of collecting blood.

### Procedure

1. Clean the RBC pipette and Neubauer's chamber thoroughly.

> Note: All glassware must be scrupulously cleaned. This is to prevent adhesion and aggregation of platelets. Anything in the pipette to which the platelets could adhere must be removed. 95 per cent ethanol is used to clean the hemocytometer. A lint-free cloth should be used.

2. Puncture the fingertip and suck the blood exactly up to the 0.5 mark of the RBC pipette.
3. Rapidly dilute the blood with the Rees–Ecker fluid to the 101 mark of the pipette.
4. Shake the pipette immediately after dilution for at least 1 minute.
5. Discard 3–5 drops of the solution from the pipette.
6. Charge the Neubauer's chamber.
7. Cover the charged chamber with a petri dish lined with moist filter paper and allow 15 minutes for the platelets to settle in the chamber.

> Note: The chamber is covered to prevent evaporation.

8. After 15 minutes, count the platelets under a high-power objective.

> Note: The platelets are bluish and must be distinguished from debris. Platelets are oval or round bodies, normally 2–4 μm in diameter and refractile in nature.

9. Count the platelets in all the 25 medium squares of the RBC square, that is, in 1 $mm^2$ area or 1/10 $mm^3$ volume.
10. Enter the results in the squares drawn on paper.

## Calculations

The cells are counted in 25 medium squares, and each of these squares has 16 smaller squares.

The area covered by the 25 medium squares is 1 $mm^2$

Platelet count/μl or $mm^3$ of blood

$$= \frac{\text{Number of platelets counted}}{\text{Volume of fluid}} \times \text{dilution}$$

Dilution is 200.

Volume of fluid in 1 $mm^2$ $= 1 \times 1/10$

$= 1 \times 0.1 = 0.1$ μl or $mm^3$

Platelet count/μl or $mm^3$ of blood = Number of platelets counted × 200/0.1

= Number of platelets counted × 2000

## Precautions and Sources of Error

1. The glassware must be scrupulously cleaned. Debris and dust are the main sources of error as they are easily mistaken for platelets.
2. The diluting fluid must be filtered just before use (to remove stained particles from the stain).
3. If venous blood is used, the platelets must be counted within 2 hours. Delay causes disintegration and clumping of platelets.
4. Blood should be rapidly diluted. This is essential because the platelets may form clumps.
5. Blood must be thoroughly mixed with the diluent by shaking the contents of the pipette for at least one minute. Inadequate mixing results in clumping of platelets.
6. The charged chamber should be kept for 15 minutes under a petri dish to prevent evaporation and for the cells to settle down.
7. Other precautions of hemocytometry (as described in Chapter 6) should also be followed.

## Important Notes

1. It is ideal to make a duplicate count to minimise errors. This is done by charging both sides of the counting chamber simultaneously, and counting both the sides separately.
2. A blood smear should be made and stained simultaneously to check and compare the value observed in the direct method.
3. If the count is low, the WBC pipette can be used for dilution for recounting. The calculation can be done by using the correct dilution factor.
4. If other hematologic tests are to be performed with platelet count, and blood is used from the same puncture, it is necessary to draw the blood for platelet count first before drawing blood for other tests.
5. The finger should not be squeezed excessively to collect blood.
6. In spite of all precautions, the error of platelet count in this method is 15–30 per cent.

# The Brecher–Cronkite Method

## Principle

This method uses phase-contrast microscopy. Ammonium oxalate is one of the constituents of the diluent that completely lyses the red cells. Platelets are then counted with a phase-hemocytometer and phase-contrast microscope to enhance the refractileness of the platelets.

## Advantages

1. Identification of platelets is easier.
2. The error involved is low (5–10 per cent).

# Platelet Count by Study of Blood Smear

## Principle

The principle is the same as that of making a blood smear.

## Procedure

1. Place a drop of 14% magnesium sulphate solution on the tip of a finger and prick through this drop of solution.

Note: Magnesium sulphate prevents clumping of blood.

2. Make a blood smear and stain with Leishman stain.
3. Count platelets per 1000 red cells.

### Normal Count

The normal ratio of platelets to RBCs is 1 : 20.

Note: Total red cell count can be done separately. If the red cell count is 5,000,000/mm$^3$, and platelet count in the indirect method is 1 : 20, the *indirect absolute count* of platelets will be 250,000/mm$^3$ of blood.

## Platelet Count by Automated Method

Automated platelet counting is done with an S Plus Coulter counter. In the S Plus model, platelets and red cells pass through the apertures. The particles that are between 2 and 10 fL are counted as platelets. A platelet graph is also plotted according to the size distribution of the platelets counted.

## DISCUSSION

Platelets participate in the coagulation of blood and are, therefore, associated with the hemostatic mechanisms of the body.

## Clinical Significance

Platelet count is usually ordered as a part of the laboratory diagnosis of a bleeding disorder. When platelet count increases in the blood, the condition is known as **thrombocytosis**, and when the count decreases, the condition is called **thrombocytopenia**. Thrombocytopenia can be caused by impaired production or increased destruction of the platelets. Prolonged bleeding time is the hallmark of thrombocytopenia. When platelet count is less than 50,000 per mm$^3$ of blood, the count is called **critical count**, as bleeding may occur spontaneously, as below this count hemorrhagic tendency appears. However, count below 20,000 leads to spontaneous hemorrhage.

The hemorrhagic tendency is proportional to the degree of thrombocytopenia and is characterised by petechiae, ecchymoses, menorrhagia and bleeding from mucous membranes into the central nervous system. To differentiate the causes of thrombocytopenia, the bone marrow should be carefully examined. If megakaryocytes are absent in the bone marrow, this implies failure of platelet production.

## Conditions that Alter Thrombocyte Count

### Thrombocytosis

1. Polycythemia vera
2. Chronic myeloid leukemia
3. Iron deficiency anemia
4. Splenectomy
5. Chronic infection
6. Surgery
7. Acute hemorrhage

### Thrombocytopenia

1. Idiopathic thrombocytopenic purpura
2. Aplastic anemia
3. Hypersplenism
4. Acute leukemia
5. Cytotoxic chemotherapy
6. Radiation treatment

## VIVA

1. Why does the platelet count produce inaccurate results unless performed very carefully?
2. What are the different methods of platelet count?
3. What is the principle of the Rees–Ecker method?
4. What are the advantages of using the Spencer–Brightline counting chamber for platelet count?
5. Why is the Rees–Ecker fluid an ideal diluent for platelet count?
6. What is the composition of the Rees–Ecker fluid and what are the functions of each constituent?
7. Why is the Rees–Ecker fluid filtered before every use?
8. Why is venous blood preferred to capillary blood for platelet count?
9. Why is glassware cleaned thoroughly for platelet count?

10. Why is the blood rapidly diluted and thoroughly mixed with the diluting fluid?
11. Why is the charged chamber covered by a petri dish for 15 minutes?
12. How do you identify platelets under the high-power objective?
13. What are the sources of error in the manual method of platelet count?
14. What is the other method of platelet count using the principle of hemocytometry and what are its advantages?
15. How is the indirect count of platelets performed?
16. What are the precursor cells for platelets?
17. What are the factors that regulate the development of platelets?
18. What is the lifespan of platelets and how are they removed from circulation?
19. What is the normal platelet count?
20. What are the properties of platelets? What are its functions?
21. What are the causes of thrombocytosis and thrombocytopenia (Refer 'Viva' of previous chapter)?

In addition, all the questions of previous chapters, especially questions related to bleeding time, may be asked here.

CHAPTER 19

# General Examination

## LEARNING OBJECTIVES

After completing this practical, you will be able to:

- Describe the importance of general examination in clinical physiology.
- List the parameters (signs) to be examined in general examination.
- Examine and elicit different signs.
- List the common causes of abnormalities of the signs.

You may also be able to:

- Explain the physiological basis of development of abnormal signs.
- Correlate the abnormal signs with the pathophysiology of the disease processes.

## INTRODUCTION

A thorough and detailed general examination is an essential part of the clinical examination of a patient and should be performed prior to any systemic examination. If meticulously performed, the general examination provides adequate clues to the diagnosis.

### Requirements

1. Patient's examination should be conducted in a comfortable, private and quiet area.
2. Preferably, examination should be done in daylight as skin changes are better appreciated in natural light. Artificial light should be avoided.
3. Usually patients will be apprehensive to be examined, especially when the environment is unfamiliar. Reassure the patient about the need for the examination for diagnosing the disease.
4. A thorough general examination requires the subject to be adequately exposed. The patient should be asked to undress maximally.
5. If a male doctor examines a female patient, especially if the private parts are to be examined, always a chaperone/female attender/female nurse should be present. This is done to reassure the patient and to protect the doctor from accusations of immodesty.
6. If covered areas and private parts need to be examined as part of the clinical examination, do not hesitate to unclothe these parts and examine properly.
7. Try to expose only the area you are examining at the time. Cover the body parts just examined as you proceed to the next.
8. Examine the subject/patient standing on his/her right-hand side, as it is easy to examine the abdominal viscera, jugular vein, apex beat from the right side.
9. Pay regular attention to the patient's comfort, especially while examining an elderly subject, such as adjustment of pillow, which usually gets disturbed during examination. This reassures the patient that you are concerned about his/her welfare.
10. Make a quick assessment of patient's illness. If the patient is very sick, the detailed examination may be postponed till acute problem has been attended. The examination should not put the ill patient to further distress.

### Steps of Examination

The general examination begins the moment the patient is seen. It should be done without unnecessary embarrassment and discomfort to the patient. It should preferably be performed in daylight. General examination is carried out under the following headings:

1. General appearance
2. Mental state and intelligence
3. Consciousness and cooperation
4. Build
5. Development (height, weight and sexual maturity)
6. State of nutrition
7. Pallor (anemia)
8. Icterus (jaundice)
9. Cyanosis
10. Clubbing
11. Edema

12. Lymphadenopathy
13. Skin condition
14. *Vital signs* Temperature, pulse, respiration, blood pressure

## General Appearance

Look at the subject, and observe whether he looks healthy, unwell or ill. If he looks ill, assess the severity of the illness: whether the patient is ill, very ill or in distress.

## Mental State and Intelligence

One should assess the mood of the patient and should try to study the mind of the patient. This is detected by observing the way the patient describes his emotional state.

The patient's level of intelligence is one of the important pieces of information to be obtained from the interview. This helps to determine the suitable treatment. An approximate assessment of intelligence is obtained from the educational and occupational history and from an assessment of his general knowledge.

## Consciousness and Cooperation

It is important to ascertain the level of consciousness of the patient. The level of consciousness can be clear sensorium, drowsiness, stupor, semicoma and coma. If he is fully conscious, assess whether he is cooperative enough to provide all information.

## Build

Build is the skeletal structure of a person. It is assessed in relation to the age and sex of the individual as compared to a normal person. It should be observed whether the patient is tall or short, lean or fat, and muscular or asthenic.

## Development

### Height

The height of each patient should be measured to find out whether he is of average height for that age and sex. If he is too tall or short, details of the measurement of span (from the tip of the middle finger of one side to the tip of the middle finger of the other side of outstretched upper limbs), upper segment (crown to the pubic symphysis), and the lower segment (pubic symphysis to foot) should be taken. Normally, in adults, the armspan is equal to the height of the person and the upper segment is equal to the length of the lower segment.

### Weight

The weight should be recorded preferably on an empty stomach, without shoes and with minimum clothing. It should be ascertained whether the patient's weight is normal for age and sex or if he is overweight or underweight.

### Body Mass Index

Body mass index (BMI) is an important index of physical development of an individual. It is assessed by the Quetlet formula,

$$\text{BMI} = \frac{\text{Weight (in kg)}}{(\text{Height in metres})^2}$$

Though there are many other anthropometric indices such as waist circumference, waist–hip ratio, waist–height ratio, skin fold thickness, neck circumference, etc., BMI is the commonly used parameter for assessment of adiposity and cardiovascular (CV) risk of the person, as degrees of obesity have traditionally been calculated by the level of BMI. As the Asian population is more prone to CV risks even at lower range of BMI, compared to European, African, American and other populations, the BMI range for grading obesity in Asian population is different. BMI range for Asian population is as follows:

Normal BMI : 18.5–22.9 (below 18.5 is underweight)
Overweight (Preobese) : 23–27.49
Obesity : 27.5 or above

## Sexual Development

Effort should be made to assess the development of secondary sexual characteristics.

In males, secondary sexual characteristics develop between 13 and 18 years. Hair grows on the face, trunk, axillae and pubic region. The pubic hair develops with the upper border convex upwards and may extend up to the umbilicus. Laryngeal growth results in thick voice. Considerable muscular development occurs.

In females, secondary sexual characteristics develop between 11 and 15 years. There is development of breasts, and the female distribution of fat gives the characteristic curves of the body. Hair also grows in the axillae and pubis. The pubic hair exhibits an upper margin, which is concave upwards.

## Nutrition

Assessment of the nutritional state of a patient is an important part of the general examination. It is done by taking dietary history, and by performing physical examination including anthropometric measurements. The physical examination includes measurement of the bulk of the muscles and body fat (skinfold thickness). Anthropometric measurements include recording of height and weight. It is performed to ascertain whether the patient is well nourished or malnourished. Malnutrition may be due to starvation, maldigestion of food or malabsorption of nutrients from the gastrointestinal tract.

## Pallor

Pallor is paleness of the skin. It depends on the thickness and quality of the skin, and the amount and quality of the blood in the capillaries. Thus, pallor is seen in persons with thick or opaque skin, in conditions where blood flow in the capillaries is diminished, such as shock, or when the hemoglobin content in the blood is decreased. Pallor is usually detected by examining the lower palpebral conjunctiva (Fig. 19.1)

The tip and dorsum of the tongue, soft palate, palms and nails should also be examined to assess pallor. The degree of pallor is expressed as plus 1 to plus 3 (Fig. 19.2):

Pallor : 0 (no anemia)
Pallor : + (mild anemia)
Pallor : ++ (moderate anemia)
Pallor : +++ (severe anemia)

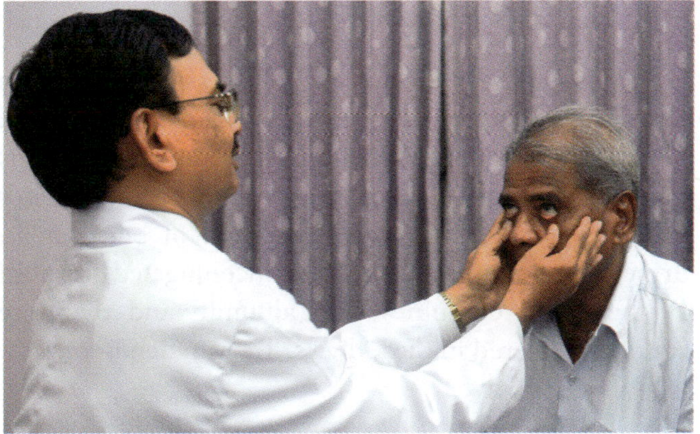

Fig. 19.1 For detection of pallor, note that lower eyelids are retracted down to assess the paleness of lower palpebral conjunctiva.

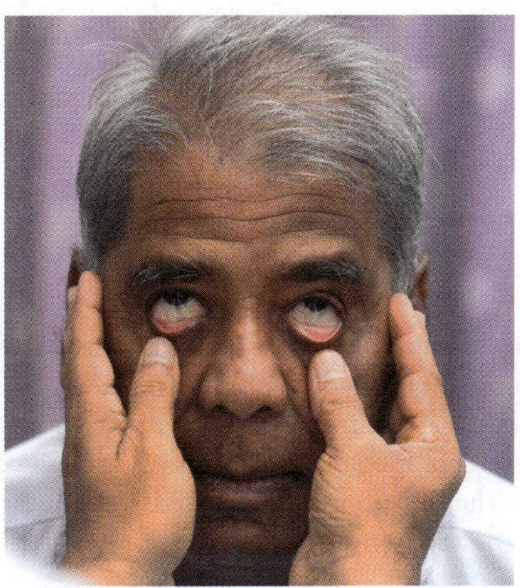

Fig. 19.2 Note the pallor as + (mild anemia) in this subject.

# JAUNDICE

Jaundice is the yellow discolouration of the sclera (Fig. 19.3), skin and mucous membranes of the body, which occurs due to the presence of excess bilirubin in the blood. Normal serum bilirubin concentration is 0.2 to 0.8 mg/100 ml of blood. When the bilirubin level exceeds 2 mg per cent, jaundice appears clinically. Hyperbilirubinemia between 0.8 and 2 mg% is called *subclinical* or *latent jaundice*.

## Types

Jaundice is classified clinically into three types: prehepatic, hepatic and post-hepatic.

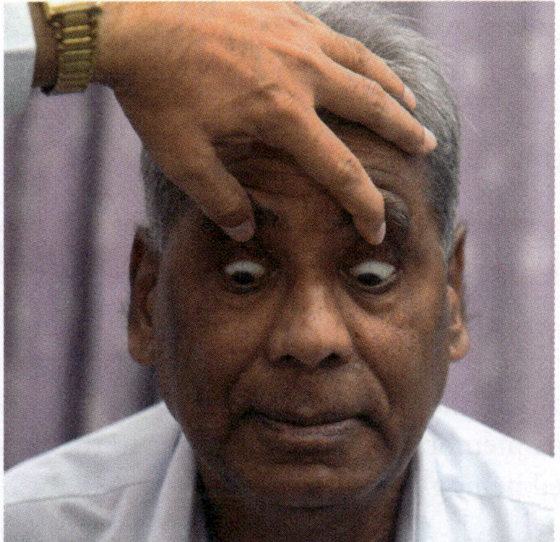

Fig. 19.3 Method of detection of icterus. Note that the upper eyelids are retracted upwards and subject is asked to look downward to assess the yellow discolouration of sclera.

## Prehepatic Jaundice

Prehepatic jaundice occurs due to excessive destruction of red cells. Therefore, it is also called *hemolytic jaundice*. Jaundice is usually mild to moderate and bilirubin is mostly unconjugated. Fecal stercobilinogen and urinary urobilinogen are increased. Excretion of bilirubin in urine is absent because the excess unconjugated bilirubin in the blood combines with albumin and therefore cannot be filtered in the kidneys. The van den Bergh test is indirect positive.

## Hepatic Jaundice

This usually occurs due to hepatitis or damage to the cells of the liver. Therefore, it is also called hepatic or *hepatocellular jaundice*. Jaundice is usually moderate to severe and may be associated with bleeding disorders. Bilirubin is both conjugated and unconjugated. Fecal stercobilinogen and urinary urobilinogen are normal or raised. Bilirubins exhibit a biphasic reaction to the van den Bergh test.

## Post-hepatic Jaundice

This occurs due to obstruction in the biliary tract. Therefore, it is called *obstructive jaundice*. Because of obstruction, no bilirubin reaches the intestine. Hence, fecal stercobilinogen and urinary urobilinogen are absent. The bilirubin is conjugated and appears in the urine. The van den Bergh test is direct positive.

**Causes of yellow discolouration of skin**

1. Jaundice
2. Carotenemia
3. Hemochromatosis
4. Picrates
5. Mephacrine

# CYANOSIS

## Definition

Cyanosis is the bluish discolouration of the skin and mucous membranes of the body due to the presence of reduced hemoglobin in more than 5 g% in the blood.

## Physiological Basis

Hemoglobin in the arterial blood is 95 per cent saturated with oxygen. Therefore, about 14.25 g (taking 15 g% of hemoglobin as the standard) in the arterial blood is oxyhemoglobin and only 0.75 g is reduced hemoglobin in a normal adult. In mixed venous blood, about 70 per cent of hemoglobin is saturated with oxygen. Hence, 10.5 g of the 15 g per cent of hemoglobin in the venous blood is oxyhemoglobin and 4.5 g is reduced hemoglobin. The amount of reduced hemoglobin in capillary blood is assumed to be the mean of arterial and venous content of the reduced hemoglobin. Thus, in a normal individual at rest, capillary blood contain 2.6 g% (0.75 + 4.5/2) of reduced hemoglobin. The colour of normal skin and mucous membrane is therefore pink. *When the concentration of reduced hemoglobin is more than 5 g per cent*, the skin and mucous membrane become blue because of the dark colour of the reduced hemoglobin. The presence of excess of other hemoglobin complexes like methemoglobin and sulfhemoglobin in the blood also produces cyanosis because of their dark colour.

> Note
> 1. Patients suffering from severe anemia with hemoglobin content less than 5 g per cent may not show cyanosis (as the total hemoglobin is less than 5 gm per cent).
> 2. Cyanosis may not be seen in carbon monoxide poisoning, because carboxyhemoglobin prevents reduction of oxyhemoglobin and the colour of carboxyhemoglobin is cherry red.

## Types

Cyanosis is of three types: peripheral, central and mixed. There is another special category of cyanosis, called differential cyanosis.

### Peripheral Cyanosis

This occurs due to slowing of the flow of blood through the tissues, thereby allowing more time for removal of oxygen by the tissues.

*Causes*

1. Decreased cardiac output, for example, heart failure
2. Local vasoconstriction, for example, extreme cold
3. Venous obstruction, for example, superior venacaval obstruction
4. Increased viscosity of blood, for example, polycythemia

### Central Cyanosis

When reduced hemoglobin concentration is more than 5 g% due to mixing of arterial blood with venous blood, or inadequate oxygenation of the arterial blood, central cyanosis results. In the early stage, cyanosis manifests in the palate, tongue and inner side of the lips. When the amount of reduced hemoglobin becomes very high, cyanosis appears in different peripheral sites too.

#### Causes

*I. Due to admixture of venous and arterial blood*

This occurs in right to left shunt in which venous blood bypasses the pulmonary circulation and directly enters into systemic circulation. It is seen in:

i) Fallot's tetralogy
ii) Pulmonary arteriovenous fistula
iii) Patent truncus arteriosus
iv) Transposition of great vessels

*II. Due to inadequate oxygenation of arterial blood*

1. Low atmospheric oxygen, for example, high altitude
2. Inadequate ventilation, for example, lung collapse, airway obstruction
3. Decreased gaseous exchange through the pulmonary membrane, for example, hyaline membrane disease

### Mixed Cyanosis

In this type of cyanosis, both central and peripheral mechanisms operate. The most common example is chronic cor pulmonale due to emphysema.

### Differential Cyanosis

This is a condition where cyanosis appears only in one half of the body. For example, in patent ductus arteriosus with reversal of shunt due to pulmonary hypertension, cyanosis is seen only in the lower limbs; both upper limbs are spared.

## CLUBBING

### Definition

Bulbous enlargement of soft parts of the terminal phalanges with over-curving of the nails both transversely and longitudinally is called clubbing.

### Detection

Clubbing is diagnosed by the presence of any of the following five signs.

1. **Fluctuation test (Nail bed fluctuation)** Normally, the nail bed fluctuates very slightly. Fluctuation increases in clubbing. This is elicited by assessing fluctuation of the nail base. Examiner holds the base of the nail from both sides and gently presses the tip of the nail (Fig. 19.4) to elicit nail bed fluctuation, if present.
2. **Curving of nails** In clubbing, the nails curve in both transverse and longitudinal directions. The curving is due to hypertrophy of nail bed tissue.
3. **Profile sign** The presence of a transverse ridge at the root of the nail due to thickening of fibroelastic tissue is called profile sign.
4. **Schamroth's sign** When two fingers are held together with their nails facing each other, a space is seen at the nail folds. This space is lost in clubbing (positive Schamroth's sign).
5. **Base angle** In a normal finger the angle between the base of the nail and the adjacent portion of the dorsum of the terminal phalanx is an obtuse angle of about 160°. In clubbing, this angle gets obliterated in the outward direction and becomes 180° or more. This is best viewed vertically from the side.

### Physiological Basis

The exact physiological basis of clubbing is not known. It may be due to any of the following causes:

1. **Dilatation of AV anastomosis** In clubbing, the AV (arteriovenous) anastomotic channels increase in the fingers (the cause is not known). This causes hypertrophy of tissues in the nail bed.
2. **Increased pressure gradient** An increase in pressure gradient between the radial artery and digital artery causes edema and increased cellularity of the

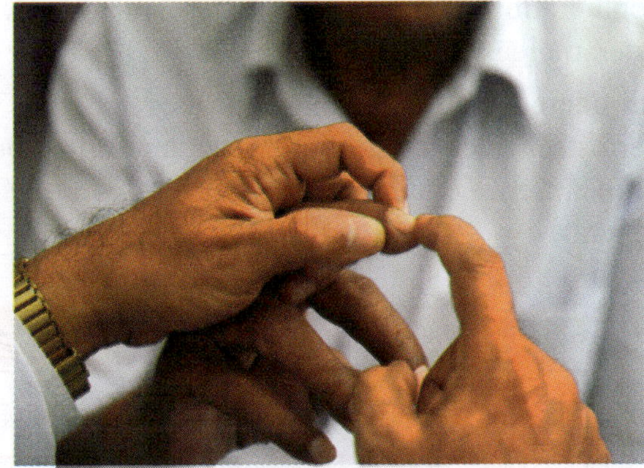

Fig. 19.4 Fluctuation test for assessing clubbing. Examiner holds the base of the nail and gently presses the tip of the nail to assess fluctuation of the nail bed.

connective tissue in the finger. This predisposes to clubbing.

3. **Capillary stasis** Capillary stasis results from back pressure, which may cause clubbing.
4. **Vitamin deficiency and hormonal disorders** These are thought to be involved in the genesis of clubbing.

## Causes

A. Bronchopulmonary diseases
   1. Bronchiectasis
   2. Lung abscess
   3. Bronchogenic carcinoma
   4. Emphysema

B. Cardiac diseases
   1. Congenital cyanotic heart disease
   2. Subacute bacterial endocarditis

C. Gastrointestinal diseases
   1. Ulcerative colitis
   2. Biliary cirrhosis of liver

D. Endocrine disorders
   1. Thyrotoxicosis
   2. Acromegaly

E. Hereditary

## Degrees of Clubbing

**First degree** When only increased fluctuation of the nail bed is present, it is first degree clubbing.

**Second degree** When curving of nail is present in addition to increased fluctuation of nail bed, there is second degree clubbing.

**Third degree** If increased fluctuation, increased curving and obliteration of base angle of the nails are present together, there is third degree clubbing.

**Fourth degree** Combination of the above changes plus subperiosteal thickening of the wrist and ankle bones with the presence of definite transverse ridge at the root of the nails.

# EDEMA

## Definition

Edema is swelling of the skin and subcutaneous tissues due to accumulation of free fluid in excess in the interstitial tissue space.

## Types

Edema is classified as localised or generalised and pitting or non-pitting.

## Method of Detection

Edema is diagnosed by pressing the skin against the bones in the dependent parts (Fig. 19.5), which leaves a pit or depression in the case of pitting edema (Fig. 19.6). Edema may be non-pitting as seen in filariasis.

## Common Causes

A. Cardiac causes
   1. Congestive heart failure
   2. Constrictive pericarditis

B. Hepatic causes
   1. Cirrhosis of liver
   2. Carcinoma of liver

C. Renal causes
   1. Nephrotic syndrome
   2. Acute nephritis

D. Anemia and hypoproteinemia

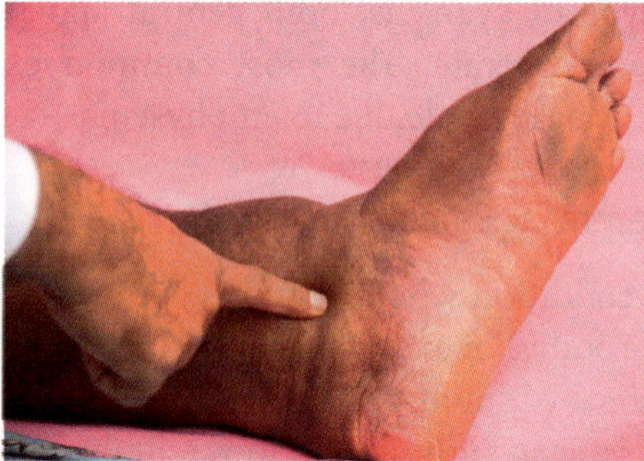

Fig. 19.5 Assessment of edema. Note that the skin against the medial malleolus (dependent part of this subject) is pressed for about 20 seconds.

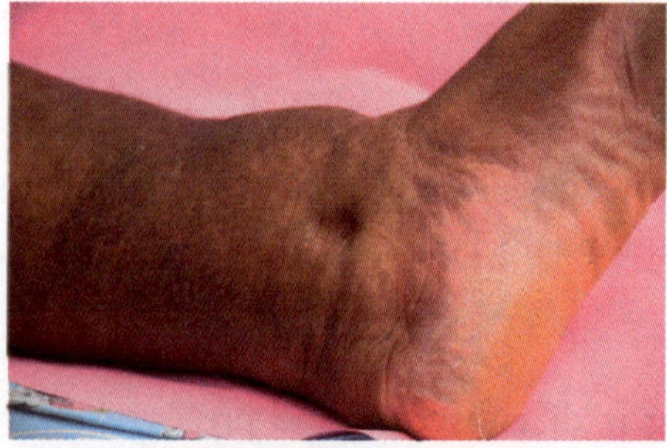

Fig. 19.6 Pitting edema. Note the presence of pit (depression) in the ankle following putting pressure over the area.

## Special Features

**Cardiac edema** It is usually seen in the dependant parts of the body. Dyspnea at rest is one of the associated features.

**Hepatic edema** Edema is prominent on the abdomen. Ascites is one of the associated features.

**Renal edema** Edema first appears in the face. Puffiness of the lower eyelid in the morning is a characteristic feature.

**Anemia and hypoproteinemia** Edema is generalised from the beginning. Severe pallor is one of the associated features.

## Physiological Basis

Edema occurs due to excess accumulation of fluid in the interstitial tissue space. Interstitial fluid is formed by filtration through the capillary walls. The capillary wall is regarded as a semi-permeable membrane. The main driving forces causing filtration of fluid through the capillaries are hydrostatic pressure within the capillaries and oncotic pressure (osmotic pressure exerted by the plasma proteins). Hydrostatic pressure favours filtration whereas oncotic pressure opposes it. Therefore, when hydrostatic pressure increases or oncotic pressure decreases, there is excess filtration of fluid into the interstitial tissue space. Normally, the fluid from the interstitial space is removed by the lymphatics. When excess filtration of fluid occurs, the lymphatics cannot remove all the fluid and more fluid accumulates in the interstitial tissue space. This leads to formation of edema.

## Physiological Mechanisms

**Cardiac failure** In congestive cardiac failure, edema develops in dependent parts of the body due to the following mechanisms.

1. Decreased cardiac output decreases blood volume and pressure, which increases renin release from the kidney. Renin forms angiotensin II which increases aldosterone secretion from the adrenal cortex. Aldosterone increases reabsorption of sodium and water from the kidney. This increases total body sodium and water, which results in edema formation.
2. Decreased cardiac output also stimulates sympathetic activity which causes renal vasoconstriction. Constriction of the renal artery causes release of renin which activates the renin–angiotensin–aldosterone axis.
3. In congestive cardiac failure, due to failure of the right ventricle (backward failure), pressure in the systemic veins increases. This increases hydrostatic pressure in the capillaries, which results in edema formation.

**Nephrotic syndrome** The main cause of edema formation in nephrotic syndrome is the loss of protein in the urine. Protein passes from the glomerulus into the tubular fluid, which results in proteinuria. Loss of protein from the kidney decreases oncotic pressure because of hypoproteinemia and results in edema formation.

**Cirrhosis of liver** In cirrhosis of liver, there is loss of liver tissue. There is decrease in the synthesis of protein by the liver. This results in hypoproteinemia which causes decreased oncotic pressure and edema formation.

**Anemia and hypoproteinemia** In anemia, hypoxia of capillaries increases capillary permeability, which results in edema formation. However, the main cause of edema in anemia is hypoproteinemia.

# LYMPHADENOPATHY

The neck, axilla, inguinal region and supratrochlear areas of both the sides should be examined thoroughly to check for enlargement of lymph nodes. The lymph nodes in the neck should be examined by standing behind the subject and with the patient's head slightly flexed. The glands should be examined in proper order starting from the submental group and proceeding to the submandibular, cervical, posterior auricular and the occipital groups. Lymph nodes in the axilla should also be examined by standing behind the subject and with the patient's arm slightly abducted. In the axilla, anterior, posterior, apical and lateral groups of lymph nodes are examined. The lymph nodes in the inguinal region are examined in a supine position with thigh extended.

## Procedure of Examination

Lymph nodes are palpated to check their size and shape, consistency, mobility and tenderness.

1. **Size and shape** The size of the enlarged lymph node is expressed in centimetres in its longest diameter. The surface of the enlarged nodes may be smooth,

irregular or lobulated. Malignant lymph nodes are often irregular.

2. **Consistency** Lymph nodes are often elastic and rubbery. They are firm in tuberculosis, firm and shotty in syphilis, and hard in carcinoma.
3. **Mobility** Nodes may be mobile or fixed. In benign conditions, nodes are usually separated and mobile. In tuberculosis, the nodes are often matted. In malignant conditions, the nodes are usually fixed to the skin and surrounding tissues.
4. **Tenderness** While palpating the lymph nodes, the patient may complain of pain or may grimace during palpation, which indicates that the lymph nodes are tender. Usually lymph nodes are tender in inflammatory conditions and non-tender (painless) in malignant diseases.

## Causes

**A. Neoplastic**

- I. Hematologic
  1. Lymphomas (Hodgkin and non-Hodgkin)
  2. Acute leukemia
  3. Chronic lymphocytic leukemia
- II. Non-hematologic
  1. Carcinoma of breast
  2. Carcinoma of lungs

**B. Inflammatory**

- I. Infections
  1. Tuberculosis
  2. Syphilis
  3. Filariasis
  4. Infectious mononucleosis
- II. Connective tissue diseases
  1. Systemic lupus erythematosus
  2 Sarcoidosis

**C. Endocrine diseases**

1. Hyperthyroidism
2. Addison's disease

**D. Drugs**

1. Carbamazepine
2. Cephaloridine
3. Meprobamate
4. Phenylbutazone
5. Phenytoin

# THE SKIN

The skin is examined carefully, preferably in daylight and the maximum surface of body should be exposed. The skin is examined for the colour, pigmentation, eruptions and secondary lesions.

## Colour of the Skin

Pallor of the skin is seen in anemia. Yellow skin is seen in jaundice. Blue skin is seen in cyanosis.

## Pigmentation

The skin looks white in albinisim. Patches of white and black pigments are seen in vitiligo. The skin is dark in Addison's disease.

## Eruptions

Different skin eruptions like macules, papules, vesicles, pustules and petechiae occur in different clinical conditions.

## Secondary Lesions

Scales, crusts, excoriations, fissures, ulcers and scars occur in different conditions.

# VITAL SIGNS

There are four vital signs that must always be checked in general examination. These are temperature, pulse, respiration and blood pressure.

## Temperature

Body temperature is usually recorded by using a clinical thermometer. The thermometer is placed either in the mouth or in the axilla for at least one minute. The thermometer can also be placed in the rectum, especially in infants and collapsed patients. The body temperature is usually expressed in Fahrenheit or in Centigrade.

### Normal Value

The normal body temperature at rest is 98–99°F (36.6–37.2°C).

Febrile : >37.2°C (99°F or above)
Mild fever : 37.2– 38.3°C (99–101°F)

Moderate fever : 38.3–40°C (101–104°F)
High fever : 40–41.2°C (104–106°F)
Hyperpyrexia : > 41.6°C (>107°F)
Subnormal : < 36.6°C (<98°F)
Hypothermia : < 35°C (< 95°F)

## Fever

### Definition

Increase in the diurnal variation of body temperature of more than 1°C (1.5°F) or rise of temperature above the maximum normal temperature is called fever.

### Types

Typically, three classical types of fever are seen in clinical practice. These are continued, remittent and intermittent fever.

**Continued fever** The temperature remains high throughout the day and at no time does it touch the baseline, and the diurnal variation of temperature is not more than 1°C. This is commonly seen in:

- Typhoid
- Subacute bacterial endocarditis
- Urinary tract infection
- Brucellosis
- Glandular fever

**Remittent fever** The temperature remains raised throughout the day and at no time does it touch the baseline, but the diurnal variation is more than 2°C.

**Intermittent fever** Fever is present only for several hours during the day and remits to normal for the rest of the day. Intermittent fever may be quotidian, tertian, quartan or irregular intermittent.

*Quotidian* When the paroxysm of intermittent fever occurs every day.

*Tertian* When the paroxysm of fever occurs on alternate days.

*Quartan* When two days intervene between consecutive attacks.

*Irregular intermittent* Paroxysm of fever occurs irregularly.

### Causes

1. Infections
   Bacterial
   Viral
   Rickettsial
   Fungal
   Parasitic
2. Immunologic
   Rheumatic fever
   Rheumatoid arthritis
   Other collagen diseases
3. Neoplastic
   Carcinoma of any organ
   Leukemia
4. Metabolic
   Gout
   Porphyria
   Addison's disease
5. Physical agents
   Heat stroke
   Radiation sickness
6. Drug-induced fever

## Hypothermia

### Definition

Hypothermia is a condition in which body temperature decreases below the normal range.

### Causes

1. Prolonged exposure to cold
2. Myxedema
3. Hypopituitarism
4. Hypoglycemia
5. Hypnosedative poisoning

### Physiological Effects

Hypothermia causes bradycardia, hypotension and shallow respiration and, in severe cases, confusion, stupor and coma. The brain is probably protected by the low temperature.

## Pulse

Count the radial pulse for a minute when the subject is at rest. Examination of pulse is not only performed as part of the examination of the cardiovascular system, but also routinely in general examination as it provides information about the functioning of the heart. It is palpated by three middle fingers with the patient's forearm semipronated and wrist slightly flexed. The pulse is examined for rate, rhythm, volume, character and condition of the arterial wall. A normal pulse rate is 60–100 per minute, regular in rhythm, and normal in volume and character. The arterial wall is neither thickened nor tortuous. (Details of the procedure and abnormalities of pulse are given in Chapter 24).

## Respiration

Rate of respiration is counted for a minute. It should preferably be counted when the subject's attention is distracted from his breathing. Rhythm and type of respiration are also noted. The normal rate of respiration in an adult is 12–20 per minute. (Details of change in respiration in different conditions are given in Chapter 21).

## Blood Pressure

The blood pressure is recorded by a sphygmomanometer, first by the palpatory and then by the ascultatory method.

Normal range of blood pressure in adults:

Systolic : 100–119 mm Hg
Diastolic : 60–79 mm Hg

(Details of blood pressure recording and the conditions affecting blood pressure are given in Chapter 25).

## VIVA

1. What is the importance of general examination in clinical medicine?
2. What are the parameters that are looked for in general examination?
3. How do you assess the development of the subject?
4. How do you assess the nutritional status of the subject?
5. Where do you look to confirm pallor clinically?
6. What is jaundice?
7. Where do you look to detect jaundice clinically?
8. What are the types of jaundice and how do you differentiate them?
9. What are the causes of the yellow colour of the skin?
10. What is cyanosis?
11. What are the types of cyanosis and how do you differentiate them?
12. What is the physiological basis of cyanosis?
13. What is clubbing?
14. What are the causes of clubbing?
15. How do you detect clubbing?
16. Define edema.
17. What are the types of edema and what are their causes?
18. What is the physiological basis of edema in heart failure, nephrotic syndrome and cirrhosis of the liver?
19. Which regions of the body are specially checked for lymph node enlargement? Why?
20. What are the common causes of lymphadenopathy?
21. What are the vital signs?
22. What is the normal body temperature?
23. What is fever?
24. What are the types of fever?
25. How do you differentiate between various types of fever?
26. What are the common causes of fever?
27. What is hypothermia?
28. What are the causes of hypothermia?
29. What is the importance of examination of pulse in general examination?
30. What is the normal rate of respiration in adults?
31. What is the normal systolic and diastolic pressure in adults?

CHAPTER 20

# Stethography

### LEARNING OBJECTIVES

After completing this practical, you will be able to:

- Define stethography.
- Tie the stethograph at the proper position around the chest of the subject.
- Record respiratory movements (normal and following different maneuvers).
- List the precautions taken during stethographic recordings.
- Define breaking point.
- List the factors that affect the breaking point.
- Define and give examples of periodic breathing.

You may also be able to:

- Explain the effects of exercise and hyperventilation on respiration.
- Explain the differences in breath-holding time following inspiration and expiration.

## INTRODUCTION

Stethography is the method by which respiratory movements are recorded. Stethography is useful in assessing breath holding time (BHT) following inspiration and expiration, and in response to different stimuli. Physiologically, BHT is a determinant of respiratory capacity of the individual. This can be used as a tool in the assessment of respiratory fitness.

## METHODS

### Method of Using a Stethograph

#### Principle

The stethograph is tied around the chest of the subject. The movement of the chest causes a change in the air pressure in the stethograph, which is recorded on a moving drum.

#### Requirements

1. **Stethograph** The stethograph (Fig. 20.1) consists of a corrugated rubber tube with a stopper at each end and an air outlet pipe connected to the tambour.
2. **Marey's tambour** It is a metallic cup with a side tube and a rubber diaphragm mounted at the top (Fig. 20.2). A writing lever is attached to a small metal disc, which rests on the rubber diaphragm.

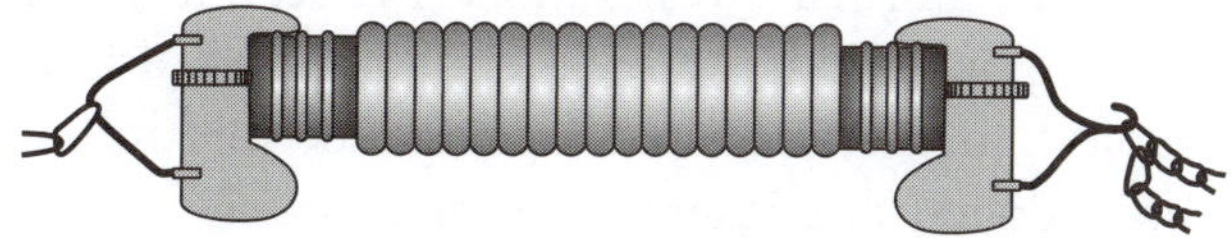

Fig. 20.1 Stethograph.

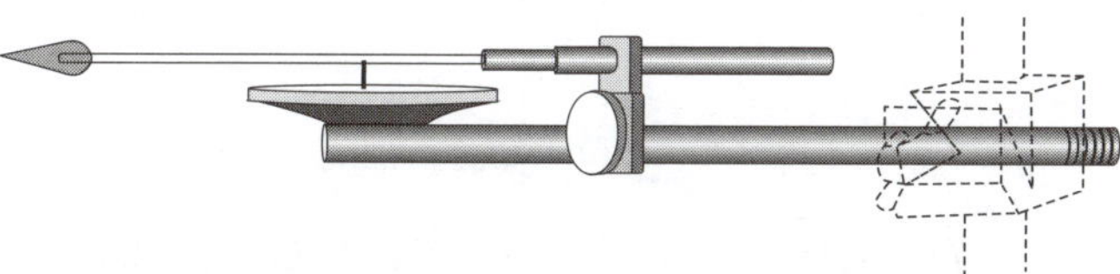

Fig, 20.2 Marey's tambour.

   The side tube of the metal cup is connected to the stethograph by a rubber tube.
3. Kymograph
4. Drinking water

#### Procedure

1. Ask the subject to sit comfortably on a stool with his/her back towards the recording apparatus.
2. Tie the stethograph around the chest of the subject at the level of the fourth intercostal space and connect it to the tambour.

> Note: Check that when the stethograph is connected to the tambour, the pressure change in the stethograph is transmitted to it. It is confirmed by movement of the lever with movement of the chest.

3. Bring the writing lever in contact with the paper of the kymograph and set the drum to move at a slow speed (2.5 mm/s).

4. Record normal respiration for about 5 cm.
5. Ask the subject to drink water and record the effect of deglutition on respiratory movement. Then take a normal tracing.
6. Take a normal tracing and ask the subject to hold his breath as long as possible after quiet inspiration and expiration and following deep inspiration and deep expiration, and record the effects.

> Note: The effects of all these respiratory maneuvers should be recorded separately. Normal tracings should be recorded before and after each recording.

7. Record normal respiration and stop the drum. Ask the subject to take deep breaths as rapidly as possible for one and a half minutes. Immediately after hyperventilation, start the drum and record the effect on respiratory movement.
8. Record normal respiration. Disconnect the stethograph from Marey's tambour and ask the subject to exercise (spot jogging) for one minute. Immediately after exercise, connect the stethograph to the kymograph and record the effect of exercise on respiratory movement.

## Precautions

1. The subject should sit comfortably and in an erect posture.
2. The tambour should be tied at the level of the fourth intercostal space because expansion of the chest is maximum at this level.
3. Before and after the recordings for each maneuver (for example, swallowing water), normal tracings should be taken.
4. The recording should not be made during the act of hyperventilation but immediately after.
5. The stethograph must be disconnected from the tambour during exercise, and recording should be made immediately after exercise.
6. For BHT, the recording should be made after quiet inspiration and quiet expiration, and forceful inspiration and forceful expiration.

## Observation

Note that downstroke is inspiration and upstroke is expiration. Note that apnea occurs during the act

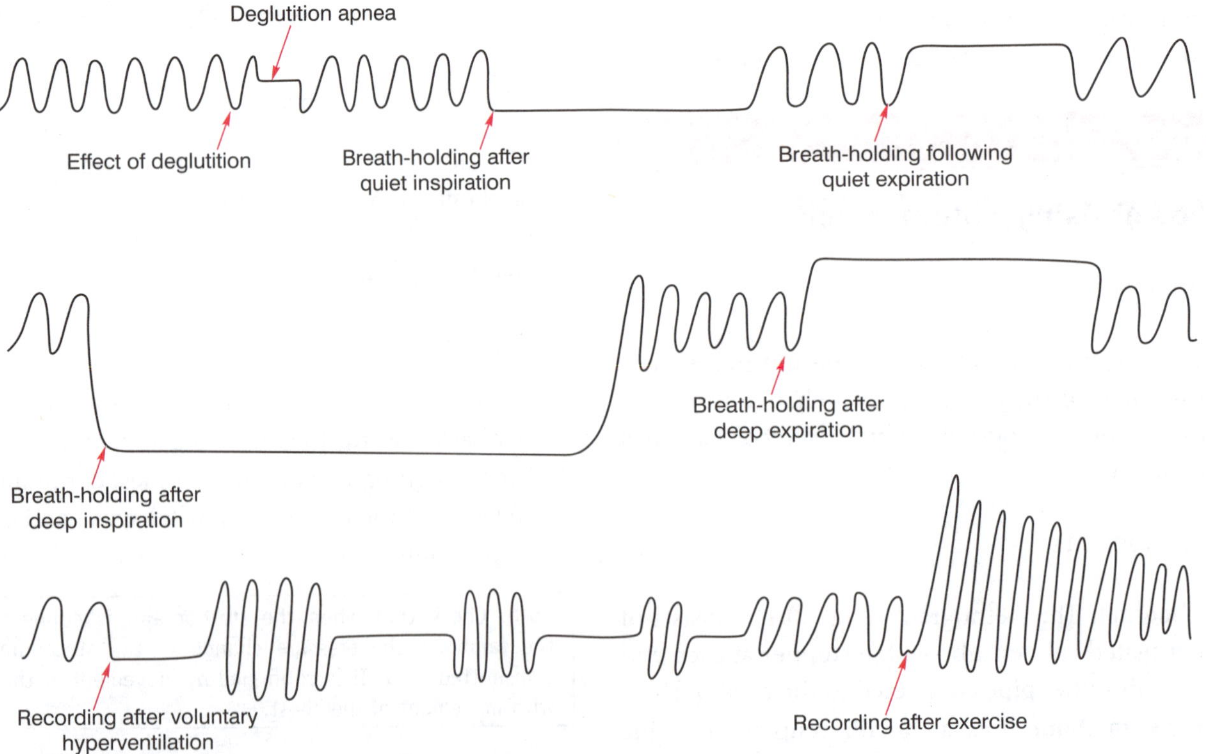


Fig. 20.3 Recording of respiratory movements to study the effect of deglutition, voluntary hyperventilation and exercise, and to determine breath-holding time (BHT).

of deglutition. Study the duration of BHT following normal and deep inspiration and expiration. Observe the breathing pattern following hyperventilation and exercise (Fig. 20.3).

## DISCUSSION

### Deglutition Apnea

During deglutition (drinking of water), respiration stops temporarily. This is called deglutition apnea. It is due to closure of the glottis, which helps in passage of food or water in the esophagus and prevents entry of food materials into the respiratory tract.

### Breath-Holding Time (BHT)

BHT is the maximum time for which the subject can hold his breath. BHT is greater following inspiration than expiration. Respiration can be voluntarily held for some time, but eventually, the voluntary control is overridden. The point at which breathing can no longer be voluntarily inhibited is called the *breaking point*. The breaking is due to rise in arterial $pCO_2$ and the fall in $pO_2$, as body tissues continue to utilise oxygen and produce carbon dioxide. The rise in arterial $pCO_2$ and fall in $pO_2$ stimulate central and peripheral chemoreceptors, which stimulate respiration. Generally, breaking point is reached at alveolar $pO_2$ of 56 mm Hg and alveolar $pCO_2$ of 49 mm Hg. It has been suggested that proprioceptive impulses from respiratory muscles and joints may be involved in the breaking point.

#### Factors Affecting Breaking Point

1. Breathing 100 per cent oxygen increases BHT. Breathing 100 per cent oxygen before holding breath increases alveolar $pO_2$, so the breaking point is delayed.
2. Hyperventilation at room air increases BHT. This is because hyperventilation removes $CO_2$ from the blood and therefore delays breaking point.
3. Psychological factors play a role. Encouragement delays breaking point.

### Hyperventilation

Periodic breathing occurs following voluntary hyperventilation. There occurs apnea followed by a brief period of hyperpnea. The apnea occurs due to removal of carbon dioxide during hyperventilation, so respiration stops temporarily. This causes accumulation of carbon dioxide, which stimulates respiration; as a result, there is hyperventilation.

Periodic breathing (**Cheyne–Stokes breathing**) is characterised by alternating apnea and hyperventilation. It is seen physiologically in sleep (especially in infants), at high altitude and following voluntary hyperventilation, and pathologically in left ventricular failure and brain damage.

### Exercise

During exercise, hyperventilation occurs due to stimulation of respiratory centres by increased discharge from the proprioceptors in the joints, ligaments and muscles. Though the increase in respiration is proportionate to the increase in oxygen consumption, the role of oxygen in stimulation of hyperventilation is still not clear. Increased body temperature, increased $K^+$ level and lactic acid concentration play a role in hyperventilation. But, as the exercise is mild to moderate here, hyperventilation is mainly due to increased proprioceptive information from the exercising muscles and joints.

Hyperventilation persists after intense exercise due to increased arterial $H^+$ concentration, which occurs due to lactic acidemia. Sometimes, a pattern of periodic breathing is also observed following exercise.

## VIVA

1. What is stethography?
2. Why is the stethograph tied at the fourth intercostal space around the chest?
3. What are the precautions taken for stethography?
4. What is deglutition apnea? What is its cause?
5. What is breaking point? What are its causes?

6. What are the factors that affect breaking point?
7. What are the causes of periodic breathing that occurs following voluntary hyperventilation?
8. What are the effects of exercise on respiratory movement?
9. What is periodic breathing? Give examples.
10. Briefly explain the effects of $pO_2$ and $pCO_2$ on respiration.

Chapter 21

# Clinical Examination of the Respiratory System

## Learning Objectives

After completing this practical, you will be able to:

- Trace the different lines, prominences, lung fissures and borders on the surface of the chest.
- Perform a clinical examination of the respiratory system, proceeding in the proper sequence.
- List the different abnormalities of the shape of the chest.
- Name the different types and causes of abnormal respiration.
- State the causes of unilateral and bilateral restriction of chest movements.
- State the causes of increased and decreased vocal fremitus.
- List the rules of percussion.
- List the differences between vesicular and bronchial breath sounds.

You may also be able to:

- Explain the common abnormalities observed in different parameters of examination of the respiratory system.
- Explain the differences between vesicular and bronchial breathing.
- Describe the types and causes of bronchial breathing.
- List the reasons for production of different bronchial breath sounds.

## INTRODUCTION

Clinical examination of the respiratory system is performed to assess the functional status of the respiratory tract and lungs. It should be carried out meticulously and methodically in a patient suffering from lung disease. The clinical examination can provide sufficient information to diagnose the exact nature of pathology in the lungs. For interpretation and correlation of the findings of the clinical examination with the disease process, one should have knowledge of the functional anatomy of the lungs.

## Anatomical Landmarks

### Different Lines

1. **Midsternal line** This is a vertical line drawn through the centre of the sternum and xiphoid.
2. **Midclavicular line** This is a vertical line, parallel to the midsternal line, which extends downwards from the centre of each clavicle. The centre of the clavicle is located between the middle of the suprasternal notch and the tip of the acromion.
3. **Anterior axillary line** This is a vertical line extending downwards from the anterior axillary fold.
4. **Posterior axillary line** This is a vertical line extending downwards from the posterior axillary fold.
5. **Midaxillary line** This is a vertical line originating at a point midway between the anterior and the posterior axillary line.
6. **Midspinal line** This is a vertical line that passes through the centre of the back as defined by the spinal processes.
7. **Midscapular line** This is a vertical line on the posterior aspect of the chest, which runs parallel to the midspinal line and extends through the apices of the scapula.

### Different Prominences

1. **Sternal angle** This is a transverse bony ridge at the junction of the body of the sternum and the manubrium. This is also known as the *angle of Louis* or *Ludwig's angle*.

   *Significance of the sternal angle*

   1. The second costal cartilage articulates the sternum at this point. Therefore, the rib that corresponds to this point is the second rib. The intercostal space below this is the second intercostal space. It helps in identifying all the intercostal spaces.
   2. The trachea bifurcates into two main bronchi at this point.
   3. The level of the upper border of the atria of the heart coincides with this point.
   4. The anterior borders of the lungs meet in the midline here.

5. The disc between the fourth and fifth thoracic vertebrae in the back coincides with this.

2. **Suprasternal notch** This is the top of the manubrium.
3. **Vertebral prominence** The spinous process of the seventh cervical vertebra is most prominent on the back and is easily seen and felt.

### Lung Fissure and Borders

1. **Oblique fissure (major interlobar fissure)** It starts from the second thoracic spine posteriorly and extends obliquely downwards and forwards to the sixth costochondral junction anteriorly.
2. **Horizontal fissure (minor interlobar fissure)** It starts from the right fourth costochondral junction and passes horizontally to meet the oblique fissure in the midaxillary line.

> Note: The lower lobe lies below the oblique fissure on either side. Above it, lies the upper lobe on the left side. On the right side the upper lobe lies above the horizontal fissure. Between the oblique and the horizontal fissures lies the middle lobe of the right lung. The greater part of the back of the chest is occupied by the lower lobe. The anterior aspect of the chest is occupied by the upper lobe in the left and upper and middle lobe in the right.

3. **Upper border of lung** It is limited to a level 5 cm above the sternoclavicular joint.
4. **Lower border of lung** It lies on the sixth rib on the midclavicular line, on the eighth rib on the midaxillary line and on the tenth rib on the posterior scapular line.

## METHODS

## Methods of Examination

### Principle

Examination of the respiratory system is carried out by inspection, palpation, percussion and auscultation of the chest. Inspection shows the configuration, the degree of movement of the chest, and the type and rate of respiration. Palpation confirms the movement of the chest, detects abnormal pulsation, areas of tenderness and the degree of vocal fremitus. Percussion demonstrates the nature of changes (if any) of the lung tissues, bronchi and the pleura, and shows whether the lung tissues contain less or more air than normal and whether the pleura contains less or more fluid than normal. Auscultation detects the type, intensity and nature of breath sounds, and the presence of any other sound.

### Requirements

1. Measuring tape
2. Stethoscope

### Procedure

It consists of examination of the chest, which follows observation of a few particular signs in general examination that are relevant to this system. It is best accomplished when the patient is standing or is comfortably seated in an erect position after complete exposure of the chest in good light.

#### *General Examination*

1. **Pallor** Presence of anemia is common in patients with chronic hemoptysis.
2. **Cyanosis** Cyanosis occurs due to the presence of excess deoxygenated hemoglobin (>5 g%). Cyanosis may occur due to inadequate ventilation of perfused lung areas as in pneumonia, or due to the decrease in the total amount of air ventilating the lungs, as seen in poliomyelitis.
3. **Clubbing** Clubbing is recognised by the bulbousness of the soft, terminal portion of the fingers and by an excessive curvature of the nail in both the longitudinal and lateral planes. It is seen in bronchogenic carcinoma, chronic suppurative diseases of the lung like bronchiectasis, empyema, and lung abscess.
4. **Lymph node enlargement** The neck and supraclavicular region should be particularly examined to check for enlargement of lymph nodes.

#### *Examination of the Chest*

**Inspection**

1. ***Shape of the chest*** Examine the shape of the chest. The chest of a normal healthy adult is bilaterally symmetrical. The transverse diameter is greater than the antero-posterior diameter, the ratio being 7 : 5. Check for abnormalities of the chest.
2. ***Symmetry of the chest*** Look for symmetry of the chest, comparing both sides. The chest may bulge or be depressed either on one or both sides.

3. ***Movement of the chest*** Observe whether the chest moves normally and symmetrically equally on both sides with respiration and whether a difference exists in the movement of the chest between the upper and lower parts.

> Note: Normally, the movements are equal on both the sides and are more in the base of the lungs than the apex. But one should keep in mind that if lesions are present in both the lungs, the movement may be equally affected on both sides.

4. ***Respiratory movement*** Look for the following points while observing the movements of the chest with respiration.
   a) *Rate* The normal rate of respiration in adults is 12–18 per minute. Respiration rate is higher in children. The increased rate of respiration is called tachypnea and the decreased rate of respiration is called bradypnea.
   b) *Rhythm* Determine whether the respiration is regular or irregular.
   c) *Depth* Look for the depth (degree) of respiration. The respiration may be decreased unilaterally or on both sides.
   d) *Type* Note whether the respiration is predominantly thoracic or abdominal. In men, respiration is abdominothoracic and in women, the respiration is thoracoabdominal.

**Palpation**

1. ***Expansion of the chest*** Expansion of the chest is assessed by placing the two palms firmly on both the sides of the chest and apposing the thumbs in the midline anteriorly (Fig. 21.1). The subject is asked to take a deep breath and the movement of the thumbs away from the midline is observed. This indicates the extent of expansion of the chest. Normally, the expansion is more than 5 cm at the base of the lungs in adults. The expansion is less at the apex of the lungs. Expansion may be less on the side where the lung is affected by disease.
2. ***Position of the trachea*** The position of the trachea can be detected in three ways.
   a) Place the tip of the index and ring finger of the right hand on the sternoclavicular joints (sternal ends of the clavicles) on either side and place the middle finger on the suprasternal notch. Then gently push the middle finger forward to feel the tracheal rings. The position of the trachea is determined by observing the spaces between the finger tips. Normally, the trachea is centrally placed or slightly deviated to the right.
   b) Place the index finger firmly into the suprasternal notch and locate the tracheal rings in relation to the sternum.
   c) Find the space between the anterior border of the sternomastoid muscle and the trachea. If the trachea has deviated to one side, the space becomes narrow on that side.
3. ***Position of the apex beat*** Locate the position of the apex beat (details of the procedure are described in Chapter 28). Displacement of the apex and the trachea to one side indicates the shifting of the mediastinum to that side.

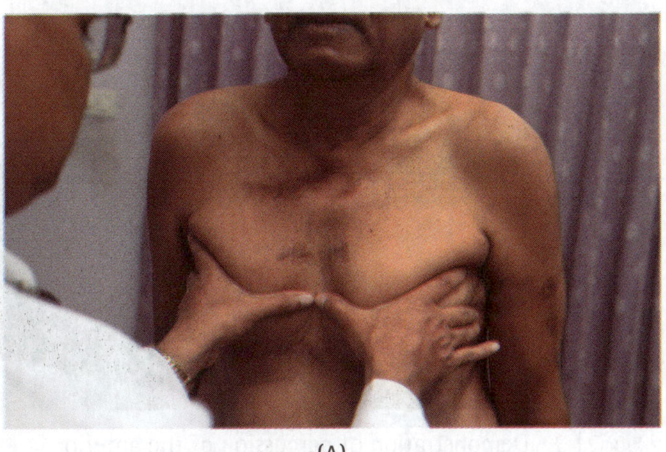

(A)

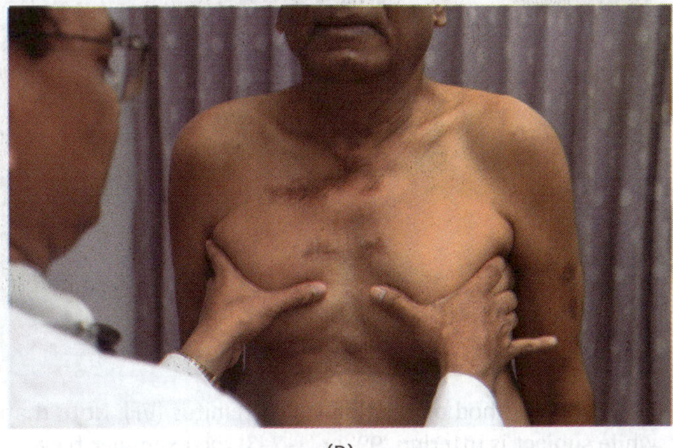

(B)

Fig. 21.1 Demonstration of chest expansion. Note that chest expansion is performed by firmly holding the chest with both palms and apposing thumbs at the centre (A). Subject is asked to take maximum inspiration possible with which thumbs move apart (B). The distance between the thumbs is noted as the degree of chest expansion.

4. ***Vocal fremitus (VF)*** Ask the subject to repeat 'ninety-nine' or 'one-two-three' and feel the vibration from the surface of the chest by placing the ulnar border of the hand on the surface of the chest, in the intercostal space (Fig. 21.2). To compare both sides (diseased and normal sides), examine the opposite side of the chest in the same intercostal space immediately.

> Note: The vibration transmitted to the chest wall from the respiratory passages represents VF. The vibration is conducted from the larynx by the trachea and bronchi to the smaller tubes within the lungs and then through the lung tissues to the chest wall. It should be elicited over symmetrical areas on both the sides of the chest alternately. It may be normal, increased, reduced or absent.

5. ***Tenderness*** Palpate all the regions of the chest wall to elicit tenderness if present. Tenderness may be seen in injury to the chest wall, inflammatory conditions of the ribs and intercostal muscles, malignant deposits in the ribs, pleurisy, a painful lung infection and so on.

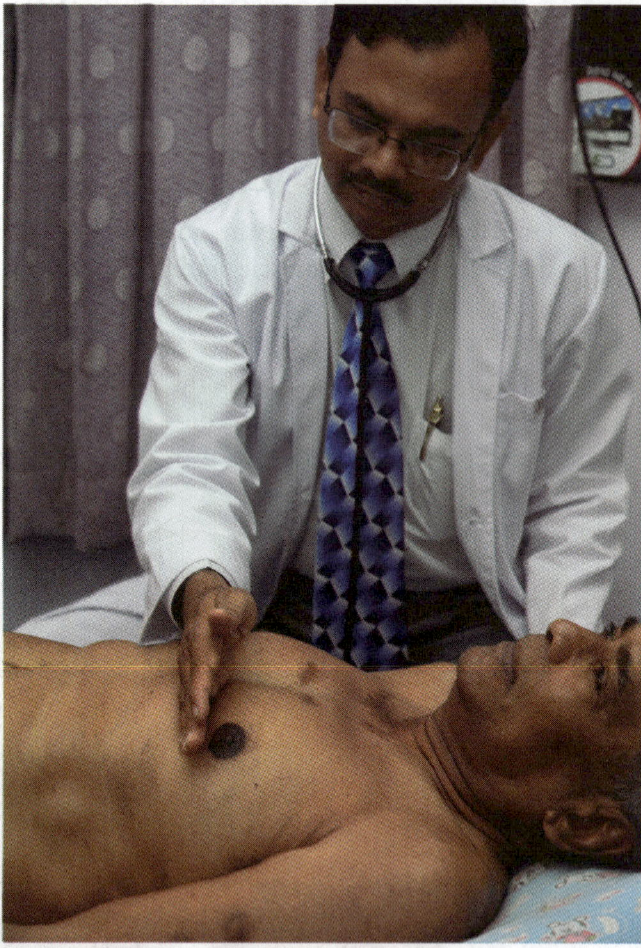

Fig. 21.2 Method of eliciting vocal fremitus (VF). Note that while subject is uttering '99' or '1-2-3' the examiner feels the vibration from the surface of the chest by placing the ulnar border of the hand firmly in the intercostal space. Opposite side of the chest in the same intercostal space is examined immediately.

**Percussion** Percuss different areas (supraclavicular, infraclavicular, mammary, inframammary, axillary, infra-axillary, suprascapular, interscapular and infrascapular) on both sides of the chest. While percussing the back of the subject, ask him to cross his arms in front of his chest, the left hand touching the right shoulder and vice versa, and to lean forward. While percussing the axillary region, ask the subject to lift his hands up on to his head. The areas are percussed keeping the pleximeter finger in the intercostal spaces. The clavicle should be percussed directly by the percussing finger without using the pleximeter finger. Percussion of corresponding regions on both sides should be performed and compared simultaneously.

***Rules of percussion***

1. Apply the pleximeter finger firmly on the surface of the chest (Fig. 21.3).
2. The percussing finger should strike the middle phalanx of the pleximeter finger perpendicularly (vertically).
3. The strokes should be delivered from the wrist and finger joints, not from the elbow.
4. The percussing finger should be lifted up immediately after striking the pleximeter finger.
5. The long axis of the pleximeter finger should be parallel to the edge of the organ being percussed.

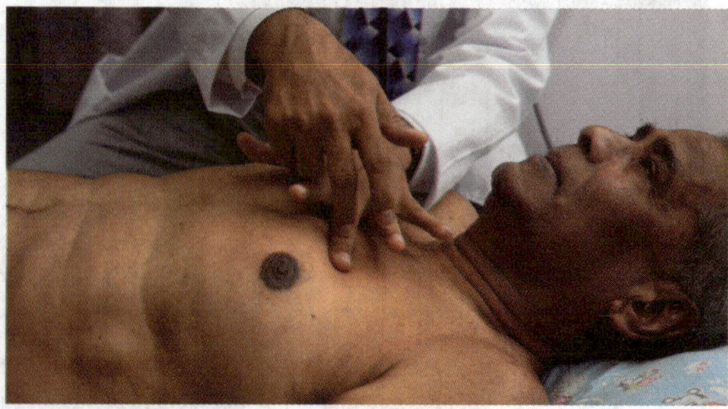

Fig. 21.3 Demonstration of percussion of the anterior aspect of the chest. Note that the pleximeter finger is placed firmly on the anterior surface of the chest in the intercostal space. Percussing finger strokes the pleximeter finger at right angle.

6. Percussion should be carried out from the more resonant to the less resonant area.

**Auscultation** Auscultate all the areas of the chest (supraclavicular, infraclavicular, mammary, inframammary, axillary, infra-axillary, suprascapular, interscapular and infrascapular) and compare both the sides immediately. While auscultating, place the chest piece of the stethoscope firmly over the chest and ask the patient to breathe regularly and deeply with mouth slightly open (Fig. 21.4).

> Note: The purpose of auscultation is to obtain information over and above what the three steps (inspection, palpation, and percussion) of physical examination furnish. Auscultation is done to detect the type of breath sound, the intensity and character of vocal resonance and presence of any adventitious sounds.

***Breath sounds*** Auscultate all the areas over the chest for breath sounds. Use the diaphragm of the stethoscope to auscultate breath sounds. Try to note the *intensity* and character of the breath sounds.

***Vocal resonance*** Vocal resonance is the auscultatory counterpart of vocal fremitus. Ask the subject to repeat 'one-two-three' or 'ninety-nine' at a constant volume and auscultate the symmetrical areas of both the sides of the chest. The intensity of vocal resonance depends on the loudness and depth of the subject's voice and the conductivity of the lungs. It may be normal, decreased or increased. Vocal resonance of normal intensity conveys the impression of being produced just at the chest piece of the stethoscope and is heard as a soft sound.

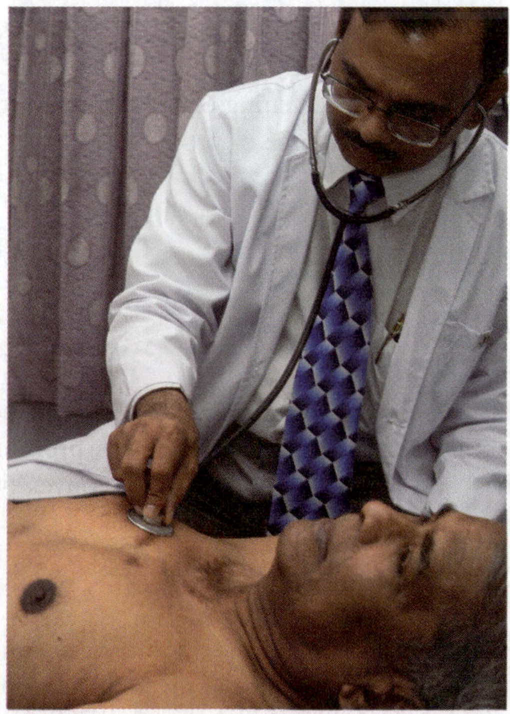

Fig. 21.4 Auscultation of breath sounds. Note that the stethoscope is firmly placed over the chest surface. If stethoscope is placed loose, chest movement during respiration causes rubbing of the skin against diaphragm of stethoscope and produces false adventitious sounds.

***Adventitious (added) sounds*** Note the presence of any adventitious sounds.

## Precautions

1. The examination should be carried out with the subject standing or seated comfortably with chest fully exposed.
2. General examination should be carried out before examining the chest.
3. Inspection of the chest should be performed without touching the subject.
4. While detecting expansion of the chest, the subject should be instructed to expand his chest as much possible.
5. While detecting the position of the trachea, palpate the tracheal rings gently. If you press hard on the trachea, the subject will feel uncomfortable.
6. Both VF and VR should be elicited on the symmetrical areas on both sides simultaneously and compared.
7. In case of percussion, the rules should be strictly followed, and the maneuver should be carried out on both sides simultaneously to compare the findings.
8. For elicting VR on different areas of the chest, the subject should be instructed to utter the words at a constant pitch and volume throughout the maneuver.

# DISCUSSION

## Inspectory Findings

### Shape of the Chest

The chest of a normal healthy adult is bilaterally symmetrical and the transverse diameter is greater than the antero-posterior diameter, the ratio being 7 : 5. The following abnormalities should be looked for at inspection (Fig. 21.5).

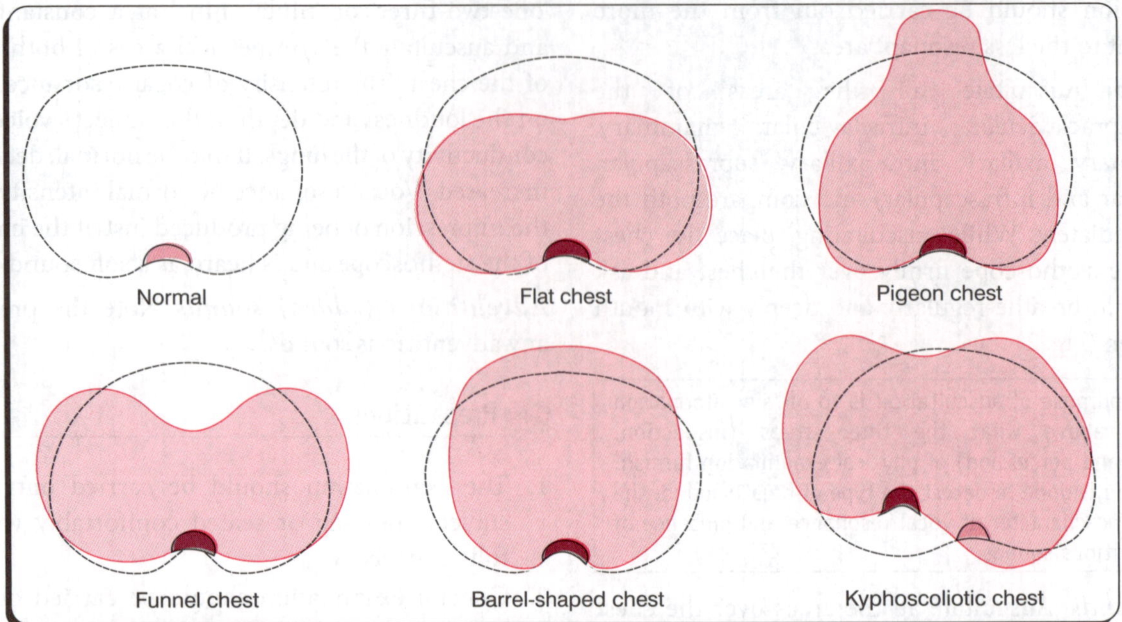


Fig. 21.5 Types (shape) of chest. Normal shape of the chest is marked by dotted lines. Note that the ratio of transverse to anteroposterior diameter of the normal adult chest is 7 : 5.

**Flat chest** This is usually associated with long neck, prominent larynx and clavicle, and long narrow chest.

*Features*

1. Exaggerated supra- and infraclavicular fossa
2. Narrow intercostal spaces
3. Acute subcostal angle

*Causes* It is seen in healthy persons, but may be associated with:

1. Rickets in childhood
2. Chronic nasal obstruction from hypertrophied adenoid
3. Bilateral tuberculosis

**Pigeon chest** The sternum is unduly prominent and projects beyond the plane of the front of the abdomen. It is seen in:

- Persons with rickets
- Recurrent lung infection in children

**Funnel chest** The features are

1. Depression at the lower end of the sternum
2. Prominent costochondral junction
3. Diminished antero-posterior diameter of the chest

   Causes could be rickets or congenital.

**Barrel-shaped chest** The features are

1. Increased anteroposterior diameter of the chest.
2. The ribs are wide apart and tend to be horizontal.
3. The spine is unduly concave.
4. The sternum is more arched.
5. Angle of Louis is more prominent.
6. Fullness of supraclavicular fossae.

*Cause* The usual cause is chronic obstructive emphysema.

**Kyphosis** This is backward bending of the vertebral column resulting in convexity posteriorly and concavity anteriorly. It causes, shortening of the chest and undue prominence of the vertebrae.

*Causes*

1. Caries spine
2. Osteoarthritis
3. Secondary osteoporosis
4. Chronic obstructive emphysema
5. Ankylosing spondylitis

**Scoliosis** This consists of lateral bending of the spine and rotation of the vertebrae resulting in undue prominence of the chest and scapula on the side of the convexity, and flattening of the chest.

**Kyphoscoliosis** In this, kyphosis is associated with scoliosis.

**Harrison's sulcus** This is a transverse groove or constriction in the chest, which begins at the xiphisternum and passes outwards and slightly downwards and may sometimes reach the midaxillary line. It is seen in rickets.

**Rickety rosary** This is characterised by the presence of a number of rounded or knob-like projections at the costochondral junctions. It is usually seen in rickets.

## Symmetry of the Chest

The chest may bulge or be depressed either on one side or on both the sides.

**Localised or unilateral fullness (bulging)**

1. Pleural effusion
2. Pneumothorax
3. Intrathoracic tumours

**Symmetrical or bilateral fullness**

1. Emphysema
2. Bilateral pleural effusion
3. Bilateral pneumothorax

**Unilateral depression**

1. Fibrosis
2. Collapse

**Bilateral depression**

1. Bilateral fibrosis
2. Bilateral collapse

## Respiratory Movements

**Rate** The normal rate of respiration in adults is 12–18 per minute. The respiration rate is greater in children than in adults. Increased rate of respiration is called *tachypnea* and decreased rate of respiration is called *bradypnea*.

**Causes of tachypnea**

A. *Physiological conditions*
   1. Newborns and infants
   2. Children
   3. Gender (rate of respiration is higher in women)
   4. Exercise
   5. Excitement and emotion
   6. Nervousness

B. *Pathological conditions*

Different disease conditions that produce hypoxia; for example, pneumonia causes tachypnea.

**Causes of bradypnea**

Bradypnea is not seen normally. It is usually seen in conditions of CNS depression, as in narcotic poisoning.

**Rhythm** Irregular respiration is commonly seen in intracranial lesions.

**Depth** The respiration may be decreased unilaterally or on both sides.

*Unilateral restriction of movement*

- Pleural effusion
- Pneumothorax
- Fibrosis
- Collapse
- Consolidation

*Bilaterial restriction of movement*

- Emphysema
- Bilateral pleural effusion
- Bilateral consolidation

**Type** Respiration may be predominantly thoracic or abdominal. In men, respiration is abdominothoracic and in women the respiration is thoracoabdominal.

### *Types of Abnormal Respiration*

**Kussmaul respiration** There is increased rate and depth of respiration (air hunger). It is seen in metabolic acidosis like diabetic ketoacidosis.

**Cheyne–Stokes respiration** In this type of respiration, a period of hyperpnea is followed by apnea. It is seen in physiological conditions like sleep (especially in infants), at high altitude, following hyperventilation, and in pathological conditions like cardiac failure, renal failure, brain tumour and narcotic poisoning.

**Biot's respiration** The respiration is irregular in depth and rhythm. Irregular pauses with occasional sighs occur. It is seen in meningitis.

# Palpatory Findings

## Expansion of the Chest

Normally, the expansion is more than 5 cm at the base of the lungs in adults. The expansion is less towards the apex of the lungs. Maximum chest expansion is detected at the fourth intercostal space. It is always less on the side of the chest that is affected by disease of the chest wall or lung.

## Position of Apex and Trachea

Displacement of the apex and trachea to one side indicates the shifting of the mediastinum to that side. But, displacement of the apex may occur without displacement of trachea, or the apex and trachea may displace in opposite directions depending on the nature of pathology.

## Shifting of Mediastinum

i) The mediastinum shifts to the side of collapse and fibrosis of the lungs.

ii) It shifts to the opposite side in pleural effusion, pneumothorax and hydropneumothorax or a mass (for example, tumour) in the thorax.

### Vocal Fremitus (VF)

VF may be normal, increased, reduced or absent.

**VF is increased in**

- Consolidation of lungs, for example, lobar pneumonia
- Large cavity near the chest surface

**VF is diminished in**

- Bronchial obstruction
- Collapse
- Fibrosis
- Thickened pleura
- Emphysema

**VF is absent in**

VF may be completely absent when the lung is separated from the chest wall by massive pleural effusion or pneumothorax.

### Tenderness

Tenderness may be present due to an injury to the chest wall, inflammatory conditions of the ribs and intercostal muscles, malignant deposits in the ribs, pleurisy, or in painful lesions of the lungs.

## Percussion Findings

### Significance

Percussion is carried out to detect the limit of lung resonance and presence of any pathology in the lungs. Percussion over a normal lung produces a resonant note. 'Resonant' is a relative term as there is no absolute standard. Cardiac dullness is noted on the left side between the third and fifth space and hepatic dullness is noted on the right side from the fifth rib downwards in the midclavicular line, eighth rib downwards in the midaxillary line and tenth rib downwards in the midscapular line. One should keep in mind that lesions more than 5 cm away from the chest wall or the lesions less than 2–3 cm in diameter will not alter the percussion note. The percussion note is expressed as normal resonance, hyper-resonance, impaired resonance or dullness, and stony dullness. When the dullness shifts from one part of the chest to the other, it is called shifting dullness.

### Hyper-resonance

Hyper-resonance occurs when the amount of air in the lungs or chest cavity is increased. This occurs in:

1. Emphysema
2. Pneumothorax
3. Over an emphysematous bulla
4. Over a large superficial cavity

### Dullness or Impaired Resonance

Dullness or impaired resonance results from any condition that interferes with the production of normal resonant vibrations within the lungs or with the transmission of these vibrations to the chest wall. This is seen in:

1. Consolidation
2. Thickened pleura
3. Fibrosis and collapse
4. Atelectasis

### Stony Dullness

When the percussion note is very dull, it is called stony dullness. It is seen in pleural effusion.

### Shifting Dullness

If the dullness shifts when the patient changes position, this is called shifting dullness. It is one of the important tests to detect the presence of air and fluid in the pleural cavity. It is a reliable sign of hydropneumothorax.

### Tidal Percussion

A dull note obtained above the upper border of liver dullness may be due to liver enlargement or due to a disorder either in the lungs or pleura. Tidal percussion is done to differentiate the pathology. Normally, there is an increase in the area of resonance downwards by 4–6 cm during full inspiration due to movement of the diaphragm, lungs and liver downwards. In upward enlargement of liver, the increase in the area of resonance in deep inspiration (in tidal percussion) remains within normal limits. In lung pathology, the area of resonance decreases on tidal percussion.

## Auscultatory Findings

Auscultation is performed to detect the type of breath sound, the intensity and character of vocal resonance and presence of any adventitious sounds.

## Breath Sounds

The breath sounds originate in the large airways due to turbulent airflow during breathing. Sounds produced in the large airways (bronchial breath sounds) are of higher frequencies, above 600 Hz. These sounds are transmitted to the lung tissue, which acts as a low-pass filter, filtering out higherfrequency sounds and converting them into low-frequency sounds (vesicular sounds) that are transmitted to the chest wall. Therefore, sounds auscultated from the chest wall in normal persons are vesicular breath sounds though the sounds originate in the large airways (bronchi).

### *Intensity*

The breath sound is produced by the repetitive movement of air into and out of alveoli that are ventilated. The intensity of the sound is directly proportional to the amount of air entering the alveoli. It may be normal, reduced or increased.

**Reduced intensity** Breath sounds decrease in intensity if there is a localised airway narrowing, if the lung is extensively damaged by the disease process or if there is interference in transmission of sound from the lung tissue to the chest wall.

1. Airway narrowing
   - Bronchial obstruction with or without collapse of the lung
   - Consolidation with an obstructed bronchus (obstructive pneumonia)
2. Damage to lung tissue
   - Fibrosis
   - Atelectasis
3. Interference in transmission of sounds
   - Thickened pleura
   - Pleural effusion
   - Pneumothorax
   - Emphysema

**Increased intensity** Breath sounds may be increased in intensity in thin subjects or when the ventilation of lung tissue is increased, as in compensatory emphysema. Loud breath sounds should not be confused with bronchial breath sounds.

### *Character*

On the basis of character, breath sounds are divided into two types: vesicular and bronchial.

**A. Vesicular breath sounds** The normal character of breath sounds is vesicular. These sounds originate in large airways, but when transmitted through the lung tissue to the chest wall they become low-pitched vesicular sounds.

These sounds have the following characteristics.

1. Duration of inspiration is more than that of expiration.
2. Intensity of inspiration is greater than that of expiration.
3. There is no gap between inspiration and expiration (Fig. 21.6A).
4. Sounds are rustling in nature.
5. They are low-pitched, with frequencies in the range of 200–600 Hz.

*Vesicular breath sound with prolonged expiration* In some diseases, the breath sound is normal in character (vesicular) but the duration of expiration is either equal to or more than that of inspiration. There will be no gap between expiration and inspiration. This is seen when there is partial obstruction of the bronchi as in asthma.

**B. Bronchial breath sounds** The bronchial breath sounds originate in the larger airways and are transmitted directly to the chest wall without passing through the alveoli. The sound passing through the lung tissue is not modified and auscultated like bronchial sounds from the chest walls. This sound resembles the sound obtained by listening over the trachea (directly placing a stethoscope on the trachea).

The following are the characteristics of these sounds:

1. Duration of expiration is equal to or longer than that of inspiration.
2. Intensity of expiration is more than that of inspiration.
3. There is a definite gap between inspiration and expiration (Fig. 21.6B).
4. Sounds are harsh or aspirate in nature.
5. They are high-pitched with frequencies above 600 Hz.

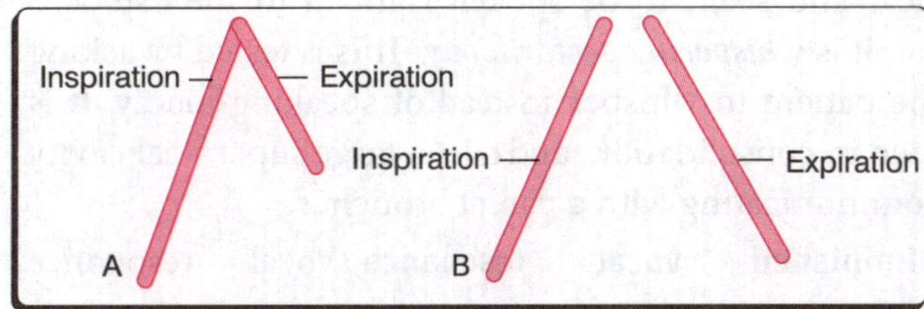


Fig. 21.6 Vesicular (A) and bronchial (B) breath sounds.

Bronchial breath sounds are of three types: tubular, cavernous and amphoric.

*The tubular bronchial breath sound* is a high-pitched sound resulting from the passage of vibrations produced in the small bronchi directly to the chest wall through a solid lung tissue. This is seen when the lung parenchyma becomes a solid mass, as in consolidation.

The *cavernous bronchial breath sound* is a low-pitched bronchial breath sound heard over a cavity, which is situated superficially and communicated to a patent bronchus. The size of the cavity should be more than 2 cm in diameter to produce a cavernous breath sound.

The *amphoric bronchial breath sound* is a high-pitched bronchial sound that resembles the sound produced by blowing air into a wide-mouthed bottle. This is heard over a very large cavity communicating pneumothorax. It is also seen in large pulmonary cysts having communication with a patent bronchus.

### Vocal Resonance

Vocal resonance is the auscultatory counterpart of vocal fremitus. The intensity of vocal resonance depends on the loudness and depth of the subject's voice and the conductivity of the lungs. It may be normal, decreased or increased.

**Increased vocal resonance** When the sounds appear to be nearer to the ear than the chest piece and louder than the normal, the vocal resonance is said to be increased. The three types of increased vocal resonance are bronchophony, aegophony and whispering pectoriloquy.

*Bronchophony* If the vocal resonance is increased and appears to arise from the earpiece of the stethoscope, it is described as *bronchophony*. It is seen in consolidation of the lungs as in lobar pneumonia.

*Aegophony* When the increased vocal resonance is high-pitched giving a nasal intonation or having a bleating character ('goat voice'), it is called *aegophony*.

*Whispering pectoriloquy* If the vocal resonance is increased to such an extent that the sounds become very clear and seem to be spoken right in to the listener's ear, it is *whispering pectoriloquy*. This is tested by asking the patient to whisper instead of speaking loudly. It is seen in consolidation, and over a large superficial cavity communicating with a patent bronchus.

**Diminished vocal resonance** Vocal resonance decreases in:

1. Pleural effusion
2. Pneumothorax
3. Collapse
4. Thickened pleura
5. Emphysema

## Adventitious (Added) Sounds

These sounds may arise from the lungs and bronchi or pleura. The sounds that arise from the lungs and bronchi are ronchi, wheeze, stridor and crepitations. The sound that originates from the pleura is the pleural rub.

### Ronchi

These are prolonged, uninterrupted musical sounds that occur due to partial obstruction to the flow of air in a narrowed bronchus or bronchiole.

The narrowing of the lumen of the airway may occur due to mucosal swelling, viscid thick secretion, spasm or infiltration of the wall.

Ronchi are of two types. Sibilant and sonorous. *Sibilant ronchi* are high-pitched, and are produced in the smaller bronchi. *Sonorous ronchi* are low-pitched, and are produced in the large bronchi.

*Causes*

1. Bronchitis
2. Bronchial asthma
3. Obstruction of bronchial tube by a tumour or foreign body

### Wheeze

Wheeze is a high-pitched musical sound, which results from partial airway obstruction. This is louder and more persistent during expiration. Sometimes the sound is so loud that it can be heard without the aid of a stethoscope. It is heard during attacks of asthma.

### Stridor

This is a jerky, high-pitched and coarse sound usually heard during inspiration. It occurs due to obstruction to inspiratory airflow due to airway obstruction. It is commonly heard in:

- Foreign body impaction
- Tumour (pressing the airway from outside)
- Diphtheria (diphtheric membrane)

### Crepitations

These are moist discontinuous crackling or bubbling sounds produced either in the alveoli, bronchi or in cavities. These are produced only in the presence of fluid or secretions.

Crepitations are of two types: fine and coarse.

**Fine crepitations** These are caused by the opening of collapsed alveoli. It occurs at the end of an inspiration and indicates the presence of exudate in the alveoli. When collapsed alveoli open, the separation of the alveolar wall produces a crackling sound. These are heard in the early stages of pneumonia, localised tuberculosis, and at the base of the lungs in heart failure.

**Coarse crepitations** These are heard in any phase of respiration and indicate the presence of secretion in the bronchi or bronchioles. It is heard in:

- bronchitis
- polycystic diseases of the lungs
- resolving stage of pneumonia
- bronchiectasis

### *Pleural Rub*

This is a rough, harsh crackling sound produced by the rubbing of the visceral and parietal pleura against each other during respiration. It indicates inflammation of the pleura and presence of inflammatory exudates. It can be confused with coarse crepitations. It disappears when the subject is asked to hold his breath and remains unaffected by coughing.

## VIVA

1. How do you draw the midsternal, midclavicular, anterior-axillary, posterior-axillary, midaxillary, midspinal and midscapular lines?
2. How do you locate the sternal angle? What is its significance?
3. How do you trace the surface anatomy of major interlobar and horizontal fissures of lungs?
4. How do you determine the lower border of the lungs on the chest?
5. What is the significance of looking for clubbing and cyanosis before examining the chest?
6. What are the common abnormalities of the shape of the chest?
7. What are the features of flat chest and in what conditions is it observed?
8. What is 'pigeon chest' and in what conditions is it observed?
9. What is 'barrel-shaped chest' and in what conditions is it observed?
10. What is kyphoscoliosis and in what conditions is it observed?
11. What is 'rickety rosary' and in what conditions is it observed?
12. What are the causes of unilateral bulging of the chest?
13. What are the causes of unilateral depression of the chest?
14. What are the causes of tachypnea?
15. What are the causes of unilateral restriction of the movement of the chest?
16. What are the types of abnormal respiration?
17. What is Cheyne–Stokes respiration? What are the causes of this abnormal respiration?
18. How do you clinically determine the expansion of the chest?
19. How do you clinically determine the position of the trachea?
20. What are the causes of shifting of mediastinum?
21. What are the causes of increased and decreased vocal fremitus?
22. What are the rules of percussion?
23. What are the causes of hyper-resonance of the lungs?
24. What are the causes of dullness of the lungs?
25. What is stony dullness and in what conditions does it occur?
26. What is shifting dullness and in what conditions does it occur?
27. What is tidal percussion and what is its significance?
28. What are the types of breath sounds and how do you differentiate between them?
29. What are the conditions that decrease the intensity of the breath sound?
30. What are the types of breath sounds and how do you differentiate between them?
31. What are the features of bronchial breath sounds?

32. What are the types of bronchial breath sounds and how are they produced?
33. What do you mean by vocal resonance?
34. Name the conditions in which vocal resonance is increased and those in which it is decreased?
35. What is bronchophony and in which condition is it seen?
36. What is aegophony and in which condition is it seen?
37. What does whispering pectoriloquy indicate?
38. What are adventitious breath sounds?
39. What is the mechanism of production of ronchi and in what conditions is it seen?
40. What is a wheeze?
41. What are the types and causes of crepitations?
42. What is the mechanism of production of crepitations?
43. What do you mean by pleural rub and in what conditions is it seen?

# CHAPTER 22

# Effect of Posture on Vital Capacity

## LEARNING OBJECTIVES

After completing this practical, you will be able to:

- Define vital capacity.
- Record the effect of posture on vital capacity.
- List the precautions taken during the recording.
- State the normal value of vital capacity.
- List the factors that affect vital capacity.

You may also be able to:

- Explain the variation in vital capacity in different conditions.
- List the reasons for alteration in vital capacity with change in posture.
- Explain the physiological significance of vital capacity.

## INTRODUCTION

Vital capacity (VC) is the maximum volume of air that can be expired from the lungs by forceful effort following a maximal inspiration. VC is computed as the sum of tidal volume, inspiratory reserve volume and expiratory reserve volume. The average value of VC is 4.5 litres in males and 3.3 litres in females. VC depends on the growth and development of the subject and the physical training he/she has received. Change of posture also affects vital capacity.

### Factors Affecting Vital Capacity

#### Physiological Factors

1. **Posture** VC is greater in an erect posture than in the sitting and lying postures (for explanation, *see* Discussion).
2. **Age** VC is high in young adults, and low in children and old people. As age advances, compliance of the lungs and chest wall decreases, and therefore vital capacity decreases.
3. **Gender** VC is greater in males because the size of the chest is larger and muscle power is more in males.
4. **Physical build** VC is low in obese and very thin persons. It is high in well-built persons. Vital capacity depends on chest size, muscle power and body surface area of the individual.
5. **Pregnancy** VC is low during pregnancy because chest expansion decreases as abdominal size increases.
6. **Physical training** VC is higher in trained athletes than in untrained individuals. It is even higher in swimmers and divers.

#### Pathological Factors

1. VC decreases in the diseases of the chest wall (for example, kyphoscoliosis), lungs (for example, emphysema, fibrosis, pulmonary edema) and pleura (for example, pleural effusion, pneumothorax).
2. VC decreases in diseases of the abdomen in which lung expansion is restricted as seen in abdominal tumours and ascites.

## METHODS

### Method to Demonstrate the Effect of Posture on VC

#### Principle

Change in posture changes the ability to carry out physical effort and the ventilatory capacity of the lungs. Therefore, posture affects the vital capacity.

#### Apparatus Required

1. Student's spirometer (vitalometer) (Fig. 22.1).
2. Mouthpiece

#### Procedure

1. Adjust the reading of the vitalometer to the zero mark.

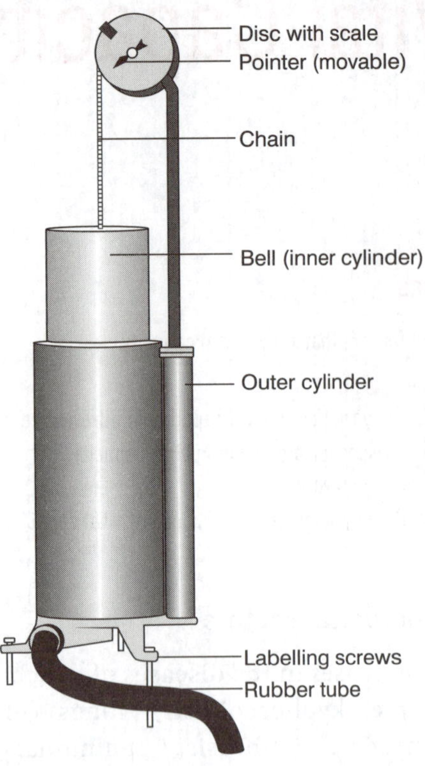


Fig. 22.1 Student's spirometer.

2. Ask the subject to lie down comfortably on a couch.
3. Connect the mouthpiece of the vitalometer to the subject's mouth.
4. Ask the subject to exhale forcefully to the maximum after taking a deep inspiration.
5. Record the vital capacity from the scale of the vitalometer.
6. Change the position of the arrow to zero and ask the subject to repeat the maneuver.
7. Record vital capacity three times, with a gap of at least two minutes between each, and record the best one.
8. Ask the subject to sit on a stool with his/her spine erect.
9. Record vital capacity (as described above) three times and record the best reading.
10. Ask the subject to stand up.
11. Record vital capacity three times and record the best reading.
12. Compare the vital capacities recorded in the three positions.

## Observation

Note that vital capacity is maximum in the erect posture, and minimum in the supine posture.

## Precautions

1. Each time, before recording vital capacity, the arrow mark of the scale should be adjusted to zero.
2. In the sitting and standing postures, the spine of the subject should be erect.
3. The subject should be trained and encouraged to put his/her maximum effort possible.
4. A minimum of three attempts should be made in all the postures and the best of the three should be taken.
5. The gap between each attempt should be a minimum of one to two minutes.
6. The test should not be performed on a full stomach.

# DISCUSSION

Vital capacity is more in the erect posture than in supine and sitting postures because of the following reasons:

1. More physical (muscular) effort is applied in the erect posture.
2. In the erect posture, the diaphragm descends; therefore, the capacity of the thoracic cage increases. In the supine position, the diaphragm is pulled upward because the abdominal viscera push the diaphragm. Therefore, the capacity of the thoracic cage decreases. Hence, vital capacity is greater in the erect posture than in the supine position.
3. In the supine position, due to elimination of the effect of gravity, the blood flow to the lungs increases. This decreases vital capacity. In the standing posture, blood is pooled in the lower extremities, therefore venous return decreases. This decreases pulmonary blood flow. Thus vital capacity increases on standing.

## Physiological Significance

The vital capacity indicates the strength of the respiratory muscles. Therefore, the maximum inspiratory and expiratory effort of the person can be assessed by determining vital capacity.

## VIVA

1. Define vital capacity.
2. What is the normal value of VC in males and females?
3. What are the factors that affect vital capacity?
4. What are the precautions for recording vital capacity?
5. Why is the vital capacity greater in the standing posture than in the sitting and supine postures?
6. What is the physiological significance of VC?

CHAPTER 23

# Electrocardiography

## LEARNING OBJECTIVES

After completing this practical, you will be able to:

- Define ECG.
- Classify ECG leads.
- Handle the ECG machine properly.
- Record ECG.
- List the precautions taken while recording ECG.
- List the uses of ECG.
- Identify the different waves and complexes of ECG.
- State the cause of production of the P wave, QRS complex and T wave.
- Calculate the heart rate and mean QRS axis.
- Define and state the normal duration and significance of PR interval, QRS complex and QT interval.

You may also be able to:

- Explain the physiological significance of different waves, complexes and intervals.
- List the conditions that cause alteration in different waves, complexes and intervals.
- Explain the physiological basis of such alterations.

## INTRODUCTION

Electrocardiography is the method of recording an electrocardiogram (ECG). ECG is the recording, and electrocardiograph is the machine that records the ECG. It is one of the most important and commonly ordered diagnostic tests in clinical practice.

ECG is the graphic recording of the electrical activities of the heart. The body is a volume conductor, that is, body fluids are good conductors of electricity. Therefore, electrical changes occurring in the heart with each heart beat are conducted all over the body and can be picked up from the body surface. The record of these electrical fluctuations during the cardiac cycle is called an electrocardiogram. Thus, the ECG recorded at the body surface represents the algebraic sum of the action potential of the individual cardiac muscle fibres.

### Uses of ECG

An ECG is useful in the diagnosis of many heart diseases. It is regularly recorded before any surgical intervention to assess the cardiac status of the patient. However, it does not give direct information concerning the mechanical performance of the heart. It may be completely normal in a patient with organic heart disease or may show some non-specific abnormalities in a normal subject. Therefore, the ECG must be interpreted with the clinical features of the patient and with the findings of other investigations.

The ECG is recorded to study the following parameters:

1. Anatomical orientation of the heart
2. Relative size of the chambers of the heart
3. A variety of disturbances of rhythm and conduction
4. To detect ischemia of the myocardium, if present
5. The location, extent and progress of myocardial infarction
6. The effects of altered electrolyte concentration
7. The influence of certain drugs like digitalis
8. Evaluation of electronic pacemaker function

## METHODS

### Electrocardiography

#### Principle

Electrical activities generated with each beat are conducted from the heart to the body surface, which are picked up and recorded by the electrocardiograph.

## Requirements

### 1. ECG Machine

In modern electrocardiography, two types of ECG apparatus are used: the string galvanometer and the radio-amplifier. The apparatus should be sensitive to potential changes of the order of microvolts and have a frequency response of 50–100 Hz. The use of the string galvanometer needs experience. This apparatus is not used in routine practice because the photographic paper used for recording needs to be developed. At present, the transistor amplifier and cathode ray tubes are used for this purpose. It has a main switch which regulates the power supply; a lead selection switch which selects various leads; a calibration switch, used for calibration; and a start–stop switch to regulate paper speed (Fig. 23.1).

### 2. Cardiac Jelly

This is a specially made paste that contains fine sand or glass particles used for placing electrodes on the body surface. It helps in establishing proper contact of the electrode plates to the body.

### 3. ECG Paper

This is the strip of graph paper which has vertical and horizontal lines 1 mm apart. The horizontal axis represents time whereas the vertical axis denotes amplitude. There is a heavy line every 5 mm in both the planes. Thus, there are small squares of 1 mm × 1 mm, and big squares of 5 mm × 5 mm. The ECG paper is a heat-sensitive, plastic-coated paper. The ECG is inscribed on this paper by a hot stylus.

**Paper speed** Conventional ECG is taken at a speed of 25 mm/s. One small square (1 mm) corresponds to 0.04 seconds, while the big square (5 mm) is equivalent to 0.20 seconds (Fig. 23.2). When the ECG paper runs through 5 big squares, one second recording has been taken.

**Sensitivity** Voltage is measured along the vertical axis. Usually, a 10 mm deflection is equivalent to 1 mV. There is provision to change the sensitivity in special circumstances, for example, when ECG complexes are too small, the sensitivity can be doubled so that a 1 mV deflection is equivalent to 20 mm. When ECG complexes are too large, sensitivity may be reduced to half from the original so that 1 mV is equivalent to 5 mm. The process of determination of sensitivity is called *standardisation*. It is displayed by pressing the calibration button before and after an ECG is recorded.

### 4. ECG Leads

The ECG leads are broadly classified into two categories, the direct and the indirect. A lead or an electrode is a metal plate (flat discs of dimension 7.5 × 5 cm, non-

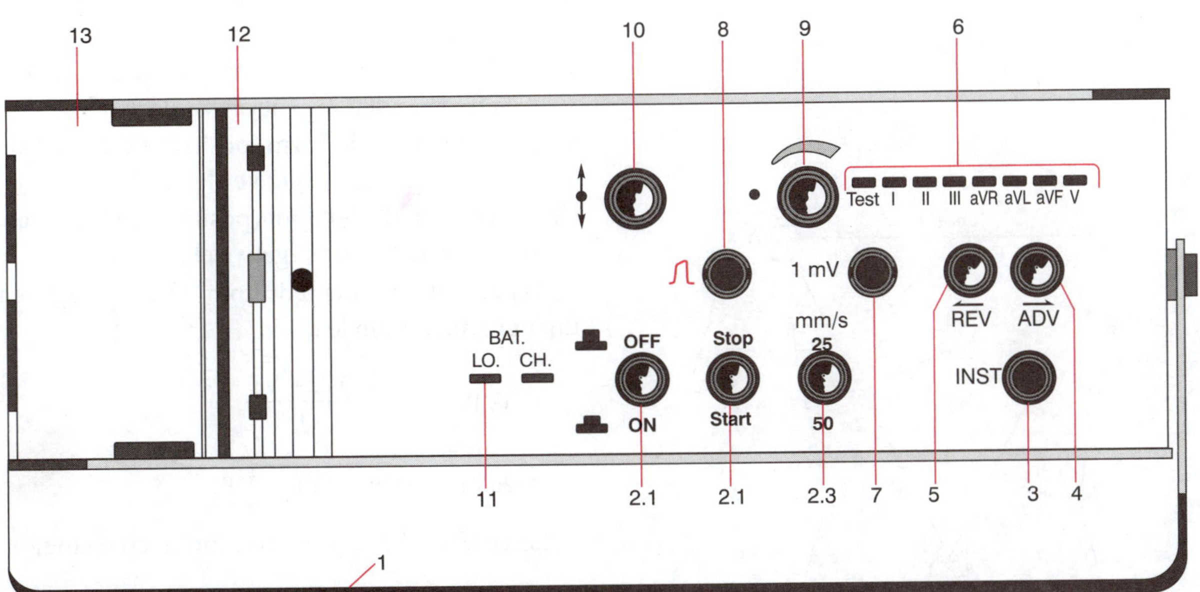


Fig. 23.1 Schematic diagram of the front view of an ECG machine.1: Handle; 2.1, 2.2 and 2.3: Control switches; 3: Stylus adjuster; 4 and 5: Lead positioners; 6: Lead selection button; 7: Voltage selection; 8: Filter A/C; 9: Gain; 10: Stylus deflector; 11: Battery strength indicator; 12 Stylus protector; 13: Table for guiding paper movement. (*Source:* Cardidat 108T/MK-VI; BPL Ltd.)

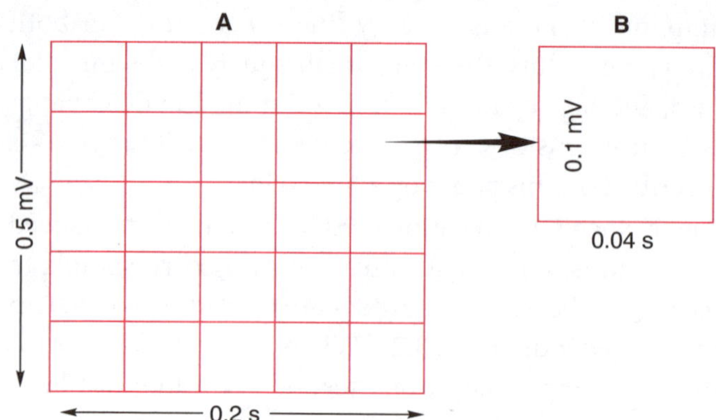


Fig. 23.2 Squares of the ECG paper. A: Large square; B: Small square. Time depicted in figures represents the time of the paper speed of 25 mm/s.

corrosive) applied snugly over an appropriate body part. For better contact of the leads, ECG jelly is applied after the skin surface is cleaned thoroughly.

**Direct leads** Leads applied directly to the surface of the heart to record ECG are called direct leads. These leads are used to record cardiac activities during cardiac surgery or during an experiment.

**Indirect leads** Leads applied away from the heart to record the cardiac activities are called indirect leads. The different indirect leads are limb leads, chest leads and esophageal leads.

**Limb leads** Limb leads are of two types, bipolar and unipolar.

*Bipolar limb leads* Bipolar standard limb leads (I, II and III) are the original leads selected by Einthoven to record electrical potential on the frontal plane. In the method of bipolar leads, two similar electrodes are placed on the body surface and the potential difference between these two electrodes is recorded. The electrodes are attached to the right arm, left arm and left foot as depicted in the Einthoven triangle (Fig. 23.3). Another electrode is applied to the right leg, which acts as a ground wire to prevent external disturbances during recording.

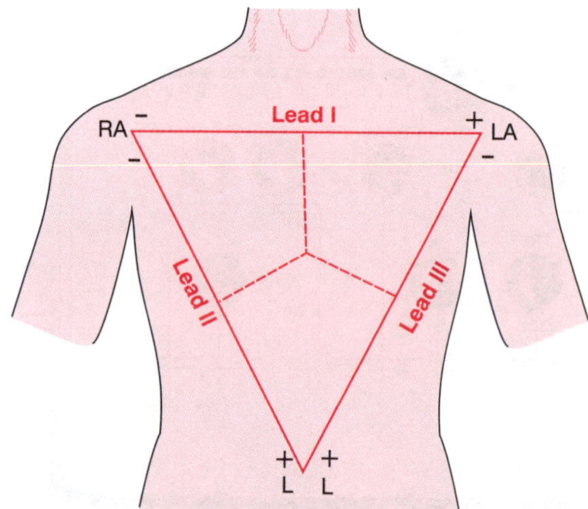


Fig. 23.3 Einthoven's triangle. RA: right arm; LA: Left arm; LL: Left leg. Note that perpendiculars drawn from the midpoint of each limb of the triangle intersect at the centre of the electrical activity.

Lead I Between the right arm (negative electrode) and the left arm (positive electrode).

Lead II Between the right arm (negative electrode) and the left leg (positive electrode).

Lead III Between the left arm (negative electrode) and the left leg (positive electrode).

*Unipolar limb leads* In this method, one electrode is active while the other is indifferent. There are three unipolar limb leads: aVR, aVL and aVF. Here 'a' stands for augmented leads. The potential recorded in aVL is one-and-a-half times that recorded in VL, and similarly for aVR and aVF. Therefore, these leads are called augmented leads. 'V' stands for voltage, and R, L and F indicate that the exploring (active) electrode is on the right arm, left arm and left foot respectively. The other (indifferent) electrode is connected to the remaining two leads through a high resistance coil. For example, while recording from lead aVL the active electrode is placed on the left arm, the indifferent electrode is connected through a high resistance to the other two electrodes placed on the left foot and fight arm.

aVR Between the right arm (positive electrode) and left arm + left leg (negative electrode).

aVL Between the left arm (positive electrode) and right arm + left leg (negative electrode).

aVF Between the left foot (positive electrode) and right arm + left arm (negative electrode).

Vector of augmented limb lead = $^3/_2$ vector of unaugmented limb lead.

$$aVR = VR - \frac{VL + VF}{2}$$

$$2aVR = 2VR - (VL + VF)$$

Since VR + VL + VF = 0 (Einthoven triangle),

$$VR = -(VL + VF)$$

$$2aVR = 2VR + VR$$

$$aVR = \frac{3}{2}\ VR$$

**Chest leads** Chest leads are of two types, bipolar and unipolar.

*Bipolar chest leads* These leads were used before the discovery of unipolar chest leads. These leads record differences of potential between any given position on the chest and on one extremity. They are not used now because the potential in the extremity appreciably alters the pattern of the chest leads.

*Lewis lead* This is a special bipolar chest lead used for recording ECG in atrial arrhythmias. This lead amplifies the waves of atrial activity.

*Unipolar chest leads* There are six chest leads that are used routinely; $V_1$ to $V_6$. There are three other chest leads ($V_7$–$V_9$). The chest leads employ an exploring electrode on the chest surface. The reference electrode is connected to the right arm, left arm and left leg through a high resistance, called Wilson's terminal, which is maintained at zero potential. The right leg is connected with a grounding electrode to avoid electrical interference. The position of the chest electrodes (positive electrodes) on the chest surface in different leads are as follows:

$V_1$ In the right fourth intercostal space at the right border of the sternum.

$V_2$ In the left fourth intercostal space at the left border of the sternum.

$V_3$ At the midpoint between $V_2$ and $V_4$.

$V_4$ In the left fifth intercostal space on the midclavicular line.

$V_5$ In the left fifth intercostal space on the anterior axillary line.

$V_6$ In the left fifth intercostal space on the midaxillary line.

$V_7$ In the left fifth intercostal space on the posterior axillary line.

$V_8$ In the left fifth intercostal space on the posterior scapular line.

$V_9$ In the left fifth intercostal space on the back just left to the spine.

**Esophageal leads** In these leads, an electrode is fixed on the tip of the esophageal catheter, which is positioned in the esophagus close to the heart chambers. The leads are designated as $E_{18}$, $E_{20}$ and so on. In this, E stands for 'esophageal', and the number indicates the distance of the electrode from the incisor teeth expressed in centimetres.

$E_{15-25}$ Used for recording the activity of the right atrium.

$E_{25-35}$ Used for recording the activity from the AV groove region.

$E_{40-50}$ Used for recording the activity from the posterior surface of the left ventricle.

## Procedure

1. Ask the subject to lie down on a couch comfortably.
2. Clean the skin thoroughly with alcohol around the left and right wrists and left and right leg just above the ankle joint and apply jelly.
3. Connect the electrodes in these positions.
4. Switch on the machine and keep the stylus at the centre of the paper.
5. Adjust the sensitivity to get a standard calibration of 1 cm / 1 mV by pressing the 'CAL' button 3 to 4 times.
6. Adjust the lead selector knob to record ECG of the 12 leads in the following order: I, II, III, aVR, aVL and aVF.
7. Place the chest electrodes in an appropriate position on the chest after thorough cleaning and application of jelly, and record the ECG from $V_1$ to $V_6$.
8. Again take the standard calibration.
9. Tear out the paper from the machine and label the record.
10. Write the name and age of the subject and the date of the recording.
11. Calculate heart rate and QRS axis as described in the 'Discussion'.
12. Study and interpret the ECG as described under 'Discussion' (Systematic Interpretation of ECG).

## Precautions

1. The subject should be totally relaxed.
2. The skin in the area where the electrodes are connected should be thoroughly cleaned and jelly should be applied to decrease skin resistance.
3. The right foot should be connected for grounding.
4. Ensure that the leads are properly applied at the appropriate places and are in good contact with the body surface.
5. Before starting the recording, ensure that the required voltage is available at the mains and that the instrument is properly earthed.
6. Standardisation should be done before and after the recording, to ensure that proper standard was maintained throughout the recording.

7. A minimum of three ECG complexes should be recorded for each lead.
8. The stylus should be adjusted so that it records at the centre of the paper.
9. Recording of 12 leads should be done in proper sequence as I, II, III, aVR, aVL, aVF and $V_1$ to $V_6$.

## DISCUSSION

### Features of a Good ECG

1. Optimal standardisation of the calibration signal forms rectangles. The corners of the signal form a right angle.
2. The base line is stable.
3. Contains a minimum of three complexes of each lead.
4. Contains a long strip of II and $V_1$ if arrhythmia is suspected or present.
5. No interference by alternating current.
6. ECG complexes are recorded at the centre of the paper and do not overshoot the margins.

### Normal ECG

The ECG tracing shows different waves, intervals and segments (Fig. 23.4).

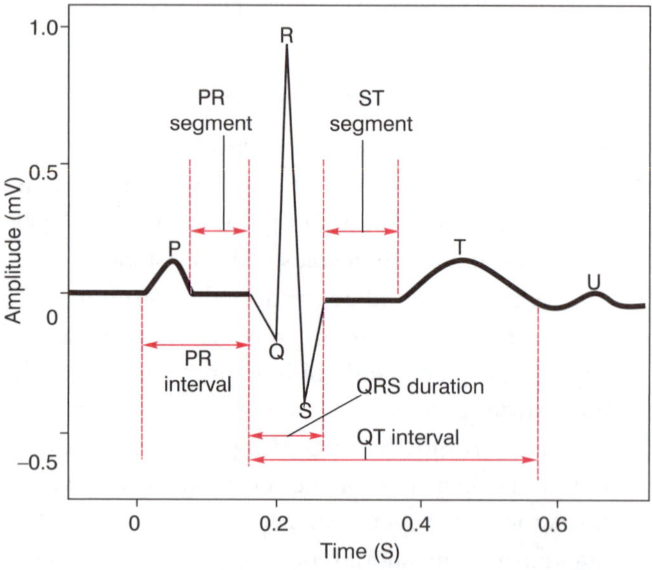


Fig. 23.4 Normal ECG showing different waves, segments and intervals.

#### Waves

**P wave** This is the deflection produced by atrial depolarisation.

**QRS complex** This consists of Q, R and S waves. The QRS complex is the deflection produced by ventricular depolarisation.

**Q wave** This is the initial negative deflection in the QRS complex.

**R wave** This is the positive deflection in the QRS complex.

**S wave** This is the second negative deflection in the QRS complex.

QS complex is the term used when the entire QRS complex is negative, without any positive deflection.

**T wave** This is the positive deflection produced by ventricular repolarisation.

**U wave** This is the final positive deflection in the ECG. This wave is not always present normally. It occurs due to slow repolarisation of the papillary muscle.

#### Segments

**PR segment** This lies between the end of the P wave and the beginning of the QRS complex.

**ST segment** This lies between the end of the QRS complex and the beginning of the T wave. The point where the QRS complex ends and the ST segment begins is called the *J point*. There is no electrical activity at the J point. Elevation of the J point (even 1 mm from the base) suggests myocardial ischemia.

#### Intervals

**PR interval**

*Definition* This is the interval between the beginning of the P wave to the beginning of the QRS complex.

*Normal duration* The range of PR interval is 0.12–0.20 seconds (average 0.18 s). PR interval shortens as the heart rate increases, from the average of 0.18 s at the rate of 70 to 0.14 s at the rate of 130.

*Significance* This represents atrial depolarisation and conduction through the AV node.

**QRS interval (QRS duration)**

*Definition* This is the interval of the QRS complex. It is measured from the beginning of the Q wave (or R wave if the Q wave is absent) to the J point.

*Normal duration* The normal range is 0.08–0.10 seconds.

*Significance* This represents ventricular depolarisation. Atrial repolarisation also occurs in this period.

### QT interval

*Definition* This is the interval of the QRS complex and T wave. It is measured from the beginning of the QRS complex to the end of the T wave.

*Normal duration* The normal range is 0.40–0.43 seconds.

*Significance* This represents ventricular depolarisation and ventricular repolarisation. It corresponds to the duration of electrical systole.

### ST interval

*Definition* This is the interval between the J point and the end of the T wave. It is calculated by deducting QRS interval from the QT interval.

*Normal duration* The average duration is 0.32 seconds.

*Significance* This represents ventricular repolarisation.

### PP interval

*Definition* This is the interval measured between either the peaks or the beginnings of two successive P waves.

*Significance* The PP interval is measured for calculating the atrial rate.

### RR interval

*Definition* This is the interval between two successive R waves. It is measured between the peaks of two successive R waves.

*Significance* The RR interval is measured for calculating the heart rate (the ventricular rate).

## Normal 12-Lead ECG

The deflection of waves in a particular lead is governed by a basic law; that is, a positive (upward) deflection is seen in any lead if electrical depolarisation spreads towards the positive pole of that lead, and a negative (downward) deflection is seen if depolarisation spreads towards the negative pole of the lead. An isoelectric or biphasic deflection is seen when the depolarisaton starts in the SA node and spreads downwards to the subject's left (towards the positive pole of lead II and away from the positive pole of lead aVR). The P wave is always positive in lead II and negative in lead aVR (Fig. 23.5). Ventricular septum depolarises from left to right (towards lead $V_1$ and away from lead $V_6$). This produces a small q wave (*septal q wave*) in $V_6$ and a small r wave (*septal r wave*) in lead $V_1$. During ventricular depolarisation, as left ventricular mass is more than right ventricular mass, the net direction of depolarisation is towards the left chest leads (Fig. 23.6). This produces tall 'R' wave in leads $V_5$ and $V_6$, and a deep S wave in leads $V_1$ and $V_2$. Chest leads

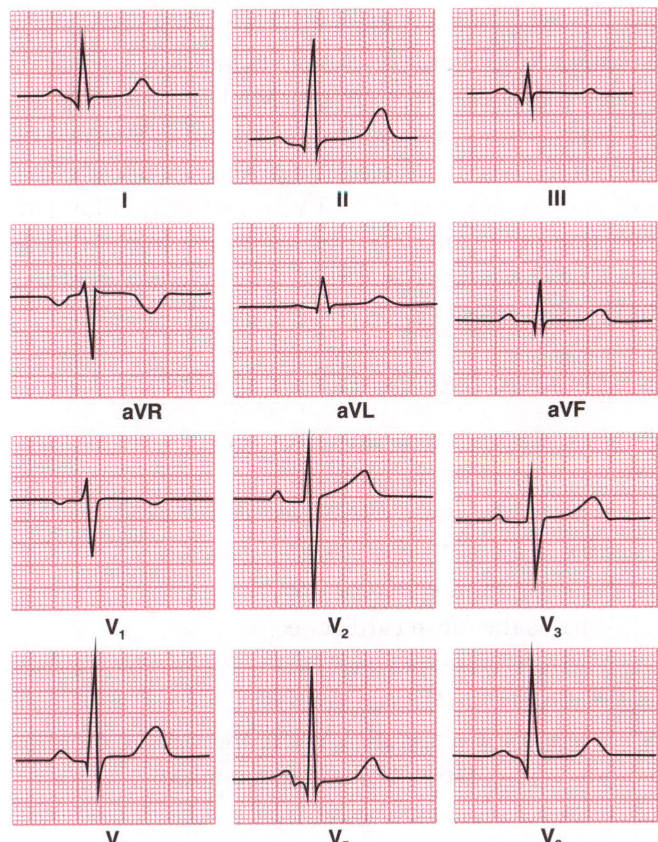


Fig. 23.5 Normal 12-lead ECG.

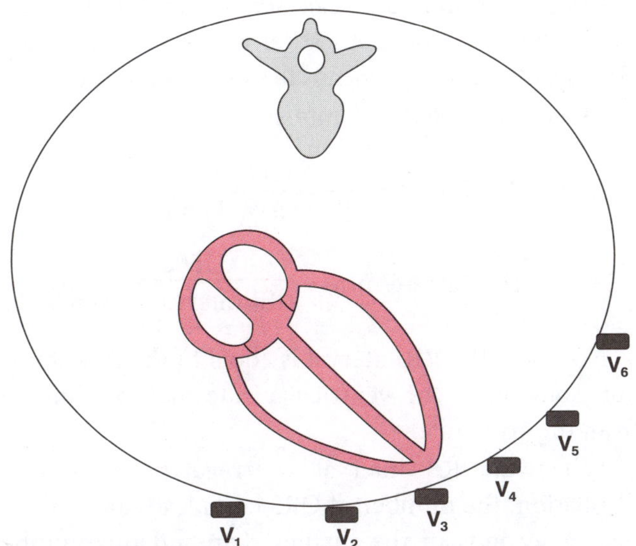


Fig. 23.6 Diagram of orientation of precordial ECG leads. Leads $V_1$ and $V_2$ overlie the right ventricle. Leads $V_3$ and $V_4$ are transitional leads between the right and left ventricles, and leads $V_5$ and $V_6$ overlie the left ventricle.

between these two positions show a transitional pattern. In extremity leads, the QRS complex varies depending on whether the heart is more horizontal or vertical. When the heart is more vertical, leads II, III and aVF show a qR pattern and when the heart is more horizontal, leads I and aVL show a qR pattern. The T wave normally follows the direction of the QRS complex deflection. In chest leads, the T wave is positive in left-sided leads (and also in $V_2$). In $V_1$, the T wave may be positive or negative.

## Systematic Interpretation of ECG

Routine screening of the ECG requires step-by-step examination of the ECG.

1. What is the heart rate? What is the atrial rate and what is the ventricular rate?
2. Is the rhythm regular or irregular?
3. What is the mean cardiac vector?
4. Are the P waves normal? Do the P waves have a fixed relation to the QRS complexes?
5. What is PR interval? What is the voltage duration and configuration of the QRS complex?
6. Is the ST segment isoelectric?
7. Are the T waves normal?
8. What is the QT interval? Is the QTc appropriate for the heart rate? (QTc is the QT interval corrected for the rate.)

#### *Rate*

The heart rate should be calculated first. The comment should be made on both atrial and ventricular rates. Usually, the heart rate means the ventricular rate.

At a paper speed of 25 mm/s:

$$\text{Atrial rate/min} = \frac{1500}{\text{PP interval in mm}}$$

$$\text{Ventricular rate/min} = \frac{1500}{\text{RR interval in mm}}$$

Normally the RR interval is equal to the PP interval but, sometimes the ventricular rate may be different from the artial rate.

When the RR interval is irregular, as in atrial fibrillation, the number of QRS complexes are counted over 5 seconds in the rhythm strip and this number is multiplied by 12 to provide the number of QRS complexes in 60 seconds (1 minute). This enables the measurement of the average ventricular rate.

The normal heart rate is 60–100 per minute.

#### *Rhythm*

Normally the rhythm is regular. It is seen by calculating successive cycle lengths (RR intervals). However, there may be minor variations of rhythm. A variation up to 10 per cent in the adjacent cycle length is considered normal.

#### *Mean QRS Axis (Cardiac Vector)*

Cardiac vector can be calculated roughly and accurately.

**Rough Estimation**

*Normal* For rough estimation of cardiac vector, QRS complexes are seen in lead I and aVF. When the QRS complexes are predominantly upright (that is, there is a dominant R in both leads), the axis is normal.

*Right axis deviation* If the QRS complex in lead I is predominantly negative (that is, dominant S in lead I) while it is predominantly positive in aVF (that is, dominant R in aVF), there is right axis deviation.

*Left axis deviation* If the QRS complex is predominantly positive in lead I but negative in aVF, left axis deviation is present. When the QRS complexes in both lead I and aVF are predominantly negative, the axis is intermediate.

**Accurate Estimation** The vector at any given moment in the two dimensions of the frontal plane can be calculated from any two standard limb leads. The height of QRS complexes in mm in lead I, II, and III are measured and an Einthoven's triangle is drawn (Fig. 23.7A). In each lead, distances equal to the height of the R wave minus the height of the largest negative deflection in the QRS complex are measured. These distances are drawn from the midpoint to the side of the triangle representing that lead. Perpendicular lines are drawn from the midpoint of the arms of the triangle to the centre and from the end of the QRS complexes drawn on the triangle. An arrow is drawn from the centre of the triangle to the point of intersection of the perpendiculars extended from the distances measured on the sides. This arrow represents the magnitude and direction of the mean QRS vector. The normal direction of the mean QRS vector is generally said to be –30 to +110 degrees (Fig. 23.7B). If the axis falls to the left of –30°, **left axis deviation** is present and if the axis falls to the right of +110°, **right axis deviation** is present.

## Waves and Intervals

### P Wave

*Duration and amplitude* Normal P wave duration does not exceed 0.10 s and P waves are not more than 2.5 mm tall.

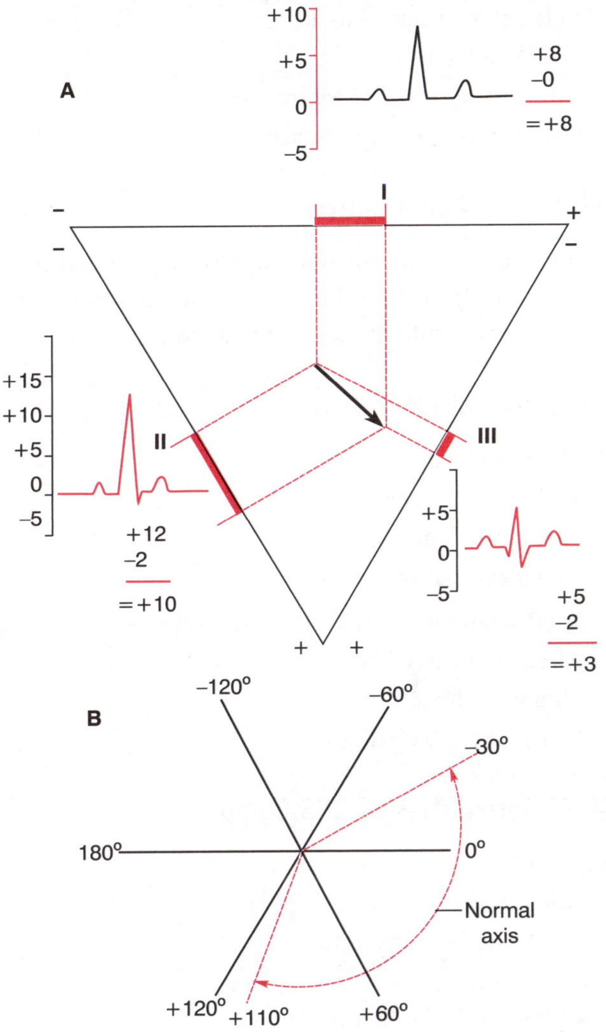


Fig. 23.7 Mean QRS axis, determination (A) and normal value (B).

*Configuration* Usually P waves are upright in lead I to aVF and $V_3$–$V_6$; inverted in aVR; and upright, inverted or biphasic in lead III, aVL, and $V_1$ and $V_6$. P wave morphology is best studied in lead II and $V_1$.

## PR Interval

Normal PR interval is 0.12–0.20 seconds, that is, 3–5 small squares. Normally, there should not be any variation in PR intervals.

## QRS Complex

*Amplitude* In limb leads, that is, in lead I, II, III, aVR, aVL and aVF, the total amplitude of QRS should be 5 mm or more. In chest leads, the amplitude of QRS complex should be 10 mm or more.

*Duration* The normal duration of the QRS complex does not exceed 0.11 seconds.

*Configuration* Normally, the R wave is dominant in leads I, II, $V_4$–$V_6$ and the S wave is dominant in aVR, $V_1$ and $V_2$. Either R or S wave may be dominant in lead III, aVL, aVF and $V_3$ depending on the position of the heart.

## Q Wave

Normally, Q waves are small in lead I, aVL, $V_5$ and $V_6$. A QS complex is commonly found in aVR. There may be deep Q waves in lead III alone in normal individuals and may become less prominent on deep inspiration. Occasionally, a deep Q wave is found in $V_1$ and $V_2$. Depth of Q wave is less than 25 per cent of the height of the ensuing R wave in most leads and may be up to 50 per cent in aVL. Any Q wave with greater amplitude is considered pathological.

## ST Segment

The normal ST segment is isoelectric. ST depression less than 0.5 mm is not abnormal. ST elevation up to 1 mm in limb leads and $V_5$ and $V_6$ and 2 mm in $V_1$–$V_4$ may be normal.

## T Wave

T waves are upright in lead I, II, $V_4$–$V_6$; inverted in aVR; and upright, inverted or biphasic in lead III, aVL, aVF and $V_1$–$V_3$.

## QT Interval

The upper limit of a normal QT interval is 0.42 s in males and 0.43 s in females. QT intervals should be measured in the lead where the end of the T wave is best discernible. QT interval varies with the heart rate. Therefore, corrected QT interval (QTc) is measured by using *Bazett's formula*.

$$QTc = \frac{QT}{\sqrt{RR}}$$

(QT is the QT interval and RR is the RR interval in seconds).

# Abnormal ECG

## Abnormalities of Heart Rate

The physiological basis for alteration in heart rate has been described in Chapter 24.

**Bradycardia**

1. Sinus bradycardia
   - Athletes
   - Sick sinus syndrome
   - Drugs (e.g., beta blockers)
   - Obstructive jaundice
   - Raised intracranial pressure
   - Myxedema
2. Junctional (nodal) rhythm
3. Complete heart block

**Tachycardia**

1. Sinus tachycardia
   - Anxiety
   - Fever
   - Hypoxemia
   - Thyrotoxicosis
   - Cardiac failure
   - Acute carditis
2. Ectopic (re-entrant) tachycardia
3. Atrial premature beats
   - Anxiety
   - Excess tea or coffee intake
   - Viral infections
   - Rheumatic heart disease
   - Digitalis toxicity
   - Cardiomyopathies
4. Paroxysmal supraventricular tachycardia
5. Atrial fibrillation
   - Rheumatic heart disease with mitral stenosis
   - Coronary artery disease
   - Cardiomyopathies
   - Thyrotoxicosis
6. Atrial flutter
   - Rheumatic heart disease
   - Coronary artery disease
7. Ventricular premature beats
8. Ventricular tachycardia

## Abnormal Axis Deviation

**Right axis deviation**

1. Right ventricular hypertrophy
2. Left posterior hemiblock
3. WPW syndrome
4. Dextrocardia

**Left axis deviation**

1. Left ventricular hypertrophy
2. Left anterior hemiblock
3. WPW syndrome
4. Inferior myocardial infarction
5. Obstructive airway disease

## P Wave Abnormalities

P wave may be abnormal due to atrial enlargement and intra-atrial conduction abnormalities. Atrial enlargement results in tall and peaked P waves.

## Abnormal PR Interval

**Short PR interval**

1. WPW syndrome
2. Nodal rhythm
3. Atrial premature beats

**Long PR interval (first degree AV block)**

1. Rheumatic carditis
2. Digitalis effect
3. Coronary artery disease

## Abnormalities of QRS Complex

**Amplitude**

1. *Low amplitude*
   - Marked emphysema
   - Myxedema
   - Pericardial effusion
   - Cardiomyopathy
2. *High amplitude*
   - Ventricular hypertrophy

**Pathological Q waves**

Depth of Q wave more than 25 per cent of the height of the ensuing R wave, or more than 0.04 s in duration, is considered pathological. Common causes are:

- Acute or old myocardial infarction
- Unstable angina
- Dilated cardiomyopathy
- Hypertrophic cardiomyopathy

## Abnormalities of ST Segment

**ST elevation**

1. Acute myocardial infarction
2. Acute pericarditis

**ST depression**

Commonly seen in myocardial ischemia.

## Abnormalities of T Wave

**Tall T wave**

1. Hyperkalemia
2. Acute myocardial infarction

**Inverted T wave**

I. Physiological
- Young children
- Deep inspiration (occasionally)
- After a heavy meal (occasionally)

II. Pathological
- Ventricular hypertrophy (due to strain)
- Bundle branch block
- Digitalis effect
- Myocardial ischemia

## Abnormal QT Interval

**Prolonged QT interval**

1. Hereditary
2. Antiarrhythmic drugs, like quinidine
3. Hypokalemia
4. Acute myocardial infarction

**Shortened QT interval**

This is of less clinical significance and may be seen in hypercalcemia.

# VIVA

1. Define ECG.
2. What are the uses of ECG?
3. What are the types of ECG machines used to record ECG in the laboratories?
4. How does the stylus write on the ECG paper?
5. What is the need for standardisation before and after the recording of ECG?
6. What are the types of ECG leads?
7. What is Einthoven's triangle?
8. Where should the different chest leads be placed?
9. What is the use of esophageal leads?
10. What are the precautions taken during recording of ECG?
11. Why is the right leg connected during ECG recording?
12. How is the main line frequency interference kept free from the ECG recording?
    Ans. Main line frequency disturbance is kept free by keeping electrode resistance below 10,000 ohms, using a single grounding electrode from the subject, and keeping all AC cords away from the subject.
13. What does a QRS complex represent?
14. What do the P, QRS, T and U waves represent?
15. What is ST segment and what is its significance?
16. What is the 'J' point? What is its significance?
17. How do you calculate the PR interval? What is its normal duration? What is its significance?
18. How do you calculate the QRS interval? What is its normal duration? What is its significance?
19. How do you calculate the QT interval? What is its normal duration? What is its significance?
20. How do you calculate the ST interval? What is its normal duration?
21. How do you calculate the PP interval? What is its significance?
22. How do you calculate the RR interval? What is its significance?
23. How do you calculate the heart rate?
24. How do you calculate ventricular rate when the RR interval is irregular?
25. How do you determine the QRS axis (cardiac vector)?
26. What do you mean by right and left axis deviation? Give examples.
27. What are the causes of tachycardia?
28. What are the causes of bradycardia?
29. What are the causes of short and long RR interval?
30. What are the causes of high and low amplitudes of QRS complex?

31. When does a Q wave become pathological? What are the conditions of pathological Q wave?
32. What are the conditions of ST depression and ST elevation?
33. What are the causes of tall T wave?
34. What are the causes of inverted T wave?
35. What are the causes of prolonged QT interval?

Chapter 24

# Clinical Examination of the Radial Pulse

## Learning Objectives

After completing this practical, you will be able to:

- Describe the importance of examination of radial pulse in clinical physiology.
- Define arterial pulse.
- List the parameters to be considered for the clinical examination of radial pulse.
- Examine the radial pulse properly (with proper sequence and procedure).
- List the common causes of tachycardia, bradycardia, irregular pulse, high and low volume pulse, water hammer pulse, pulsus paradoxus and pulsus alternans.

You may also be able to:

- Define and describe different abnormal pulses.
- Explain the causes of variation of different parameters of the arterial pulse.
- State the physiological basis of changes in different parameters of arterial pulse in different conditions.
- Explain the mechanism of genesis of tachycardia, bradycardia, irregular pulse, high- and low-volume pulse, water hammer pulse, pulsus paradoxus and pulsus alternans in different conditions.

## INTRODUCTION

Examination of the radial pulse is an important and essential part of the clinical examination of a patient. It is not only important for examination of the cardiovascular system but also for any systemic examination of the patient, because arterial pulse is one of the vital signs that must be checked along with the general examination.

### Definition

Arterial pulse is defined as the rhythmic expansion of the arterial wall due to transmission of pressure waves along the walls of the arteries, which are produced during each systole of the heart.

### Importance

Examination of the arterial pulse provides physiological information regarding:

1. The working of the heart
2. The circulatory state and hemodynamics (blood volume, blood pressure and so on)
3. The condition of the blood vessels
4. The state of autonomic activity in the body at that moment
5. The mental state of the subject
6. The state of body metabolism and temperature

### The Radial Pulse

The pulse recorded from the radial artery shows the following waves (Fig. 24.1). The pulse wave has an upstroke and a downstroke. The 'p' wave (*percussion wave* or *tidal wave*) occurs due to ejection of blood from the ventricle during systole. The 'd' wave (*dicrotic wave*) occurs due to rebound of blood against the closed aortic valve during diastole. 'n' (dicrotic notch) represents the closure of the aortic valve. Sometimes, in the upstroke of the pulse wave, a small 'a' or *anacrotic* wave is seen, which occurs due to change in the velocity of ejection of blood from the ventricle towards late systole.

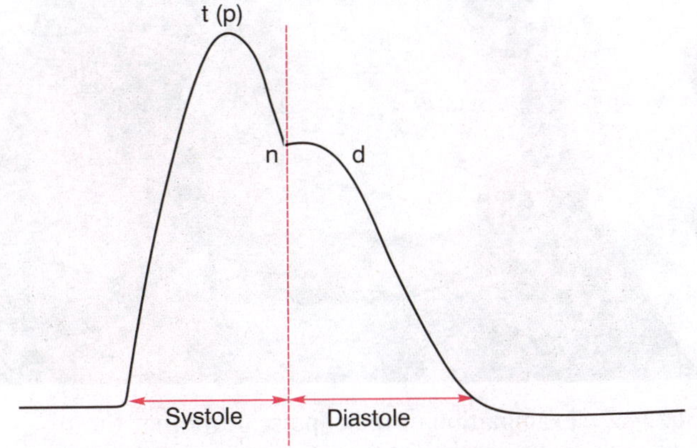


Fig. 24.1 The radial pulse. t: tidal (percussion: p) wave; n: dicrotic notch; d: dicrotic wave.

# METHODS

## Method of Examination of Radial Pulse

### Principle

With each ventricular contraction, not only is the blood pumped into the aorta but also pressure waves that are transmitted along the walls of the vessels are generated. These pressure waves expand the arterial wall, and the expansion is palpated as a pulse.

### Procedure

The arterial pulses are detected by gently compressing the vessel against the bone. The radial pulse is examined by compressing the radial artery against the head of the radius. For better elicitation of the pulse, the forearm of the subject should be semipronated and the wrist slightly flexed (Fig. 24.2).

The following aspects (parameters) of the pulse are studied.

1. Rate
2. Rhythm
3. Volume (amplitude)
4. Character
5. Condition of the arterial wall
6. Radiofemoral delay (presence or absence of delay of the femoral pulses compared with the radials)
7. Other peripheral pulses

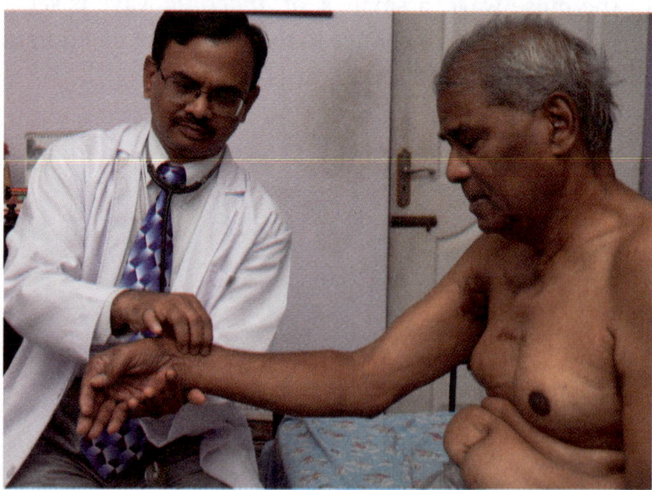

Fig. 24.2 Examination of radial pulse. Note that the subject's hand is supported by the examiner's left hand, subject's forearm is semiflexed and semipronated, and the wrist is slightly flexed.

#### *Rate*

Count the rate of the pulse, not immediately after placing the finger on the artery, but when the nervousness of the patient subsides. Count the pulse completely for one minute.

> Note: Pulse rate should be counted only when the pulse resumes its normal rate. Therefore, it is advised to feel the radial pulse gently while eliciting the history of the patient. The pulse should be counted for a minimum of one minute. The counting of pulse for 5 or 10 seconds and multiplying it by 12 or 6 to get the rate per minute is not correct, at least for beginners. The ideal time is 3 minutes and the average of the three may be taken.

In conditions of irregularities of the heart, the counting of radial pulse may not reflect the true ventricular contractions. In these conditions, the heart beat should be counted by auscultating the apex. The difference between the pulse rate and the heart rate is called *pulse deficit.* It should also be noted that the pulse rate can never be more than the heart rate.

#### *Rhythm*

Rhythm is the spacing order at which successive pulse waves are felt. When spacing between all the waves is constant, the pulse is said to be regular. When spacing is not constant, the pulse is said to be irregular. The irregular pulse may have a fixed pattern of irregularity (irregular at regular intervals) or the irregularity may not have any pattern (irregularly irregular).

#### *Volume*

It is the degree of expansion of the arterial walls during each pulse wave. Usually in physiological conditions, the volume is normal and equal on both the sides. Normal volume cannot be described but only be appreciated by palpating the artery of a normal individual. The pulse volume gives an indication of the stroke volume of the left ventricle.

#### *Character*

Study the character of the arterial pulse waves. The character of a normal pulse is described as 'normal' when no abnormalities are detected. The abnormalities may be seen in rate, rhythm or amplitude of the pulse. Depending on these changes, various types of abnormal pulses are described. It should be noted that the character of the pulse is best appreciated by palpating the carotid artery in the neck.

### *Condition of the Arterial Wall*

Place three middle fingers on the artery to assess the condition of the arterial wall. Obliterate the flow of blood into the artery by pressing the index finger, and empty the vessel by the ring finger. Then palpate the artery with the middle finger. Roll the artery against the bone to assess the thickness of the arterial wall.

Normally, the arterial wall is not palpable or is just palpable. But, in old age, it is well palpable (thickened) and may be tortuous.

### *Delay*

Compare the appearance of the femoral pulse with the appearance of the radial pulse and mark if any delay is present between them. Normally there is no radiofemoral delay. Also compare with the radial pulse of the opposite side.

### *Other Peripheral Pulses*

Palpate the femoral, popliteal, posterior tibial and dorsalis pedis artery of both the sides and see if the pulses are well felt and appear simultaneously on both sides.

## Precautions

1. The subject should relax and rest for a minimum of five minutes.
2. The subject's forearm should be semipronated and the wrist should be semiflexed.
3. Pulse rate should be counted for a minimum of one minute. If irregularity is detected, the pulse should be counted for a minimum of three minutes and the average of the three should be taken as the pulse rate.
4. If the pulse is irregularly irregular, heart beats must be auscultated to detect pulse deficit, if present.
5. Pulses of both the sides should be examined and compared.
6. Femoral artery must be examined simultaneously with radial artery to detect radiofemoral delay, if present.
7. The radial pulse should be examined with the middle three fingers to check the condition of the arterial wall. The index finger should be used to obliterate the flow of blood, the ring finger should be used to empty the vessel and the middle finger should be used to palpate and roll the artery against the bone.
8. If the artery is thickened and tortuous, the brachial artery should be examined for locomotor brachii.
9. The condition of the other peripheral pulses should be assessed.
10. If alternating pulses appear to be strong and weak, sphygmomanometry should be done to confirm the presence of pulsus alternans.

# DISCUSSION

## Pulse Rate

The normal pulse rate is 60–100 per minute. The heart rate is primarily under the control of the autonomic nervous system. The heart rate increases with increased sympathetic activity and decreases with increased parasympathetic activity. A heart rate of more than 100 is called *tachycardia*, and less than 60 is called *bradycardia*. Normally, the heart rate is higher in children and low in elderly persons. The heart rate is higher in inspiration and lower in expiration.

### Conditions that Alter Heart Rate

#### *Tachycardia*

**I. Physiological**

- Exercise
- After eating
- Anger
- Emotion and excitement
- Infants and children
- Pregnancy
- High environmental temperature

In exercise, the heart rate increases due to sympathetic stimulation and due to increased body temperature. Increased sympathetic discharge to the SA node causes tachycardia. Tachycardia occurs following eating due to increased body metabolism that increases body temperature. The heart rate increases in anger, emotion and excitement due to increased sympathetic activity. The exact cause of tachycardia in pregnancy is not known, but it may be due to the direct action of progesterone on the SA node.

**II. Pathological**

- *Fever* Increased body temperature causes tachycardia by directly stimulating the SA node.

- *Anemia* Tachycardia occurs in anemia as a compensatory mechanism to improve blood (oxygen) supply to the tissues.
- *Thyrotoxicosis* Thyroxine increases the number of beta receptors in the heart and also increases the sensitivity of the beta receptors to catecholamines.
- Beriberi
- Paget's disease
- Arteriovenous fistula
- Heart failure
- Paroxysmal atrial tachycardia
- Ventricular or supraventricular tachycardia
- Other tachyarrhythmias
- Shock as seen in hemorrhage

#### *Bradycardia*

**I. Physiological**

- *Athletes* Heart rate is lower in athletes because of their increased vagal tone
- Fear
- Grief
- Very old age
- Meditation and pranayama

**II. Pathological**

- *Myxedema* In hypothyroidism, the number and sensitivity of beta receptors to catecholamines decreases.
- *Increased intracranial pressure, as in brain tumours* Increased intracranial pressure decreases heart rate by activating Cushing's reflex.
- *Obstructive jaundice* In obstructive jaundice, the concentration of bile salt increases in the blood. The toxic effect of bile salt inhibits the SA node, and therefore produces bradycardia.
- Different types of heart block.
- *Drugs like propranolol and digitalis* Propranolol is a non-specific β-receptor blocker. Therefore, it produces bradycardia by inhibiting β-receptors of the SA node. Digitalis produces bradycardia by stimulating vagal nuclei (increases vagal activity) in the medulla.

## Rhythm

The normal rhythm is regular. Irregular rhythms may be regularly irregular or irregularly irregular. Irregular rhythm may be due to sinus irregularity or premature contraction.

### Sinus Irregularity

This is called *sinus arrhythmia*. In this type of irregularity, the pulse rate constantly changes with respiration. Normally, the pulse rate is greater in inspiration than in expiration. In sinus arrhythmia the variation of heart rate in expiration and inspiration is more marked.

### Premature Contraction

This is called *extrasystole*. It occurs due to generation of impulse from an ectopic focus present in the ventricle. Therefore, this is also called *ectopic beat*.

### Irregularly Irregular Pulse

This is commonly seen in atrial fibrillation. In this condition, irregularity occurs not only in the interval between the beats, but also in the volume of the beats.

### Irregularity Associated with Heart Blocks

1. Partial heart block with dropped beat
2. Atrial flutter with irregular block

In these conditions, irregularity occurs due to block in conduction, which occurs irregularly.

### Pulse Deficit

This is the difference between the pulse rate and the heart rate. Normally, there is no pulse deficit. However, in conditions of irregular rhythm some of the heart beats may be weak. The heart may beat but the contraction may not be sufficient enough to generate pressure waves in the walls of the arteries. Therefore, the pulse rate may be less than that of the rate of heart contraction. Pulse deficit is usually seen in atrial fibrillation in which the deficit is more than ten. Pulse deficit seen in other types of heart blocks is usually less than ten.

## Volume

The volume of the pulse is a rough guide to the pulse pressure. Pulse pressure is the difference between the systolic and diastolic pressure. The systolic pressure mainly depends on the stroke volume and the diastolic pressure on the compliance of the arteries. Therefore, the volume of the pulse gives an indication of the stroke volume and the compliance of the vessels. In normal conditions, where the compliance of the vessels is normal, the volume of the pulse mainly reflects the stroke volume.

When the volume of the pulse decreases, the pulse is called *low volume pulse* and when the volume increases, the pulse is called *high volume pulse*.

### Conditions that Alter the Volume of the Pulse

#### *Low Volume Pulse*

The low volume pulse is also known as *pulsus parvus* (Fig. 24.3D). It occurs when the stroke volume of the heart decreases or when the pulse pressure decreases.

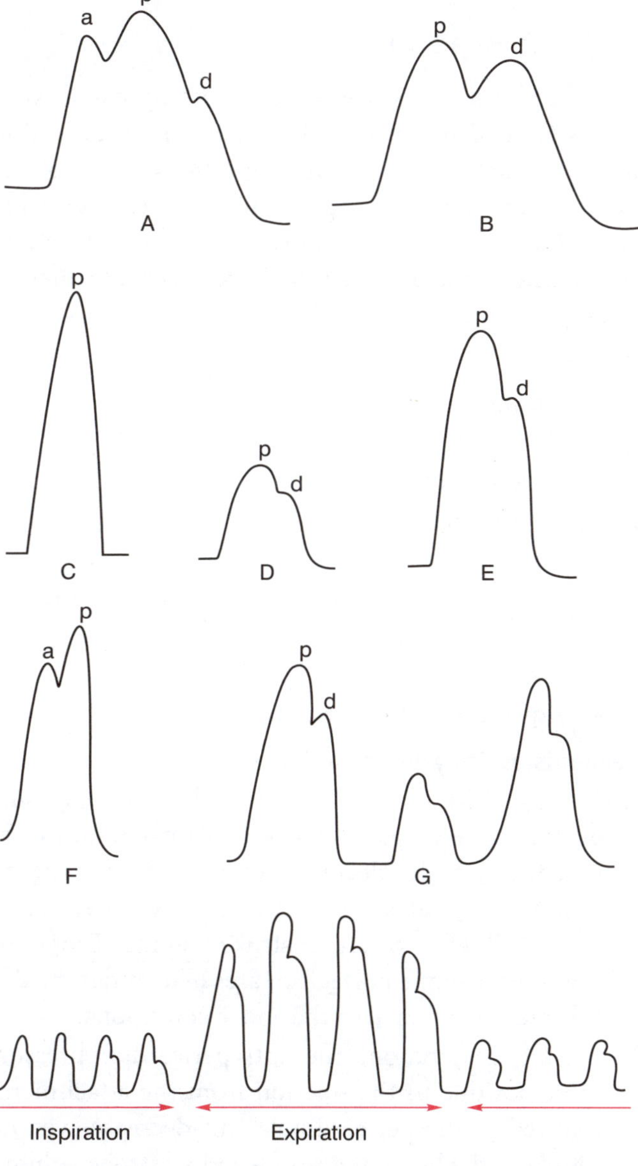


Fig. 24.3 Abnormal pulses. A: Anacrotic pulse (note that the anacrotic wave is prominent); B: Dicrotic pulse (note that the dicrotic wave is abnormally large); C: Collapsing pulse (dicrotic notch absent); D: Pulsus parvus; E: Pulsus magnus; F: Pulsus bisferiens; G: Pulsus alternans; H: Pulsus paradoxus.

Pulsus parvus is seen in:

- Aortic stenosis
- Obstructive cardiomyopathy
- Pericardial effusion
- Constrictive pericarditis
- Pulmonary stenosis
- Tight mitral stenosis
- Shock due to any cause

#### *High Volume Pulse*

The high volume pulse is called *pulsus magnus* (Fig. 24.3E). It is seen in conditions in which the stroke volume is greater and there is widening of the pulse pressure. Pulsus magnus is seen in:

- Aortic incompetence
- Thyrotoxicosis
- Patent ductus arteriosus
- Beriberi
- Anemia
- Fever
- Old age (due to increased pulse pressure)
- Exercise

## Character

The character of a pulse is described as normal when no abnormalities are detected. Different types of abnormal pulses are described in clinical medicine. Common among these are anacrotic pulse, dicrotic pulse, water hammer pulse, pulsus bisferiens, pulsus paradoxus and pulsus alternans.

### Anacrotic Pulse

This is also called anadicrotic pulse, which means two upbeats. A secondary wave occurs in the upstroke of the pulse. It is commonly found in aortic stenosis. The upstroke is slow and sloping (Fig. 24.3A). The anacrotic wave is exaggerated and has 2 upbeats. Therefore, this pulse is called anacrotic pulse.

### Dicrotic Pulse

A better name for this is 'twice-beating pulse'. The dicrotic wave is prominent in this pulse and gives the impression of two beats. Therefore, this is called dicrotic pulse (Fig. 24.3B). It is commonly seen in febrile states, especially in typhoid fever.

## Water Hammer Pulse

This is also called *collapsing pulse* or *Corrigan's pulse*. This is typically seen in aortic regurgitation. The collapsing pulse is characterised by a rapid upstroke and a rapid downstroke (descent) of the pulse wave. A dicrotic notch is usually absent (Fig. 24.3C). The rapid upstroke is due to greatly increased stroke volume and the rapid descent is due to the collapse of the pulse. The pulse pressure is therefore very high, sometimes as high as 100 mm Hg.

**Causes**

1. Common causes
   - Aortic incompetence
   - Patent ductus arteriosus
2. Less common causes
   - Arteriovenous fistula
   - Ventricular septal defect (VSD)
   - Hyperkinetic circulatory states, for example, thyrotoxicosis, severe anemia and beriberi.

> Note: The collapsing pulse is better appreciated when the patient's arm is elevated and the wrist is grasped with the palm (of the examiner's hand) against the palmar surface of the wrist.

**Physiological basis** The collapsing pulse occurs due to rapid upstroke and rapid downstroke of the pulse wave. The rapid upstroke is due to a forceful, high-amplitude and steep-rising percussion wave which gives a sharp tap to the palpating hand and the rapid downstroke is due to a rapid fall of the descending limb of the pulse wave, which results in sudden disappearance of the pulse from the palpating hand.

The steep rise of the ascending limb of the pulse wave is due to increased end diastolic volume (EDV) of the left ventricle, which causes forceful ejection of blood during systole. This is because during diastole, in addition to the ventricular filling from the left atrium, the filling also occurs from the aorta through the incompetent aortic valve. The aortic valve does not close completely, so blood from the aorta enters into the left ventricle during diastole. This increases the total EDV of the left ventricle. So, during systole, the force of contraction of the left ventricle increases due to the Frank–Starling mechanism. Therefore, there is a steep rise in the percussion wave during systole.

The steep fall of the descending limb of the pulse wave is due to the collapse (sudden disappearance) of the pulse wave from the palpating hand. This occurs due to two factors:

1. the diastolic run-off of blood into the left ventricle and
2. rapid run-off of blood into the periphery because of decreased systemic vascular resistance.

## Pulsus Bisferiens

Pulsus bisferiens is a combination of the low-rising pulse (anacrotic pulse) and the collapsing pulse (Fig. 24.3F). This is typically seen in aortic stenosis associated with aortic incompetence.

## Pulsus Paradoxus

This is a misnomer since there is nothing paradoxical in this type of pulse. Actually this is an accentuation of the normal phenomenon where the volume of the pulse decreases during inspiration and increases during expiration. In pulsus paradoxus, during inspiration, the volume of the pulse is grossly decreased, or may be absent in severe cases (Fig. 24.3H).

**Causes**

1. Common causes
   - Constrictive pericarditis
   - Pericardial effusion
2. Less common causes
   - Emphysema
   - Asthma (in the acute phase of severe asthma)
   - Massive pleural effusion
   - A mass in the thorax
   - Advanced right ventricular failure

**Mechanisms (physiological basis)**

1. During inspiration, the intrathoracic pressure becomes more negative. Blood pools in the pulmonary vascular bed. This decreases venous return to the left atrium. So, left atrial filling decreases, which results in decreased left ventricular stroke volume. Therefore, the volume of the pulse decreases in inspiration. This is more accentuated in the above conditions.
2. During inspiration, the intrapericardial pressure increases due to the traction from the attachments referred to the pericardium. This decreases venous return to the heart and results in low stroke volume. This is accentuated in pericardial effusion and constrictive pericarditis.
3. In constrictive pericarditis and pericardial effusion, the filling of the atria and ventricles decreases due to restriction to the expansion of the heart chambers.

The limitation in the diastolic filling of the atria and the ventricles during inspiration results in lowering of left ventricular stroke volume.

4. In advanced stages of right ventricular failure, increase in lung volume in inspiration accommodates more blood than normal due to much decreased pulmonary vascular resistance. There is as such decreased right ventricular output. Therefore, these two factors result in decreased left ventricular stroke volume (due to decreased venous return to left atrium).
5. In acute and severe bronchial asthma, the increased respiratory effort makes intrathoracic pressure more negative during inspiration. So, there is more pooling of blood in the pulmonary veins, which results in decreased left ventricular stroke volume.

### Pulsus Alternans

The pulse is regular, but alternate beats are strong and weak (Fig. 24.3G). It is difficult to appreciate pulsus alternans by palpating the artery. Diagnosis is confirmed while measuring blood pressure. There will be a difference of 5–20 mm Hg in the systolic pressure between two alternate beats. When the mercury is being lowered, the stronger beats are heard first, and on further lowering, the weaker beats also become audible, thus suddenly doubling the number of audible beats.

**Causes**

1. *Left ventricular failure* This is the commonest cause of pulsus alternans.
2. Toxic carditis

**Physiological basis** In left ventricular failure, because of the decreased myocardial contractility, the left ventricular stroke volume decreases. This results in low pulse volume. So, the amount of blood left in the ventricle at the end of systole (end systolic volume of the left ventricle) increases. Therefore, prior to the next ventricular contraction, the ventricular volume (EDV) is also increased. This increases the force of contraction of the left ventricle in the next beat due to the Frank–Starling mechanism. Hence, the second beat becomes stronger. Likewise, the strong beats alternate with the weak beats.

## Condition of the Arterial Wall

Normally, in young individuals, the arterial wall is soft and elastic or may not be palpable. In the elderly, it is palpable, hard and may be tortuous. This is due to thickening of the arterial wall by atherosclerosis. In such a condition, the brachial and temporal arteries may be quite prominent and tortuous. The brachial artery may exhibit a typical dancing movement with each beat, called *locomotor brachii.*

## Radiofemoral Delay

Normally, there is no delay between the appearance of pulse in the radial and femoral artery. Radiofemoral delay is typically seen in coarctation of the aorta (especially when the constriction is present distal to the origin of the left subclavian artery).

## Other Peripheral Pulses

In the absence of any pathology, all the peripheral pulses are well felt and appear simultaneously on both sides. Peripheral pulses may not be felt properly in peripheral vascular diseases.

## VIVA

1. Define arterial pulse.
2. What is the importance of examination of the radial pulse in clinical medicine?
3. What are the precautions taken during examination of the radial pulse?
4. What are the different aspects of the pulse, which are examined during clinical examination of the radial pulse?
5. Why are the three middle fingers used for examining the radial pulse?
6. What is pulse deficit and what is its most common cause?
7. What is the normal pulse rate and what is the main factor that regulates it?
8. What are the physiological conditions that cause tachycardia?
9. What is the cause of tachycardia in exercise?
10. Why does tachycardia occur after eating?

11. What are the causes of tachycardia in pregnancy?
12. Name the pathological conditions in which tachycardia occurs.
13. What is the cause of tachycardia in thyrotoxicosis?
14. What is the cause of tachycardia in anemia?
15. What is the cause of bradycardia in trained athletes?
16. Why is the heart rate reduced during sleep?

    Ans. Sympathetic activity decreases and parasympathetic activity increases during sleep. Therefore, the heart rate is lower in sleep than in the awake state.
17. What is the cause of bradycardia in increased intracranial pressure?

    Ans. When intracranial pressure increases as seen in a brain tumour, the blood flow to the vasomotor centre (VMC) in the medulla decreases because of the compression of intracranial blood vessels. This causes local hypoxia and hypercapnia, and stimulates VMC, which results in intense vasoconstriction. This is called *Cushing's reflex.* Vasoconstriction increases blood pressure, which stimulates baroreceptors, and the activation of baroreceptor reflex results in bradycardia. Therefore, bradycardia rather than tachycardia is one of the important clinical features of raised intracranial pressure.
18. What is the relationship between pulse rate and blood pressure?

    Ans. Pulse rate is inversely proportional to the blood pressure but not vice versa. This is called *Mary's law.* When blood pressure increases, the baroreceptors present in the arterial side of the circulation are stimulated. This activates the baroreceptor reflex, which results in bradycardia and hypotension. Conversely, when blood pressure decreases, there is tachycardia. Therefore, heart rate is inversely proportional to the blood pressure. But, blood pressure may not change with change in heart rate.
19. What is sinus arrhythmia?
20. What are the causes of high-volume and low-volume pulses?
21. What is the physiological significance of examining the volume of the pulse?
22. What do you mean by the collapsing pulse and what is its physiological basis?
23. What is pulsus paradoxus and what are the conditions that produce it?
24. What is the physiological basis of pulsus paradoxus in constrictive pericarditis and pericardial effusion?

    Ans. In constrictive pericarditis and in pericardial effusion, the filling of the atria and ventricles decreases due to restriction to the expansion of the heart chambers. The limitation in the diastolic filling of the atria and the ventricles during inspiration results in lowering of left ventricular stroke volume.
25. What is pulsus alternans and what is the physiological basis of this pulse?
26. What is the significance of examining the femoral artery simultaneously with the radial artery?

CHAPTER 25

# Measurement of Blood Pressure

## LEARNING OBJECTIVES

After completing this practical, you will be able to:

- Define blood pressure; define systolic, diastolic, mean arterial and pulse pressure.
- State the normal values of systolic, diastolic, mean arterial and pulse pressure.
- Tie the BP cuff properly around the arm of the subject.
- Raise the mercury column and decrease the mercury column of the sphygmomanometer at required speed, during BP recording.
- Detect the appearance and disappearance of the sounds by placing a stethoscope on the brachial artery while measuring blood pressure.
- Record BP by palpatory and auscultatory methods, and list the precautions of recording BP.
- List the physiological variations of blood pressure.
- Define hypertension and hypotension.
- Name the reflexes involved in regulation of BP.
- State the importance of baroreceptor reflex.

You may also be able to:

- List the merits and demerits of different methods of measuring blood pressure.
- Explain the mechanism of alteration in blood pressure in different physiological conditions.
- Explain the physiological basis of different types of hypertension and hypotension.
- Explain the mechanism of short-term and long-term regulation of blood pressure.
- Correlate the change in BP in some common clinical conditions.

## INTRODUCTION

Blood pressure (BP) is defined as the lateral pressure exerted by the column of blood on the walls of the arteries. Blood pressure usually means arterial pressure. The pressure in the arteries fluctuates during systole and diastole of the heart.

### Systolic BP

**Definition** Systolic blood pressure (SBP) is defined as the maximum pressure produced during the cardiac cycle. It is recorded during systole. Therefore, it is called systolic blood pressure.

**Significance** SBP depends mainly on the cardiac output. Thus, SBP increases in conditions in which cardiac output is more.

### Diastolic BP

**Definition** Diastolic blood pressure (DBP) is defined as the minimum pressure recorded during the cardiac cycle. It is recorded during diastole. Therefore, it is called diastolic pressure.

**Significance** DBP depends mainly on peripheral resistance. Thus, DBP changes in conditions in which there is change in peripheral resistance. Peripheral resistance depends mainly on the diameter of the blood vessels and viscosity of the blood.

### Pulse Pressure

**Definition** Pulse pressure (PP) is the difference between the systolic and diastolic blood pressures.

**Significance** This is the pressure that maintains the normal pulsatile nature of the flow of blood in the vascular compartment. The pulsatile nature of the flow is required for the perfusion of the tissues.

### Mean Arterial Pressure

**Definition** Mean arterial pressure (MAP) is the average pressure produced during the cardiac cycle. It is calculated by adding one-third of the PP to the diastolic pressure.

$$MAP = DBP + 1/3\ PP$$

Because the duration of the systole is less than the duration of the diastole, the MAP is slightly less than the value halfway between systolic and diastolic pressure. MAP also determines tissue perfusion.

**Significance** The MAP is the pressure that helps in the forward movement of blood in the lumen of blood vessels. MAP also determines tissue perfusion.

## Casual Blood Pressure

Blood pressure measured at any time of the day is called casual blood pressure.

## Basal Blood Pressure

Blood pressure recorded in the basal state is called basal blood pressure. It is recorded following complete physical and mental rest, after 12 hours of fasting.

## Normal Values

Normal values of different pressures in the adult male are as follows.

SBP : 100–119 mm Hg (120 to 139 mm Hg is prehypertension)

DBP : 60–79 mm Hg (80 to 89 mm Hg is prehypertension)

PP : 20–50 mm Hg

MAP : 75–105 mm Hg

## Factors Affecting BP

Blood pressure = Cardiac output × Peripheral resistance

Thus, factors that affect cardiac output and peripheral resistance also affect blood pressure. Alteration in cardiac output mainly affects systolic pressure and alteration in peripheral resistance mainly affects diastolic pressure.

## Factors Affecting Cardiac Output

Cardiac output = Stroke volume × Heart rate

Therefore, any factor that affects stroke volume or heart rate alters cardiac output. The stroke volume is affected by preload, afterload and myocardial contractility, and the heart rate is mainly affected by parasympathetic and sympathetic activities.

### 1. Preload

Preload is the end diastolic volume (EDV), that is, the amount of blood present in the ventricle at the end of the diastole. When the EDV increases, the cardiac output increases and when EDV decreases, the cardiac output decreases. This occurs due to the operation of the Frank–Starling mechanism. EDV depends on the venous return to the heart.

*Factors that increase preload*

- Increased total blood volume
- Increased venous tone
- Increased pumping action of skeletal muscle
- Increased negative intrathoracic pressure
- Increased atrial contraction

*Factors that decrease preload*

- Decreased blood volume
- Venodilation
- Increased intrapericardial pressure
- Decreased ventricular compliance

### 2. Afterload

Afterload is peripheral resistance. When peripheral resistance increases as in hypertension, the cardiac output decreases and when peripheral resistance decreases as in anemia, the cardiac output increases.

### 3. Myocardial Contractility

The contractility of the myocardium exerts a major influence on the cardiac output. The strength of the cardiac contraction is called *inotropic state* of the heart. The factors that increase the strength of contraction are said to be positively inotropic and the factors that decrease the strength of contraction are said to be negatively inotropic.

*Factors that are positively inotropic*

- Sympathetic stimulation
- Digitalis
- Glucagon
- Caffeine and theophylline

*Factors that are negatively inotropic*

- Parasympathetic stimulation
- Hypoxia, hypercapnea and acidosis
- Loss of myocardium
- Drugs like propranolol, quinidine and barbiturate

### 4. Heart Rate

Increase in heart rate increases cardiac output, and decrease in heart rate decreases cardiac output. However, a change in heart rate cannot significantly alter the cardiac output unless it is associated with a change in ventricular filling.

## Factors Affecting Peripheral Resistance

### 1. Diameter of Blood Vessels

The decrease in vessel diameter (vasoconstriction) increases peripheral resistance and increases blood pressure. Vasodilation decreases peripheral resistance and decreases blood pressure. The diameter of the blood vessels depends mainly on the *vasoconstrictor tone*, which is the rate of discharge in the vasoconstrictor nerves (sympathetic tone). Increase in vasoconstrictor tone causes arteriolar constriction and increases blood pressure and, conversely, decrease in vasoconstrictor tone decreases blood pressure. When the wall of the blood vessel becomes stiff (less compliant), peripheral resistance increases and, therefore, blood pressure increases.

### 2. Viscosity

Viscosity of blood depends on the composition of plasma, total number of cells in the blood, and resistance of the cells to deformation and temperature.

*Factors that increase viscosity*

- Polycythemia
- Hyperproteinemia
- Hereditary spherocytosis
- Decreased temperature

*Factors that decrease viscosity*

- Anemia
- Hypoproteinemia
- Increased temperature

# METHODS

Blood pressure is measured by two methods, direct and indirect.

## Direct Method

The blood pressure is measured directly by placing a cannula in the lumen of the artery and connecting the cannula to a mercury manometer or a pressure transducer. This method is used for recording blood pressure in experimental animals. In humans, blood pressure can be measured directly during open thoracic surgeries. In clinical practice, the blood pressure is measured by the indirect method.

## Indirect Method (Sphygmomanometry)

The instrument used in this method is the sphygmomanometer. Therefore, the method of measurement is called sphygmomanometry.

### Principle

The cuff of the sphygmomanometer is wrapped around the arm of the subject. The bag is then inflated until the air pressure in the cuff overcomes the arterial pressure and obliterates the arterial lumen. This is confirmed by palpating the radial pulse that disappears when the cuff pressure is raised above the arterial pressure. The pressure is then raised further by about 20 mm Hg and then slowly reduced. When the pressure in the cuff reaches just below the arterial pressure, blood escapes beyond the occlusion into the peripheral part of the artery and the pulse starts reappearing. This is detected by the appearance of sounds in the stethoscope and is taken as the systolic pressure. Subsequently, the quality of the sound changes and finally, disappears. The level where sound disappears is taken as the diastolic pressure. The sound disappears because the flow in the blood vessels becomes laminar.

### Requirements

1. Sphygmomanometer
2. Stethoscope

**Sphygmomanometer** The sphygmomanometer (Fig. 25.1) consists of a mercury manometer, cuff and air pump.

*Mercury manometer* The mercury manometer has two limbs. One limb is broader and shorter than the other. The broader limb is the reservoir for mercury. The narrow limb is graduated from 0 to 300 mm, with a smallest division of 2 mm Hg. The mercury reservoir is connected to a rubber tube.

*Cuff* The cuff is called a Riva–Rocci cuff. It consists of an inflatable rubber bag covered by non-distensible cotton fabric. Two tubes are attached to the bag, one transmits air pressure to the mercury manometer and the other is connected to the air pump. The width of the cuff is usually 12 cm. The length and width of the cuff are different for different age groups and body build.

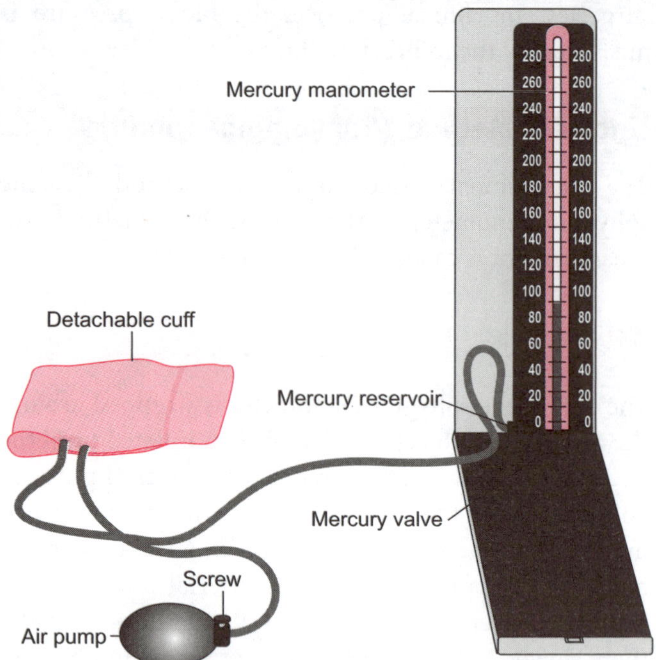


Fig. 25.1 Sphygmomanometer (1: Mercury manometer; 2: Mercury reservoir; 3: Detachable cuff; 4. Air pump; 5: Screw; 6: Mercury valve).

Roughly, the length of the rubber bag should be two-thirds and the width should be one-third of the mid-arm circumference of the subject. The width of the cuff should be 12.5 cm for measuring BP in adults, 8 cm for children up to 8 years, 5 cm for children up to 4 years and 2 to 3 cm for newborns and infants.

*Air pump* It is a rubber hand bulb provided with a one-way valve at its free end and a leak valve arrangement at the other (Fig. 25.1). A rubber tube connects the air pump to the rubber bag. The rubber bag is inflated by turning the screw clockwise and repeatedly compressing the bulb. Deflation of the bag is achieved by turning the screw anti-clockwise.

**Stethoscope** There are two types of stethoscopes, the bell type and the diaphragm type. Modern stethoscopes are a combination of the bell and diaphragm types (Fig. 25.2). The bell type chestpiece detects low-pitched sounds like heart sounds, whereas high-pitched sounds such as aortic diastolic murmurs are better heard with the diaphragm of the stethoscope. For recording blood pressure, the diaphragm type chest piece is used.

### Pre-recording Instructions

Before recording blood pressure, satisfy the following conditions.

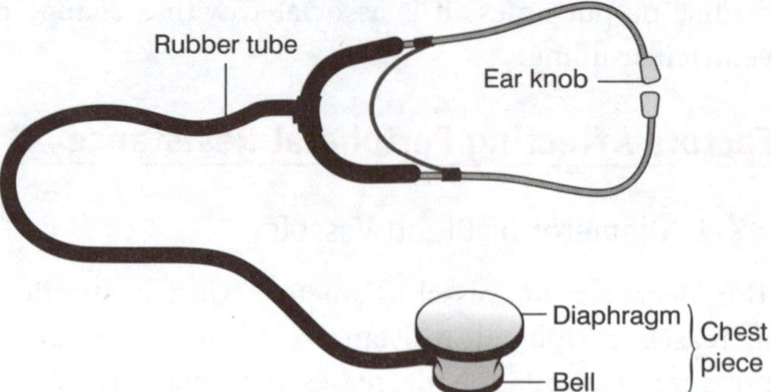


Fig. 25.2 Stethoscope.

1. The subject should be physically and mentally relaxed, free from excitement and apprehension.
2. The subject should lie down or sit comfortably.
3. The 'zero' of the sphygmomanometer and the cuff should be at the level of the heart.

The blood pressure can be measured by three methods: palpatory, auscultatory and oscillatory. Ideally, blood pressure should be measured first by the palpatory and then by the auscultatory method.

## Palpatory Method

### Procedure

1. Check the level of the mercury column in the sphygmomanometer.

> Note: Before recording the blood pressure, it should be ensured that the upper meniscus of the mercury coincides with the 'zero' of the mercury manometer. If the mercury column is higher than the zero level and cannot be readjusted, the difference should be noted and deducted from the final result. But, if the mercury column is below the zero level and cannot be brought up to the zero level, the apparatus should be discarded.

2. Expose the arm up to the shoulder.
3. Wrap the cuff around the middle of the arm (middle of the cuff lies over the brachial artery) in such a way that the lower edge of the cuff remains at a minimum distance of one inch above the cubital fossa.
4. Palpate the radial artery at the wrist by placing the middle three fingers over it.
5. Hold the rubber bulb in the other hand in such a way that your thumb and index finger remain free to manipulate the leak-valve screw.
6. Raise the pressure of the mercury manometer by repeatedly compressing the rubber bulb, and

continue to feel the radial pulse simultaneously. Note the level of the mercury in the manometer scale where the pulse disappears.

7. Raise the mercury column to about 10 mm Hg above the point of disappearance of the pulse.
8. Reduce the pressure gradually by 2–4 mm Hg per second. However, reduction in this pressure may further be slowed if there is significant bradycardia. Note the mercury level where the pulse reappears.

Note: The pulse reappears at the same level where it had disappeared.

9. Reduce the pressure rapidly to the zero level.
10. Note your observation and express the result in mm Hg.

Note: The point of disappearance (or appearance) of the pulse is the blood pressure recorded by the palpatory method. This blood pressure is the systolic pressure.

### Precautions

1. The subject should be mentally and physically relaxed.
2. The subject should lie down or sit comfortably for a minimum of five minutes before the recording.
3. The zero level of the mercury should be checked. If the mercury is not at the zero level, the difference should be noted and deducted from the result.
4. The arm of the subject should be completely exposed and kept at heart level.
5. The cuff should be tied neither very tightly nor loosely around the arm.
6. The width of the cuff should be according to the circumference of the arm to overcome the tissue resistance. The width of the cuff in adults is 12.5 cm. If a narrower cuff is used in adults, the recorded pressure will be falsely high. The narrower cuff is used for children.
7. The cuff and the equipment should be kept at the level of the heart to avoid the effect of gravity. The pressure in any vessel above the heart level is lower and in any vessel below the heart, higher.
8. The level of disappearance or reappearance of the pulse should be noted accurately.

### Advantages

1. A stethoscope is not required for measuring BP.
2. As auscultation is not required, this method can be used by less experienced medical personnel.
3. Recording is not time-consuming.
4. It gives a rough indication of the systolic pressure before recording BP by the auscultatory method.
5. An auscultatory gap, if present, is not missed in the auscultatory method when the blood pressure is first recorded by the palpatory and then by the auscultatory method.

### Disadvantages

1. This method records only the systolic pressure. Diastolic pressure cannot be determined.
2. The systolic pressure recorded is about 2–5 mm Hg less than the actual pressure.

## Auscultatory Method

### Procedure (Fig. 25.3)

1. Record blood pressure by the palpatory method as described above.
2. Raise the pressure to 30 mm Hg above the palpatory level, that is, 30 mm Hg above the level at which radial pulsation is no longer felt.

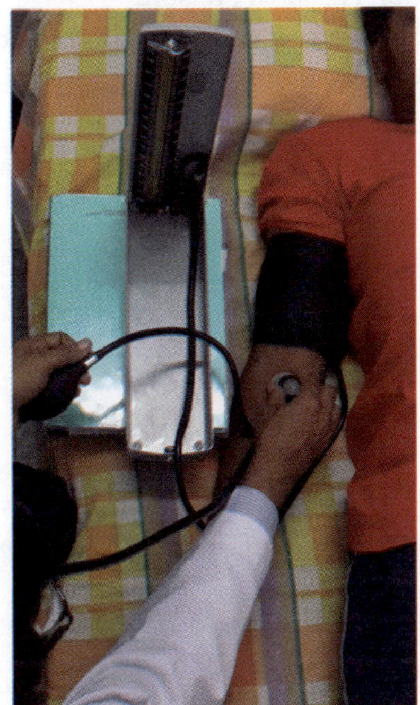

Fig. 25.3 Measurement of blood pressure by auscultatory method. Note that the sphygmomanometer is placed at the level of the heart.

3. Place the diaphragm of the stethoscope lightly on the brachial artery in the cubital fossa, that is, over the upper part of the forearm medial to the tendon of the biceps.
4. Lower the pressure at the rate of 2–4 mm Hg per second. Note the appearance of the sound, the change in character of the sound and finally the cessation of the sound, while the pressure in the cuff is progressively lowered.
5. Note the level where the sounds are first heard as the systolic pressure, and the level where the sounds cease as the diastolic pressure.

> Note: When pressure in the cuff is progressively lowered, the sounds undergoes a series of changes in their quality and intensity. These sounds are known as Korotkoff sounds (described by the Russian scientist Korotkoff in 1905). They are heard in five different phases (Fig. 25.4).

Phase I : Sudden appearance of faint tapping sounds which become gradually louder and clearer during the succeeding 10 mm Hg fall in pressure.

Phase II : The sound becomes murmurish in the next 10 mm Hg fall in pressure.

Phase III : The sound changes a little in quality but becomes clearer and louder in the next 15 mm Hg fall in pressure.

Phase IV : Sounds become muffled in character during the next 5 mm Hg fall.

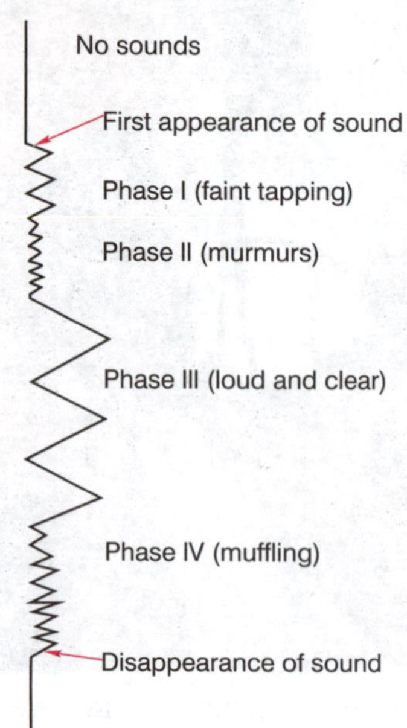


Fig. 25.4 Phases of Korotkoff sounds.

Phase V : Sounds completely disappear.

Appearance of the sound is recorded as systolic blood pressure and disappearance of sound as diastolic blood pressure. In persons with severe hypertension and in children, muffling rather than the disappearance of the sound is taken as the diastolic pressure.

## Precautions

1. The subject should be mentally and physically relaxed.
2. The size of the cuff should be proportionate to the circumference of the arm of the subject.
3. The zero reading of the manometer should be kept at the level of the heart.
4. Blood pressure should be detected first by the palpatory method before recording by the auscultatory method.
5. Pressure must be raised by 30 mm Hg above the palpatory level.
6. The cuff pressure should be decreased to the zero level between successive trials.
7. While reading the manometer, the eye should be at the level of the mercury column to avoid parallax.
8. If coarctation of the aorta is suspected, blood pressure should also be recorded in the thigh.

> Note: A cuff of greater width (about 18 cm) is used for measuring blood pressure in the thigh. The patient lies face downwards, the cuff is applied above the knee and auscultation is carried out over the popliteal artery.

Blood pressure should ideally be checked by the palpatory method before recording by the auscultatory method.

> Note: Blood pressure is checked by the palpatory method before the auscultatory method to include the auscultatory gap in the pressure range. In severely hypertensive patients, after the appearance of the sounds, occasionally the sounds disappear at a point below 200 mm Hg for a range of 20–50 mm Hg and then reappear and finally disappear at the level of diastolic pressure. The period of first (temporary) disappearance of sounds is called silent gap or auscultatory gap. The auscultatory gap is never missed if the pressure is measured first by the palpatory method because the auscultatory gap comes within the range of the systolic pressure recorded by the palpatory method. If the BP is directly measured by the auscultatory method, the auscultatory gap may be missed and the systolic value may be reported as lower than the actual value. The exact cause of the auscultatory gap is not known. It is thought to be due to the transient hyper-responsiveness of the vessel to compression.

9. The cuff and the equipment should be kept at the level of the heart to avoid the effect of gravity (Fig. 25.5).

### Disadvantages

1. Unless followed by the palpatory method, the auscultatory method may miss the auscultatory gap.
2. Needs adequate experience of detecting sounds by the stethoscope.

### Advantages

1. Gives the accurate value of systolic pressure.
2. Detects diastolic pressure.

### Special Notes

1. Diastolic pressure recorded in the sitting posture is about 5 mm Hg more than in the supine posture.
2. Arm position above and below heart level gives lower and higher BP values, respectively.
3. If BP values are different between two arms, higher value should be used.

## Oscillatory Method

### Procedure

The procedure is the same as that in the palpatory method, but instead of palpating the artery, the oscillations of the mercury column in the sphygmomanometer is noted to record BP. The pressure in the cuff is raised and the appearance and the disappearance of the oscillations of the mercury column are noted while lowering the mercury column. The point of appearance of the oscillation gives the systolic pressure, and the point of disappearance of the oscillations gives the diastolic pressure.

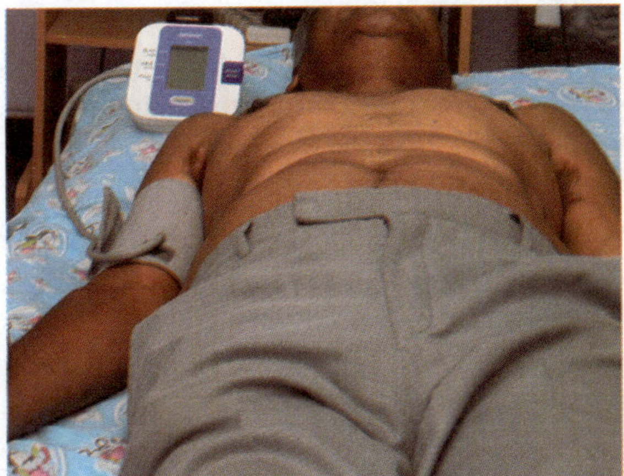

Fig. 25.5 Recording of BP using automatic BP monitor. Note that the cuff and the equipment are approximately at the level of the heart.

### Disadvantages

1. This method does not give accurate systolic and diastolic pressure.
2. Needs adequate experience to detect the exact level of the appearance and disappearance of oscillation.

# DISCUSSION

## Clinical Significance

### Physiological Conditions Altering BP

1. **Age** Blood pressure increases with age.
   In children : Systolic pressure is 90–119 mm Hg.
   Diastolic pressure is 50–79 mm Hg.
   In adults : Systolic pressure is 100–119 mm Hg.
   Diastolic pressure is 60–79 mm Hg.
   In elderly : The upper limit of systolic is considered to be 160 mm Hg, but diastolic 90 mm Hg or above is always considered abnormal.
2. **Gender** BP is less in females due to the effect of progesterone that relaxes the smooth muscles of the blood vessels. Also, cardiac vagal drive is relatively more in females compared to males. Therefore, the heart rate is comparatively less in females. Consequently, the systolic BP is less in females compared to males. This difference in females disappears after menopause.
3. **Eating** BP increases after a meal. This may be due to increased body metabolism that increases the circulation.
4. **Sleep** BP is less during sleep than in the waking state. This is because the human being is under constant stress which is absent in sleep.
5. **Emotion and excitement** In emotional and excited states, increased sympathetic discharge increases the blood pressure.

6. **Exercise** During exercise, the systolic pressure always rises because of increased cardiac output due to sympathetic stimulation which causes tachycardia and increased myocardial contractility. Diastolic pressure depends on the degree of exercise. Diastolic pressure increases in mild exercise due to vasoconstriction, remains unchanged or may even fall in moderate exercise, but always falls in intense exercise because of metabolic vasodilation and increased body temperature.
7. **Posture** On immediate standing from the supine posture, BP decreases and then returns to normal or increases due to correction by the baroreceptor reflex.
8. **Temperature** BP decreases in a hot environment due to vasodilation and increases in a cold environment due to vasoconstriction.
9. **Pregnancy** Increase in cardiac output due to increased blood volume increases systolic pressure during pregnancy, but diastolic pressure falls due to decreased peripheral resistance. Peripheral resistance decreases due to the effect of progesterone which relaxes the smooth muscle of blood vessels (causes vasodilation). Therefore, pulse pressure increases in pregnancy.

### Pathological Conditions Altering BP

Blood pressure increases (hypertension) and decreases (hypotension) in different pathological conditions.

## Pathophysiology of Hypertension

Hypertension is defined as sustained elevation of systemic arterial pressure. Usually, hypertension means rise in diastolic BP. Hypertension is broadly classified as essential and secondary.

### Essential Hypertension

This is the commonest cause of hypertension and is seen in 90 per cent of patients with hypertension. The cause of essential hypertension is not known, but is thought to be due to a hereditary defect that predisposes a person to hypertension.

### Secondary Hypertension

This is the hypertension secondary to a disease elsewhere in the body. The following are the causes of secondary hypertension.

1. Adrenocortical diseases
   - Hyperaldosteronism
   - Cushing syndrome
   - Hypertensive form of congenital virilising tumour
2. Renal diseases
   - Glomerulonephritis
   - Pyelonephritis
   - Polycystic disease
   - Tumours of JG cells
3. Pheochromocytoma
4. Severe polycythemia
5. Oral contraceptives

## Pathophysiology of Hypotension

Systolic pressure less than 90 mm Hg in adults is known as hypotension. Clinically, there are three types of hypotension: (1) chronic hypotension, (2) acute hypotension and (3) postural hypotension.

### Chronic Hypotension

Chronic hypotension is characterised by persistent low blood pressure. Usually, the patients are asymptomatic, but sometimes they complain of lethargy, weakness and giddiness.

**Causes**

- Primary adrenocortical insufficiency
- Hypopituitarism
- Malnutrition and anemia
- Chronic diarrhea
- Prolonged bed rest

### Acute Hypotension

The sudden fall of blood pressure is called acute hypotension. Usually, if severe, it is associated with fainting.

**Causes**

- Acute hemorrhage
- Acute diarrhea
- Severe vomiting
- Acute myocardial infarction
- Excessive diuresis
- Acute vasodilation

### Postural Hypotension

If systolic blood pressure falls by 20 mm Hg or more when a subject assumes an erect posture (from the supine posture), the condition is called postural or *orthostatic hypotension*. This usually results from autonomic imbalance. It may be of chronic or acute variety.

**Acute postural hypotension** This is due to temporary fall in blood pressure, which results in transient fainting. It is usually seen in the following conditions:

- Prolonged standing
- Rising from bed after a prolonged illness
- Strenuous physical exercise

**Chronic postural hypotension** Chronic postural hypotension can be primary or secondary. *Chronic primary postural hypotension* is called idiopathic postural hypotension. The cause of this hypotension is not known. It usually occurs in the elderly and may be due to the degeneration of peripheral autonomic nerves. Chronic secondary postural hypotension has following causes:

- Polyneuropathy as seen in diabetes, amyloidosis and beriberi
- Autonomic neuropathy as seen in syringomyelia, tabes dorsalis and subacute combined degeneration of spinal cord
- Patients receiving sympatholytic drugs
- Surgical sympathectomy

## Regulation of Blood Pressure

The mechanisms involved in regulation of blood pressure can be divided into two broad categories: (1) Short-term regulation and (2) Long-term regulation. Short-term regulation is mainly neural and long-term regulation is mainly hormonal.

### Short-term Regulation

**Baroreceptor reflex** Baroreceptors are present in the carotid sinus and aortic arch, and respond to stretching. They detect any change in pressure in the vessels in which they are situated. Increase in blood pressure causes distension of the carotid sinus and aortic arch, which stretches the baroreceptors and increases the firing rate in the afferent nerves (IX and X cranial nerves). This leads to excitation of the nucleus tractus solitarius (NTS) in the medulla, which in turn inhibits the vasomotor centre via interneurons. The inhibition of the vasomotor centre decreases the sympathetic output and causes vasodilation, bradycardia, decrease in cardiac output and fall in blood pressure. The excitation of NTS also stimulates the vagus nerve, which decreases the heart rate and cardiac output.

Conversely, when blood pressure falls, less distension of the carotid sinus and aortic arch inhibits the receptors and decreases the discharge rate in the afferent nerves. Due to decreased activity in the IX and X cranial nerves, NTS is inhibited, which in turn causes disinhibition (stimulation) of the vasomotor centre, which increases sympathetic output. Inhibition of NTS also inhibits the vagus nerve. This finally results in vasoconstriction, tachycardia, increased cardiac output and increase in blood pressure. The baroreceptor reflex regulates blood pressure in the pressure range of 70–150 mm Hg.

**Chemoreceptor reflex** Chemoreceptors are located in the aortic and carotid bodies. They respond to the change in chemical composition of blood, which occurs in conditions like hypoxia, hypercapnea and acidosis. Stimulation of these receptors results in bradycardia and vasoconstriction. This also causes pulmonary hyperventilation and secretion of catecholamines from the adrenal medulla, which increase heart rate. Therefore, the net effect of stimulation of chemoreceptors is no change in heart rate or mild tachycardia, and hypertension. Chemoreceptors regulate blood pressure in the pressure range of 40–70 mm Hg.

**Cushing's reflex** In severe hypotension, blood flow to the brain decreases. Hypoxia and hypercapnea of vasomotor centre occur. This causes stimulation of vasomotor centre to the maximum, which results in intense vasoconstriction that attempts to bring the pressure back to normal. This response is called *CNS ischemic response* and is a life-saving mechanism when blood pressure falls below 40 mm Hg.

When intracranial pressure increases, blood flow to the vasomotor centre decreases due to compression of blood vessels. This stimulates the vasomotor centre and causes intense vasoconstriction, which results in increased blood pressure. This is called *Cushing's reflex*. The increase in blood pressure activates the baroreceptor reflex and causes bradycardia. Therefore, bradycardia rather than tachycardia is an outstanding feature of brain tumours.

**Capillary fluid shift** When blood pressure increases, the hydrostatic pressure in the capillaries increases. This causes a shift of fluid from the intravascular compartment to the extravascular space. As a result the circulating blood volume decreases and blood pressure falls to normal.

**Stress relaxation** When blood pressure increases suddenly, the smooth muscles of the blood vessels relax in response to sudden stretching. This decreases the vascular tone and brings the pressure back to normal.

**Hormonal mechanisms** Catecholamines are released from the adrenal medulla when sympathetic discharge increases, as in hemorrhage and hypotension. The norepinephrine is a potent vasoconstrictor. The renin–angiotensin system is also activated when blood pressure falls. Angiotensin II is a potent vasoconstrictor.

## Long-term Regulation

Long-term regulation is mainly achieved by hormonal mechanisms that involve changes in the fluid volume of the body. The kidneys also play a role in long-term regulation of BP.

### *Hormonal Mechanism*

1. **The renin–angiotensin system** Fall in blood pressure releases renin from the JG cells of the kidney. Renin converts angtiotensinogen to angiotensin I, which is further converted to angiotensin II. Angiotensin II causes vasoconstriction and increases blood pressure. Angiotensin II also increases synthesis and secretion of aldosterone, which increases sodium and water reabsorption from the kidney,which in turn assists in restoration of pressure.
2. **Vasopressin (ADH)** Decrease in extracellular fluid volume increases the release of ADH from the posterior pituitary. ADH increases water reabsorption from the kidneys and causes vasoconstriction.
3. **Catecholamines** Stimulation of sympathetic fibres to the adrenal medulla causes the release of catecholamines. These hormones (especially norepinephrine) are potent vasoconstrictors.

### *Renal Mechanism*

When alteration in blood pressure occurs, the kidneys try to restore the pressure by changing the excretion of sodium and water. This mechanism is independent of other factors and is intrinsic to the kidneys.

## VIVA

1. Define blood pressure.
2. Define systolic and diastolic blood pressure and give their normal values.
3. What is mean arterial pressure and what is its significance?
4. What is pulse pressure and what is its significance?
5. What are the methods of measurement of blood pressure?
6. What are the conditions that must be satisfied before recording blood pressure?
7. Why are the zero level of the sphygmomanometer and the cuff kept at the heart level of the subject while recording blood pressure?
8. Why is the blood pressure ideally recorded by the palpatory method before recording by the auscultatory method?
9. What are the precautions for measuring blood pressure by the palpatory method?
10. Why is the pressure in the cuff raised by about 30 mm Hg above the palpatory level for recording blood pressure by the auscultatory method?
11. What is auscultatory gap and what is its significance?
12. What is the cause of the appearance, change in quality and disappearance of the sounds at various phases of blood pressure measurement?
13. What is the ideal size of the cuff for different age groups?
14. What are the precautions taken for recording blood pressure by the auscultatory method?
15. What is the oscillatory method of measurement of blood pressure?
16. In which condition is the blood pressure measured in the lower limb and what is the size of the cuff used for this purpose?
17. What are the factors that affect blood pressure?
18. Why is the pressure lower in females?
19. Why is the pressure lower during sleep?
20. What is the mechanism of alteration of systolic and diastolic pressure during exercise?
21. What happens to blood pressure on immediately standing from the supine position?

22. What is the baroreceptor reflex and what is its significance?
23. What is essential hypertension?
24. What are the causes of secondary hypertension?
25. What are the causes of acute hypotension?
26. What is postural hypotension and what are the causes of postural hypotension?
27. What are the mechanisms of short-term regulation of blood pressure?
28. Why is bradycardia a feature of raised intracranial pressure?
29. What is the role of the renin–angiotensin system in the genesis of hypertension?

Chapter 26

# Effect of Posture on Blood Pressure and Heart Rate

### Learning Objectives

After completing this practical, you will be able to:

- Record the effect of change in posture on heart rate and blood pressure.
- List the precautions to be taken while recording this effect.
- Enumerate the changes in response to standing.

You may also be able to:

- Explain the compensatory mechanisms in response to standing.
- Describe the physiological and clinical utility of this practical.

## INTRODUCTION

Change in body posture affects the functions of the cardiovascular system. The changes are more marked when a person immediately stands up from the supine posture. The cardiovascular changes are different on immediate standing and on prolonged standing.

### Cardiovascular Changes on Immediate Standing

#### Effect

When a person assumes an erect posture, the blood is pulled to the lower parts of the body due to the effect of gravity. About 200–500 ml of blood is immediately pulled in the capacitance vessels of the lower extremities. This decreases venous return, which results in decreased cardiac output. This is the cause of immediate fall in blood pressure on standing. The effects of a change in posture are more marked if it is done passively with the help of a tilting table, as the muscular activity of the act of standing is absent in passive tilt. The muscle activity after assuming the posture is also lower in passive tilting. The mean arterial pressure in the feet in the standing posture is 180–200 mm Hg and at the head level is 60–80 mm Hg, the venous pressure at feet level is 85–90 mm Hg and at the head level is 0.

#### Compensatory Mechanisms

The immediate compensatory mechanisms on standing are vasoconstriction, tachycardia and increased cardiac output. These compensatory mechanisms are triggered by a fall in blood pressure, and are mediated by the baroreceptor reflex. Decreased pressure in the carotid and aortic sinus decreases the rate of discharge from the baroreceptors, which in turn decreases stimulation of nucleus tractus solitarius (NTS). This in turn decreases vagal activity and increases sympathetic activity, which results in restoration of blood pressure.

### Cardiovascular Changes on Prolonged Standing

#### Effect

If the individual does not move (stands still) for a longer period, more than 500 ml of blood is pulled in the capacitance vessels of the lower extremities. This increases the capillary hydrostatic pressure in the lower limbs. The fluid from the intravascular compartment moves into the interstitial tissue spaces and accumulates there, as a result of which venous return to the heart significantly decreases. This decreases the stroke volume by up to 40 per cent. Therefore, cardiac output is considerably reduced, which decreases cerebral blood flow. The subject may become unconscious and fall. Fainting is a homeostatic mechanism to restore venous return, cardiac output and cerebral blood flow in the horizontal position by automatic change of posture.

#### Compensatory Mechanisms

The baroreceptor reflex restores blood pressure to normal. Activation of sympathetic fibres leads to release of catecholamines from the adrenal medulla. Catecholamines increase heart rate, cardiac output and blood pressure. The renin–angiotensin–aldosterone axis is also activated. Angiotensin II causes vasoconstriction and increases blood pressure. Aldosterone increases reabsorption of sodium and water from the kidneys and maintains blood volume and pressure. But, if the subject continues to stand for a much longer period, the compensatory mechanisms may fail and the subject may develop features of hypotension.

## METHODS

### Method to Measure the Effect of Posture on Heart Rate and BP

#### Principle

On resuming an erect posture, changes occur in cardiovascular function. The change in heart rate and blood pressure is noted immediately on standing and after two, five and ten minutes of standing. These changes are compared with the heart rate and blood pressure recorded in the supine position prior to the change in posture.

#### Requirements

1. Sphygmomanometer
2. Stethoscope

#### Procedure

1. Ask the subject to lie down in the supine position on the couch, minimum for 5 minutes.
2. Tie the BP cuff properly at the proper position of the arm of the subject.
3. Record blood pressure and pulse rate in the supine position.
4. Do not remove the BP cuff; ask the subject to stand up, and immediately record the pulse rate and blood pressure of the subject.

> Note: The subject should stand with the support of the wall (leaning against the wall) to prevent the effect of muscle–heart reflex. The increase in heart rate due to contraction of skeletal muscles is known as muscle–heart reflex. If the subject stands without support, the muscles in the lower limb and trunk contract more, which affects the heart rate. Therefore, maximum possible relaxation should be achieved during the procedure by asking the subject to stand passively.

5. Record pulse rate and blood pressure two, five and ten minutes after standing.
6. Calculate pulse pressure, mean pressure and rate pressure product from the heart rate and blood pressure.
7. Enter your observation in a tabular form.

#### Observation

Enter your observation in a format as given in Table 26.1. Note that BP falls immediately on standing. Within 15–30 seconds, systolic pressure returns to normal (or remains slightly elevated), but diastolic pressure remains elavated and tachycardia persists.

#### Precautions

1. The subject should relax for 5 minutes before recording blood pressure and pulse rate in the supine position.
2. Pulse rate and blood pressure should be recorded as soon as the patient stands up (within 15 seconds if possible).
3. The BP cuff should not be removed while changing the posture of the subject.
4. The subject should stand passively (leaning against the wall).

## DISCUSSION

The immediate result of standing is that the cardiac output decreases due to pooling of blood in the lower extremities. Therefore, a fall in blood pressure is noted immediately (if possible within 15 seconds). The fall in pressure (through baroreceptor reflex) results in tachycardia, increased cardiac output and vasoconstriction. Therefore, within 15–30 seconds the blood pressure reverts to normal. But, because of vasoconstriction peripheral resistance increases, which in turn increases the diastolic pressure. Heart

Table 26.1 Change in posture observation.

| Posture | PR | SBP | DBP | PP | MP | RPP |
|---|---|---|---|---|---|---|
| **Supine (after 5 min)** | | | | | | |
| On standing: | | | | | | |
| 1. Immediate | | | | | | |
| 2. After 2 min | | | | | | |
| 3. After 5 min | | | | | | |
| 4. After 10 min | | | | | | |

PR = Pulse rate; SBP = Systolic blood pressure; DBP = Diastolic blood pressure; PP = Pulse pressure; MP = Mean pressure; RPP = Rate pressure product (RPP = systolic pressure × heart rate × $10^{-2}$).

rate increases and systolic pressure remains normal or slightly raised.

## Physiological Significance

A change in posture initiates changes in cardiovascular function, which can be detected by various tests. These changes reflect the integrity of the autonomous nervous system, because the compensatory mechanisms are dependent on the intactness of the reflex activities, especially the baroreceptor reflex. Therefore, the heart rate and blood pressure response to standing is among the important tests to assess autonomic functions. This test detects the efficiency of cardiovascular and autonomic functions.

## Clinical Significance

### 1. Postural Hypotension

In some individuals, sudden standing causes a significant fall in blood pressure (fall in systolic pressure of more than 20 mm Hg and fall in diastolic pressure of more than 10 mm Hg), which results in fainting. This is called postural or *orthostatic hypotension*. It is usually seen in patients with autonomic neuropathy like diabetes or syphilis. It also occurs in patients receiving sympatholytic drugs. This is also seen in *primary autonomic failure* and sometimes in *primary hyperaldosteronism*, because the baroreceptor reflex is abnormal in these conditions.

### 2. Therapeutic Uses

Acute change of postures are part of the practice of different asanas. Regular practice of change of postures (asanas) improves autonomic functions. Persons practising asanas regularly keep good health, as it improves their cardiac, respiratory, neuromuscular, autonomic, mental and physiological functions. Of late, asanas have become popular because of their beneficial effects.

### 3. Problems of Traffic Personnel

Traffic police personnel stand (without activity) for hours together. This causes accumulation of fluid in the lower parts of the body and may cause hypotension and pedal edema, and sometimes results in fainting. Therefore, instead of standing at one place, these people are advised to walk around so that the skeletal muscle pump activity increases the venous return and maintains cardiac output and blood pressure.

## VIVA

1. What are the physiological changes that occur on suddenly standing up and why?
2. What are the physiological changes that occur on prolonged standing and why?
3. Why should the pulse rate and blood pressure ideally be recorded within 15 seconds to record the immediate cardiovascular response to standing?
4. What is the significance of RPP (rate pressure product)?
   Ans. As RPP is the product of heart rate and systolic BP, it reflects the myocardial work load. RPP is the index of myocardial oxygen demand and work stress. Chronically elevated RPP is a known cardiovascular risk.
5. What is the physiological and clinical utility of this practical?

# Chapter 27

# Effect of Exercise on Blood Pressure and Heart Rate

## Learning Objectives

After completing this practical, you will be able to:

- Describe the importance of study of the effect of exercise on blood pressure and heart rate.
- List the types and degrees of exercise.
- Record the effect of exercise on heart rate and blood pressure.
- List the precautions of recording this effect.
- Explain the effects of exercise on heart rate and blood pressure.

You may also be able to:

- Explain the differences between isotonic and isometric exercise.
- Describe and explain the various effects of acute and chronic exercise on different body systems.
- State the therapeutic uses of exercise in common diseases.

## INTRODUCTION

Regular exercise improves health. Exercise affects all the body systems and improves the functioning of almost all the organs of the body. The body's response to exercise can be a short-term response to an acute exercise or a long-term response to chronic exercise. Long-term response to regular exercise makes the exercise easier and improves performance. What has been described in this chapter is the body's response to acute exercise; the short-term heart rate and blood pressure response to a single bout of exercise (acute exercise). The immediate response to acute exercise depends on the degree and type of exercise, and the exercise training that the individual has received. Exercise training means the regular practice of exercise for months or years together. The cardiovascular response to exercise is different in trained and untrained individuals.

### Degree of Exercise

Depending on the rate of oxygen consumption, work done and rate of rise in heart rate, exercise is classified into three categories: mild, moderate and severe.

**Mild exercise** In this case, oxygen consumption is 0.5–1 litre per minute, work done is 150–350 watts, and rise in heart rate is about 25 per cent, that is, if the basal heart rate is 80, the heart rate will increase to about 100 per minute.

**Moderate exercise** In this case, oxygen consumption is 1–2 litres per minute, work done is 350–550 watts and rise in heart rate is about 50 per cent, that is, it rises from a basal heart rate of 80 to 120 per minute.

**Severe exercise** In this, oxygen consumption is more than 2 litres per minute, work done is more than 550 watts and rise is heart rate is about 75–100 per cent, that is, from a basal heart rate of 80 per minute it increases to 150 per minute or more.

### Types of Exercises

Exercise may be isotonic or isometric.

**Isotonic exercise** In isotonic exercise, there is a change in muscle length and the exercise is phasic in nature. Common examples are walking, jogging and running.

*Cardiovascular changes in isotonic exercise*

- Heart rate increases proportionately with the severity of exercise.
- Cardiac output increases markedly due to increase in heart rate and stroke volume.
- Systolic pressure increases.
- Diastolic pressure increases in mild exercise, does not change or decreases slightly in moderate exercise and always decreases in severe exercise.
- Blood flow to exercising muscle increases.

**Isometric exercise** Isometric exercise is the exercise in which there is no change in the length of the muscles. The exercising muscle remains contracted throughout the maneuver (e.g., pushing against the wall). Therefore, this type of exercise is called tonic exercise.

*Cardiovascular changes in isometric exercise*

- Heart rate rises at the start of exercise. This is mainly due to decreased vagal tone. Increased discharge of cardiac sympathetic fibres may also contribute.
- Stroke volume changes relatively little.
- Systolic and diastolic pressures rise sharply.
- Blood flow to the exercising muscle decreases.

The cardiovascular response to isometric exercise is different, because the exercising muscles are tonically contracted during exercise. Peripheral resistance increases, which increases diastolic pressure significantly in isometric exercise.

# METHODS

## Method to Study Effect of Exercise on Pulse Rate and BP

### Principle

Cardiovascular functions alter during exercise. Pulse rate and blood pressure are recorded before and immediately after the exercise. The results are compared to study the effect of exercise on these parameters.

### Requirements

1. Stethoscope
2. Sphygmomanometer

### Procedure

1. Record the blood pressure (by using sphygmomanometer) and the pulse rate of the given subject after 5 minutes of rest.
2. Ask the subject to perform spot jogging for a period of 5 minutes.
3. Record the pulse rate and blood pressure immediately, 2, 4, 6, 8 and 10 minutes after the exercise.
4. Calculate pulse pressure, mean pressure and rate pressure product and compare the pre- and post-exercise values.

> Note: Rate pressure product = Systolic pressure × Heart rate × $10^{-2}$. RPP is a good index of myocardial function.

5. Record your observation in a tabular form.

### Observation

Record your observation in the format given in Table 27.1. Note that heart rate and systolic pressure rise significantly immediately after exercise. As 5 minute spot jogging is a mild exercise, diastolic pressure also rises (or may not change). Pulse pressure changes accordingly. Also note that blood pressure returns to normal within 5–7 minutes of termination of exercise, whereas the heart rate takes a longer time to return to normal.

### Precautions

1. The pre- and post-exercise heart rate and blood pressure should be recorded in the same position. Note: To eliminate the effect of posture on BP, it should be recorded in the standing position both before and after exercise. If BP is recorded in the supine or sitting posture before exercise, then post-exercise BP should also be recorded in the same position. As exercise is done in the erect posture, it is better to record BP in the standing posture.
2. The subject should be encouraged to exercise properly for five minutes.
3. For the first recording following exercise (immediately after exercise), blood pressure and pulse rate should be recorded as quickly as possible.

# DISCUSSION

## Effect of Acute Exercise

### Cardiovascular Changes

**Heart rate** Heart rate increases and the degree of increase depends on the severity of the exercise. The maximum heart rate achieved during exercise decreases

Table 27.1 Exercise observation.

| | PR | SBP | DBP | PP | MP | RPP |
|---|---|---|---|---|---|---|
| 1. Basal (before exercise) | | | | | | |
| 2. Immediately after exercise | | | | | | |
| 3. Two minutes after exercise | | | | | | |
| 4. Four minutes after exercise | | | | | | |
| 5. Ten minutes after exercise | | | | | | |

PR = Pulse rate; SBP = Systolic blood pressure; DBP = Diastolic blood pressure; PP = Pulse pressure; MP = Mean pressure; RPP = Rate pressure product.

with age. In children, the heart rate can rise up to 200 beats per minute or more; in adults it seldom rises above this and in elderly subjects, it rarely goes beyond 150.

**Cardiac output** There occurs a marked increase in cardiac output. Cardiac output may increase even up to 25 litres per minute or more. Increase in cardiac output is due to increase in heart rate and stroke volume.

**Systolic blood pressure** Systolic pressure rises markedly. This occurs due to increased cardiac output.

**Diastolic blood pressure** Diastolic pressure may remain unchanged or may fall. This occurs due to decreased peripheral resistance, which is due to vasodilation in the exercising muscle.

**Muscle blood flow** Blood flow to the skeletal muscle increases due to vasodilation in the skeletal bed. There occurs vasoconstriction in the cutaneous and splanchnic circulation. So, the blood is diverted from the cutaneous and visceral circulation to the skeletal vascular bed.

#### *Physiological Basis of Cardiovascular Changes*

- Cardiac output increases due to increased heart rate and stroke volume. Tachycardia and increased stroke volume occur due to increased activity in the noradrenergic sympathetic nerves to the heart. Sympathetic activity increases by psychic stimuli and stimulation of receptors in the muscles, joints and tendons. Inhibition of vagal tone also contributes to tachycardia. Stroke volume increases due to increased myocardial contractility by sympathetic stimulation and also due to increased venous return. Venous return increases due to sympathetic venoconstriction and increased skeletal muscle pump activity. Increased thoracic pump and mobilisation of blood from the splanchnic and cutaneous beds also contribute to increased venous return.
- The systolic pressure increases due to increase in cardiac output.
- The diastolic pressure increases in mild exercise due to sympathetic vasoconstriction. But in moderate exercise, diastolic pressure remains normal or falls and in severe exercise it always falls. This occurs due to vasodilation in the exercising muscle. The blood vessels in the skeletal vascular bed receive sympathetic vasodilator fibres. Therefore, vasodilation occurs in the skeletal bed. In addition, the systemic blood vessels also dilate in severe exercise due to: (i) rise in body temperature (thermal vasodilation), and (ii) deposition of metabolites like lactic acid, $K^+$ and $CO_2$ in the active tissues (metabolic vasodilation). Total peripheral resistance decreases due to vasodilation. Therefore, in spite of increased sympathetic activity diastolic pressure falls during severe exercise.
- Muscle blood flow increases to a great extent. This happens even before the start of exercise. The initial increase in blood flow is due to neural mechanisms and continued blood flow is due to local mechanisms. The neural mechanism is the activation of the sympathetic vasodilator system and a decrease in tonic vasoconstrictor discharge. The local mechanisms are accumulation of metabolites and rise in temperature in the active muscles. Vasodilation opens up many closed capillaries.

### Respiratory Changes

- There is hyperventilation and increased oxygen supply to the tissues. Hyperventilation also removes excess $CO_2$ and heat produced by the active tissues.
- Respiratory minute volume increases linearly with work rate.
- Pulmonary blood flow increases and this increases perfusion of alveoli.

### Other Changes

- The body metabolism increases.
- The body temperature increases.
- Catecholamine secretion from the adrenal medulla and glucocorticoid secretion from the adrenal cortex increase.
- Glycogenolysis is stimulated in the liver and skeletal muscles.
- Lipolysis occurs in prolonged aerobic exercise.

## Effect of Regular Exercise (Training) on Health

### On the Cardiovascular System

There is profound improvement in cardiovascular function. The basal heart rate decreases due to increased vagal tone. Stroke volume increases due to increased myocardial muscle mass. A trained subject achieves the required cardiac output during exercise mainly by increasing the stroke volume rather than by heart rate, whereas an untrained individual achieves the same cardiac output mainly by increasing the heart rate. The blood pressure is usually maintained within the normal range. Hypertension usually does not occur unless associated with some secondary pathology.

### On the Respiratory System

There is increase in breathing capacity and $VO_{2max}$. $VO_{2max}$ is the product of maximal cardiac output and maximal oxygen extraction by the tissues. Both these parameters increase with training.

### On the Skeletal Muscles

The size of the muscles and work capability increase. The number of mitochondria and the enzymes involved in oxidative metabolism increases. The number of capillaries increases, which increases extraction of oxygen.

### On the Mind

Exercise improves memory and intellectual mental functions.

## Clinical Significance

Exercise is becoming popular nowadays because of its visible therapeutic advantages. It is regularly prescribed as part of treatment for patients suffering from cardiovascular diseases, especially hypertension and myocardial infarction. It has been seen that isotonic exercise (mild to moderate) performed regularly, decreases blood pressure significantly in otherwise resistant cases of hypertension. Exercise also improves cardiac performance in patients suffering from myocardial infarction, and prevents infarction in subjects at risk. Exercise also improves joint functions, and is therefore prescribed in patients suffering from chronic joint diseases.

## Exercise Stress Testing

Measurements of cardiovascular functions during rest are poor predictors of cardiac performance as there is substantial cardiovascular reserve capacity. Exercise is currently used as the most convenient way of stimulating the myocardium to demand maximal blood flow so that even a moderate impairment of coronary blood flow capacity becomes detectable.

**Indications for exercise testing**

1. Evaluation of patients with chest pain.
2. Evaluation of functional capacity of the heart.
3. Evaluation of patients after myocardial infarction.
4. Evaluation of patients after coronary artery by-pass surgery.
5. Screening for latent coronary artery disease.
6. Evaluation of patients with valvular heart disease.
7. Evaluation of arrhythmias.

**Contraindications to stress test**

1. Impending or acute myocardial infarction.
2. Unstable angina.
3. Severe hypertension.
4. Congestive heart failure.
5. Severe aortic stenosis.
6. Uncontrolled arrhythmias.

### Basic Principle and Procedure

The patient is made to exercise to 90% of his estimated maximal heart rate. The maximal heart rate is calculated from the age, sex, and physical training of the subject. The cardiac efficiency is tested by analysing the patient's ability to achieve the target heart rate.

The methods of exercise stress testing can be divided into two broad categories: the dynamic lower extremity testing, and the dynamic upper extremity testing. The lower extremity tests include treadmill, bicycle ergometry, and Master's step test and upper extremity testing includes arm ergometry.

### Dynamic Lower Extremity Testing

*Treadmill*

Treadmill testing is a most widely used method for exercise testing. This includes simultaneous recordings of multiple leads of ECG in a computerized treadmill. The person exercises until he achieves his target heart rate or is unable to continue because of chest pain, dyspnea and intolerable fatigue. There are different protocols like Bruce protocol, Naughton protocol, and Balke and Ware protocol. In different protocols analyses of the heart rate achievement is different.

*Bicycle Ergometry*

This is used when a patient is unable to do treadmill exercise. It is the method of chaos during radionuclide ventriculography and for dynamic testing during cardiac catheterization. Details of the procedure is described in the chapter of 'Bicycle ergometry'.

*Master's Step Test*

In this, the subject walks up and down over a device two steps high with three steps, two of which are 9 inches above the floor and a top step 18 inches high. The exercise is carried out for a prescribed number of ascents. The workload achieved in this test is usually too low to be of any significant clinical use. Therefore, after the advent of treadmill and bicycle ergometer this method of exercise testing has lost its popularity and is seldom used now.

## Dynamic Upper Extremity Testing

### *Arm Ergometry*

This is sometimes used in patients with peripheral vascular disease or in orthopedic abnormalities. Arm ergometry is less sensitive than leg ergometry for eliciting exercise-induced ischemia.

## Exercise Test Response

Exercise responses are mainly assessed by ECG changes. When the heart rate increases with exercise, a number of predictable changes occur in normal ECG. The PR interval shortens, the P wave becomes taller, and the atrial repolarisation rate becomes prominent causing depression of PQ segment. This results in J point (junction between S wave and ST segment) depression, which is usually of short duration. The ST segment becomes upsloping and slightly convex and returns to baseline within 0.04 second after the J point. The abnormal changes in ECG are analysed with recordings obtained before, during and after the termination of the test and interpreted accordingly.

## VIVA

1. What are the various types of exercise?
2. How do you determine the severity of exercise?
3. What are the differences between isotonic and isometric exercise?
4. What are the cardiovascular responses to acute exercise?
5. What are the causes of increased cardiac output in exercise?
6. What is the cause of systolic rise in blood pressure in exercise?
7. Why does diastolic pressure not change or decrease in moderate to severe exercise?
8. Why does heart rate take more time than blood pressure to come back to normal level following exercise?
   Ans. Heart rate increases in exercise due to increased sympathetic activity. Sympathetic activity takes time to return to normal, therefore the heart normalises slowly. BP returns to normal in 5–7 minutes due to muscle relaxation with stoppage of exercise, which produces vasodilation.
9. What are the effects of exercise on the respiratory system?
10. What are the benefits of performing regular exercise?
11. List the indications and contraindications for exercise stress testing.
12. Name the dynamic tests for upper extremity and lower extremity testing.
13. How is the exercise stress response interpreted?

Chapter 28

# Clinical Examination of the Cardiovascular System

## Learning Objectives

After completing this practical, you will be able to:

- Describe the importance of examination of the cardiovascular system (CVS) in clinical physiology.
- List the parameters to be examined in clinical examination of CVS.
- Define precordium and apex beat.
- Draw the midclavicular line on the precordium.
- Localise the apex of the subject.
- Locate the different auscultatory areas on the precordium.
- Auscultate the heart sounds.
- Examine the neck veins.
- List the common causes of impalpable apex beat
- Enumerate the types and causes of heart sounds.
- Name the waves in JVP and their mechanism of production.

You may also be able to:

- Draw different anatomical lines and borders of the heart.
- Locate the position of the heart valves and auscultatory areas.
- Elicit parasternal heave and appreciate the thrill, if present.
- Percuss to define the border of the heart.
- List the different conditions in which JVP is raised and prominent 'a', `c' and `v' waves are seen in the JVP tracing.
- Explain the different conditions in which apex is not palpable.
- List the causes, character and significance of heart sounds.
- Explain the mechanism and causes of split of first and second heart sounds.

## INTRODUCTION

The examination of the cardiovascular system (CVS) comprises the examination of the precordium and blood vessels. Careful assessment of the arterial and venous pulses should always precede examination of the precordium. Auscultation of the heart should be taken up only after the precordium has been thoroughly examined. Many students do not give enough time to the examination of arterial and venous pulses and the precordium, and directly auscultate the heart to diagnose heart diseases. Beginners especially, become anxious to hear the heart sounds and neglect other aspects of the CVS examination. Before one auscultates the heart, one should have some idea of what abnormalities one expects to detect with the stethoscope. One should also have a minimum knowledge of the physiological basis of production of the heart sounds.

### Anatomical Landmarks

The precordium is defined as the anterior aspect of the chest wall, which overlies the heart. Different borders of the heart and the positions of the valves are demarcated on the precordium to make clinical examination of the cardiovascular system convenient.

#### Different Lines

1. **Midclavicular line** This is defined as the vertical line dropped from the centre of the clavicle. The midpoint of the clavicle is determined by taking a point on the clavicle midway between the middle of the suprasternal notch and the tip of the acromion.
2. **Anterior axillary line** This is defined as the vertical line descending from the anterior border of the axilla.
3. **Midaxillary line** This is defined as the vertical line descending from the centre of the axilla.
4. **Posterior axillary line** This is defined as the vertical line descending from the posterior border of the axilla.
5. **Parasternal line** This is defined as the vertical line passing through the costochondral junction close to either side of the sternum.

#### Borders of the Heart

1. **Base of the heart** This is represented by a line joining the right third sternocostal articulation to a point at the level of the left second intercostal space, just internal to the parasternal line.
2. **Right border of the heart** This extends from the right third sternocostal articulation above, to the

right seventh intercostal articulation below. It is slightly curved with convexity to the right.

3. **Left border of the heart** This is traced by a line joining the point at the level of left second intercostal space just internal to the parasternal line above and the apex beat below.

## Position of the Heart Valves

**Mitral valve** This is obliquely placed behind the inner end of the left fourth costal cartilage and the adjoining part of the sternum.

**Tricuspid valve** This is situated obliquely behind the right fifth costal cartilage.

**Pulmonary valve** This is placed horizontally at the upper border of the left third costal cartilage.

**Aortic valve** This lies obliquely across the left half of the sternum at the level of the lower border of the left third costal cartilage.

## Auscultatory Areas

**Mitral Area** This area corresponds to the apex beat of the heart. The first heart sound is best heard over the mitral area. Normally, this is present in the left fifth intercostal space half an inch medial to the midclavicular line (Fig. 28.1). But in different pathological conditions, the position of the apex changes. Therefore, the auscultatory area of the mitral valve changes with the position of the apex.

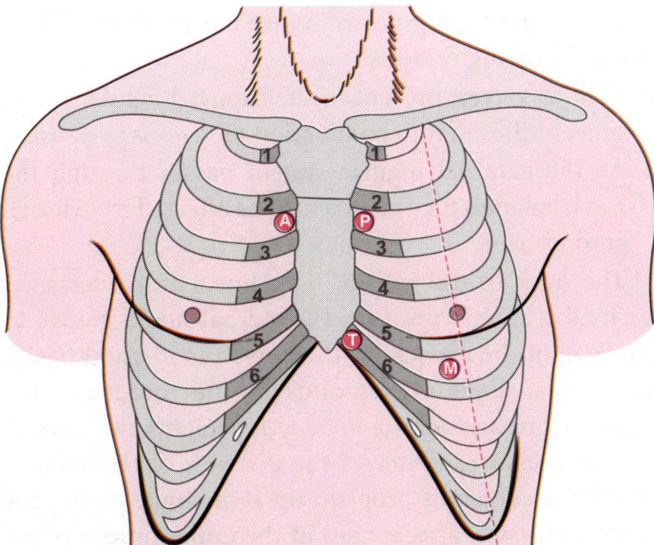


Fig. 28.1 Auscultatory areas on the precordium. A: Aortic area; P: Pulmonary area; T: Tricuspid area; M: Mitral area (apex of the heart); MCL: Midclavicular line. Note that the second rib is attached to the manubrium sterni.

**Pulmonary area** This area is half an inch in diameter with its centre in the left second intercostal space close to the parasternal line.

**Aortic area** This area is half an inch in diameter with its centre in the right second intercostal space close to the parasternal line.

Aortic murmurs are often best heard in the left third intercostal space close to the sternum. Therefore, this area is called second aortic area or Erb's point.

**Tricuspid area** This area is half an inch in diameter with its centre on the left side close to the sternum towards its lower end.

# METHODS

## Method for Examining the Cardiovascular System

### Principle

The process of examination of the cardiovascular system consists of inspection, palpation, percussion and auscultation of the precordium that follows the examination of arterial and venous pulses, recording of blood pressure and a brief general examination of the subject. The functions or any alteration in functions of the CVS are detected by thorough examination of the precordium and blood vessels.

### Requirements

1. Stethoscope
2. Cardiac bed or a couch with provision to lift the head end.

### Procedure

The examination of CVS includes (1) general examination (emphasising a few particular signs) including examination of radial pulse and the recording of blood pressure, (2) examination of the neck veins, and (3) examination of the precordium.

### General Examination in Relation to CVS

*Anemia*

Check for the degree of pallor. The degree of anemia gives a rough idea of the dynamics of circulation, heart rate and blood pressure.

### Cyanosis

Check for the presence of cyanosis. This may be present in conditions where there is mixing of arterial blood with venous blood, as seen in Fallot's tetralogy or patent truncus arteriosus.

### Edema

Check for the presence of edema in the dependent parts of the body. In cardiac patients, the location of edema depends on the posture of the patient. It is detected by applying pressure over the distal end of the tibia if the patient is mobile. But, if the patient is confined to bed, the sacral area should be examined for the presence of edema.

### Clubbing

Nail beds should be examined for the presence of clubbing. If cyanosis is present along with clubbing, this suggests right to left shunt. Clubbing may be present in congenital cyanotic heart disease and in subacute bacterial endocarditis.

### Dyspnea

Breathlessness is a feature of heart failure. Dyspnea may be present even at rest.

### Abdominal Signs

1. **Hepatomegaly** A tender hepatomegaly may be present in congestive cardiac failure.
2. **Splenomegaly** The spleen may be enlarged in bacterial endocarditis.
3. **Ascites** Ascites may be present in heart failure.
4. **Epigastric pulsation** Epigastric pulsation may occur due to the following cardiovascular disorders:
   - Aortic pulsation usually in thin and nervous patients
   - Aneurysm of abdominal aorta
   - Hypertrophy of the heart (especially the right ventricle) may give an epigastric systolic thrust

### Pulse

Examine the radial pulse for at least one minute. The arterial pulses of both the sides should be examined to check the bilateral symmetry, and the femoral arteries should be examined to detect radiofemoral delay, if present. Brachial, carotid, temporal, popliteal, posterior tibial and dorsalis pedis arteries should also be examined (also see Chapter 24).

### Blood Pressure

Blood pressure (BP) should be detected by sphygmomanometry, preferably by using a mercury manometer. It should be recorded on both sides in cardiac patients. BP should also be recorded by both palpatory and auscultatory methods, especially, if the patient is hypertensive (see Chapter 25).

## The Venous Pulse

Venous pulses are examined especially in the neck region.

### Examination of the Neck Veins

Examine the neck veins in daylight with the patient reclining at an angle of about 45°. If the patient is lying on a cardiac bed or a couch, the head end of the bed can be raised to 45° for this purpose. Otherwise, the back of the subject can be supported so that the neck muscles are relaxed and the subject reclines at 45° (Fig. 28.2B). Study the level of pressure in the internal jugular veins (jugular venous pressure (JVP)). The pressure is expressed in terms of centimetres for the vertical distance between the top of the column of the blood and the sternal angle, which corresponds to the upper border of the clavicle with the subject reclining at 45° (Figs. 28.2 A and B). It may be easier to recognise the pulsation in the external jugular veins, but pulsation in the internal jugular vein is more reliable, because it directly reflects the pressure changes in the right atrium. External jugular veins are not reliable because of the following reasons:

- Venous valves, present in the external jugular veins, prevent the smooth conduction of venous pressure.
- As the external jugular system passes through the fascial planes, they are likely to be affected by external compression.

The neck of the subject is reclined to 45° because, normally, in this position the sternal angle comes to the level of the clavicle. If the person is in good health the sternal angle corresponds to the middle of the right atrium and approximately represents the normal venous pressure, whatever the position of the subject. When the subject is propped up at an angle of 45°, the venous pressure appears just at the upper border of the clavicle, as in this position the sternal angle and clavicle remain at the same level horizontally. Therefore, venous pressure above the clavicle in this position is considered as raised JVP.

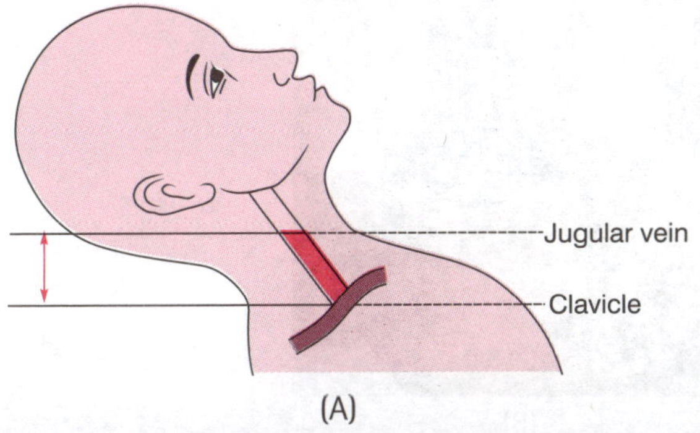


(A)

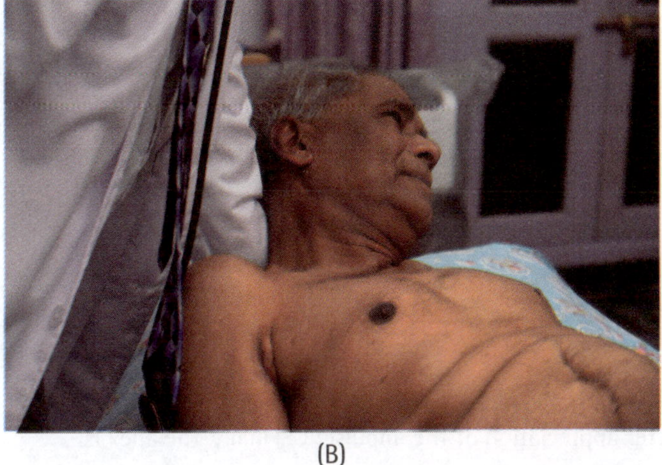

(B)

Fig. 28.2 A. Method of clinical assessment of jugular vein pressure (JVP). It is measured as vertical height of JVP above the clavicle with the patient reclining at 45°. B. Examination for neck veins for JVP. With the support of examiner, subject has reclined at 45°.

> Note: In the neck, the arterial pulsation may be confused with venous pulsation. The venous pulses can be differentiated from the arterial pulses by the following parameters.

i) The venous pulse is better seen than felt whereas the arterial pulse is better felt than seen.

ii) The venous pulse has a definite upper level, which falls during inspiration when blood is drawn into the heart.

iii) By exerting moderate pressure above the clavicle with a finger, the venous pulse can be obliterated, but not the arterial pulse.

iv) If carefully observed, two to three waves can be seen in the venous pulse.

## Examination of the Precordium

The process of examination of the precordium consists of inspection, palpation, percussion and auscultation. The subject should lie down on a couch and the examination should be carried out in adequate daylight with the precordium fully exposed.

### Inspection

1. **Skeletal deformity** Look for any precordial bulging or depression. The former is usually seen in congenital heart disease.
2. **Dilated and engorged superficial veins** Look for the presence of any dilated and engorged superficial veins over the precordium. This may be seen in superior or inferior venacaval obstruction.
3. **Pulsation**

   *Apical pulsation* Look for pulsation of the apex. Normally, the pulsation of the cardiac apex is visible. Presence of all other pulsations over the precordium is considered abnormal.

   *Other pulsations* Look for pulsation in the other areas of the precordium, especially on the pulmonary and aortic area and in the left parasternal area. Pulsations are seen in the following conditions.

   - Pulsation on the pulmonary area is seen in pulmonary hypertension or pulmonary artery dilatation.
   - Pulsation on the aortic area may be seen in the aneurysm of the aorta.
   - Pulsation on the left parasternal area indicates right ventricular hypertrophy.
   - Pulsation over the suprasternal notch indicates aneurysm of the arch of the aorta or coarctation of the aorta.

### Palpation

1. **Apex beat** Describe the position and character of the apex.

   *Position* Locate the position of the apex of the heart. This is done by first placing the palm on the precordium to feel the apical impulse (Fig. 28.3A) and then by placing the ulnar border of the palm on the pulsation area horizontally (Fig. 28.3B). Finally, the apex is localised by the tip of the middle or index finger (Fig. 28.3C). If the apex is not palpable in the supine position, ask the subject to sit down and try to locate the apex in the sitting posture. If the apex is still not palpable, ask the subject to lean forward as much as he can in the sitting posture and try to locate the apex in this leaning position. If the apex is still not palpable, palpate the corresponding area of the chest on the right side (in

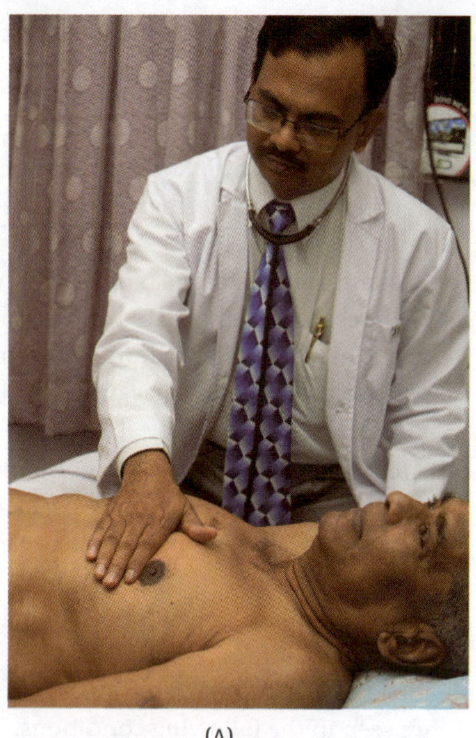

(A)

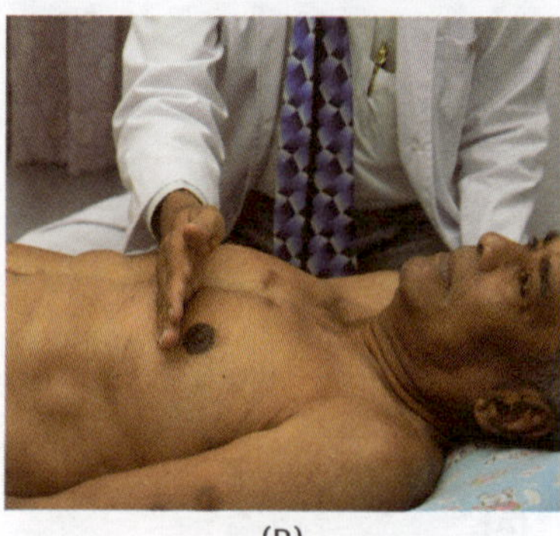

(B)

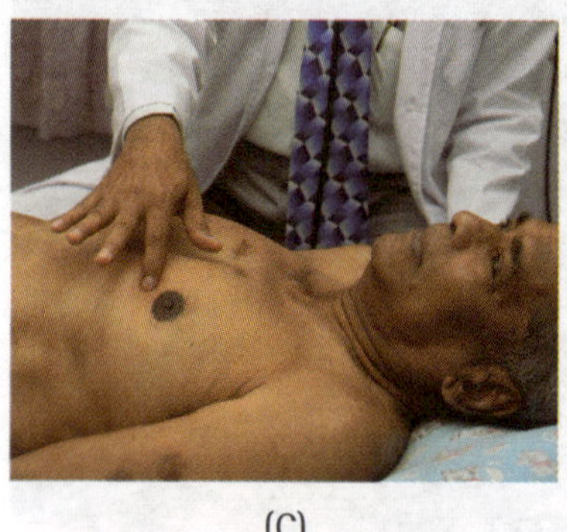

(C)

Fig. 28.3 Localisation of apex of the heart. A: Palm is gently placed on the precordium to feel the apical impulse; B: Ulnar border of the palm is placed in the intercostal space to have a better appreciation of the impulse; C: Finally, the apex is localised by the tip of the middle or index finger.

dextrocardia or dextroversion, the apex of the heart may shift to the right). Ideally, apex should not be palpated in the left lateral position because it shifts the apex laterally, and there is variation in shifting.

Note the position of the apex in the intercostal space in relation to the midclavicular line. The intercostal spaces are counted by palpating the manubrium sterni (the most elevated point on the sternum). The second rib joins the manubrium sterni. The space below the second rib is the second intercostal space and accordingly other intercostal spaces are counted.

> Note: 1. The apex is defined as the lowermost and outermost definite cardiac impulse. Therefore, if other pulsations are present on the precordium, the apex can be easily identified. 2. The apex beat is normally located in the left fifth intercostal space half an inch medial to the midclavicular line. When students are asked to locate the apex, before they palpate and localise it, they start counting the intercostal spaces and put the tip of the finger medial to the midclavicular line in the fifth space to feel the apex. This is wrong, because the apex may not always be present exactly in that position. Moreover, you do not know if the subject has any pathology in the heart. Therefore, the apex must be first localised as described above and then its position should be demarcated.

*Causes of impalpable apex*

1. Left-sided pleural effusion
2. Pneumothorax
3. Hydropneumothorax
4. Pericardial effusion
5. Shift of mediastinum to the right (right-sided lung fibrosis and collapse)
6. Obesity (thick chest wall)
7. Apex lying under a rib
8. Dextrocardia (the apex will be palpable on the right side)

*Character* Try to describe the character of the apex.

> Note: Normally, the apex beat just touches and slightly elevates the examining finger. The common abnormal characters are:
>
> - *Tapping apex* Seen in advanced mitral stenosis.
> - *Forceful and well-sustained apex* Seen in gross left ventricular hypertrophy due to chronic systemic hypertension, as it causes pressure overload and increases wall thickness.
> - *Forceful but ill-sustained apex* Seen in right ventricular hypertrophy or mild to moderate left ventricular hypertrophy. In left ventricular hypertrophy due to volume overload (as in aortic regurgitation), there is increase in the ventricular cavity size rather than wall thickness. Therefore, the apex is forceful but ill-sustained.

2. **Parasternal heave** Place the ulnar border of the palm firmly on the left parasternal line and feel for pulsations and whether the hand is lifted with each pulsation (Fig. 28.4).

> Note: Presence of parasternal heave suggests right ventricular hypertrophy.

3. **Thrills** Palpate all over the precordium for thrills.

> Note: A thrill is a palpable murmur. The thrills are best appreciated when the patient holds his breath in expiration. Thrills may be present in valvular defects or in aneurysm of great vessels.

4. **Tender points** Palpate the precordium for presence of any painful points over it.

> Note: A tender point over the precordium may be due to costochondritis, myalgia, fracture of ribs or pleuritis.

5. **Direction of flow in veins** If the veins are dilated and engorged over the precordium, detect the direction of flow in the veins. In superior venacaval obstruction, the direction of blood flow in the veins is from above downwards. In inferior venacaval obstruction, the direction of blood flow in the veins is from below upwards.

> Note: The position of the trachea should be checked along with the position of the apex to assess the position of the mediastenum.

### Percussion

Percussion is of less significance in the examination of the CVS. But percussion is carried out sometimes to detect the extent of cardiac dullness in conditions like pericardial effusion. Cardiac dullness is detected by performing a light percussion. The details of the rules of the percussion are discussed in examination of the respiratory system.

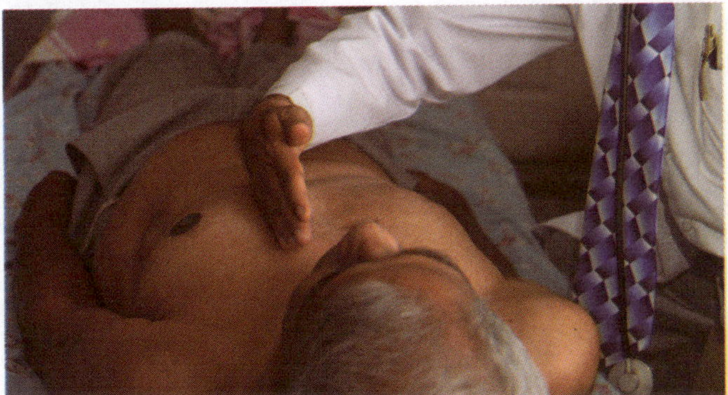

Fig. 28.4 Method of elicitation of parasternal heave. The ulnar border of the hand is firmly placed on the left parasternal line to feel the pulsations, if any, and note if the hand is lifted with each pulsation.

### Auscultation

With the help of the stethoscope, auscultate the different areas in the following sequence: mitral area, pulmonary area, aortic area and tricuspid area. The diaphragm of the stethoscope should be placed firmly on different areas to hear the heart sounds (Fig. 28.5).

In each area, the following points should be noted during auscultation.

1. **First (S1) and second (S2) heart sounds** Note their quality, intensity, duration and character. S1 is heard better on the mitral area, and S2 is heard better over pulmonary and aortic area.

> Note: The first and second heart sounds can be differentiated by their pitch and duration. The first heart sound is heard as 'lub' and the second sound as 'dub'. For beginners, it is difficult to differentiate these sounds. They can palpate the carotid artery in the neck while auscultating the heart sounds. The heart sound that coincides with the carotid pulsation is the first heart sound and the sound that follows the pulsation is the second heart sound.

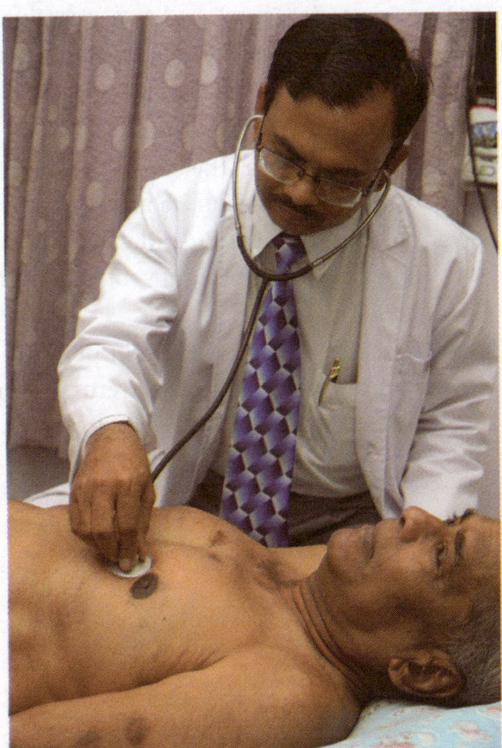

Fig. 28.5 The method of auscultation for heart sounds. Note that the diaphragm of the stethoscope is placed firmly on the apex (mitral area).

2. **Other sounds (if present)**
   - Third heart sound (S3)
   - Fourth heart sound (S4)
   - Murmurs
   - Opening snap
   - Ejection click

   If murmur is present, note the site of origin, timing, character, radiation and its relation with respiration.

## DISCUSSION

## Clinical Significance

### Arterial Pulse

Detailed discussion on arterial pulse is given in Chapter 24.

### Venous Pulse

The pulsation of internal jugular veins in the neck is examined clinically to determine the atrial pressure activity. Jugular venous pulse (JVP) has five waves: three positive waves (ascents) and two negative waves (descents). The positive waves are a, c and v waves, and negative waves are x and y descents (Fig. 28.6).

a wave : Due to atrial contraction

c wave : Coincides with the onset of ventricular systole and results from the movement (bulging) of the tricuspid valve ring into the right atrium as the right ventricular pressure rises.

v wave : Indicates the passive rise in pressure in the right atrium as venous return continues while the tricuspid valve is closed.

x descent : Caused by a fall in right atrial pressure due to relaxation of the right atrium.

y descent : Occurs due to fall in right atrial pressure when blood enters into the right ventricle as the tricuspid valve opens.

### *Conditions that Alter JVP*

**Raised JVP**

1. Right ventricular failure
2. Obstruction of superior vena cava
3. Increase in circulating blood volume
   - Pregnancy
   - Acute nephritis
   - Over-judicious treatment with IV fluids
4. Constrictive pericarditis
5. Tricuspid incompetence

Note: Persistent elevation of JVP is one of the earliest sign of congestive cardiac failure and is probably the most reliable sign of the failure.

**Prominent 'a' wave**

1. Pulmonary stenosis
2. Pulmonary hypertension
3. Tricuspid stenosis (usually in this condition there is atrial fibrillation, so, the a wave may not be seen).
4. Myxoma of right atrium
5. Distended right atrium in atrial septal defect
6. Cardiomyopathy

*Physiological basis* A prominent 'a' wave occurs due to increased force of right atrial contraction associated with right atrial hypertrophy or hypertrophy of right ventricle. When the right atrium contracts against increased resistance, the 'a' wave becomes prominent.

**Cannon wave** When the amplitude of the 'a' wave is very high, it is called cannon wave (giant 'a' wave). It is

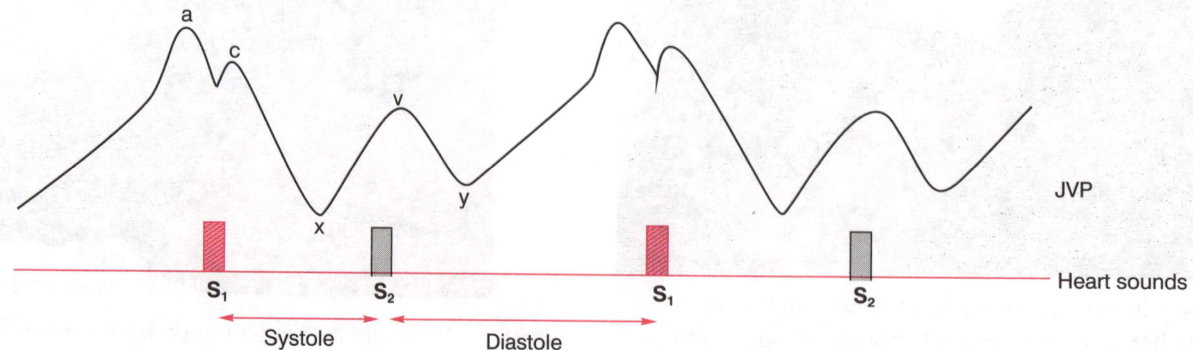


Fig. 28.6 JVP and heart sounds. JVP: Jugular venous pressure; S1: First heart sound; S2: Second heart sound.

seen when the right atrium contracts against a closed tricuspid valve. It occurs in:

1. Complete heart block when atrial and ventricular systole coincides.
2. Nodal rhythm when the atrium and ventricle are activated simultaneously.

**Absence of 'a' wave** The 'a' wave disappears in atrial fibrillation.

**Prominent 'v' wave** It is seen in tricuspid regurgitation, because when the ventricle contracts during systole, blood enters into the right atrium through the incompetent tricuspid valve. It is also seen in constrictive pericarditis and heart failure.

## Precordial Examination

The two most important parameters in precordial examination are (1) character and position of the apex of the heart and (2) heart sounds.

### *Apex of the Heart*

The position of the apex beat is a valuable physical sign in the examination of the CVS. The apex of the heart is formed by the left ventricle. Therefore, in left ventricular hypertrophy the apex becomes more forceful. Displacement of the apex occurs due to push or pull from the surrounding viscera. Pushing may be due to pleural effusion and pneumothorax, and pulling may be due to pulmonary fibrosis and collapse. Apical displacement also occurs due to cardiac diseases like enlargement of the left ventricle. It can also occur due to deformity of the thoracic cage like scoliosis.

### *Heart Sounds*

Four heart sounds have been described. These are first heart sound (S1), second heart sound (S2), third heart sound (S3) and fourth heart sound (S4). S1 and S2 are heard normally.

**First heart sound** The first heart sound represents the beginning of the systole.

*Causes* It occurs due to vibration set up by:

- Sudden closure of the AV valves.
- Rapid increase in tension in the ventricular muscles during isometric contraction acting on full ventricles.
- Turbulence created in the blood due to ventricular contraction.

*Character* It is a soft sound, heard as 'lub'.

Duration : about 0.15 seconds
Frequency : 25–45 Hz

*Significance* It signifies the beginning of the ventricular systole and AV valve closure.

a) Accentuation of first heart sound
   - Exercise
   - Hyperkinetic circulatory states like anemia and beriberi
   - Hypertension
b) Diminution of first heart sound
   - Shock
   - Acute myocardial infarction
   - Constrictive pericarditis
   - Pericardial effusion
   - Cardiomyopathy (advanced stage)
   - Obesity
   - Emphysema

***Splitting*** The first heart sound has two components: the mitral and the tricuspid components. The mitral valve closes just before the tricuspid valve. This gives rise to splitting of the first heart sound. But this splitting cannot be detected by auscultation, because both the components are very low pitched and merge into each other. Therefore, when splitting of the first heart sound is heard, it is always considered as pathological.

**Second heart sound**

*Causes*

- The second heart sound is primarily caused by the closure of the semilunar valves.
- Rushing of blood into the ventricles due to opening of the AV valves also contributes.

*Character* This is heard as 'dub'.

Duration : about 0.12 seconds
Frequency : 50 Hz

*Significance* It signifies the end of clinical systole and closure of the semilunar valves.

Loud A2 (increased aortic component) is seen in:

- Systemic hypertension

Diminished A2 is seen in:

- Aortic stenosis
- Aortic incompetence

Loud P2 (increased pulmonary component) is seen in:

- Pulmonary hypertension

Diminished P2 is seen in:

- Pulmonary stenosis

***Splitting*** Splitting of the second sound is due to the gap between the aortic and pulmonary components. It is easy to detect because aortic and pulmonary valve closure sounds are high pitched and can be separated. Aortic valve closure is audible in all areas whereas pulmonary valve closure is audible only in the pulmonary area. Splitting is most easily heard in children and may not be audible in elderly subjects.

*Mechanism of splitting* The splitting of the second heart sound is due to the separation between the closure of aortic and pulmonary valves. The closure of pulmonary valve always follows the closure of aortic valve (aortic valve closes first). The splitting is distinctly heard during inspiration. During inspiration more blood is drawn into the thorax. Therefore, venous return to right atrium increases and right ventricular stroke volume increases. This increases the duration of right ventricular systole. Thus, P2 is slightly delayed. Also, during inspiration left ventricular stroke volume decreases, because blood is pooled in the dilated pulmonary vessels and dilated left atrium (this dilatation occurs due to increased negative intrathoracic pressure). Therefore, left ventricular systole is shortened and A2 comes earlier. Therefore, during inspiration A2 occurs earlier and P2 occurs later. Hence, splitting of the second sound widens during inspiration. Exactly the opposite happens during expiration and splitting narrows.

*Reverse splitting* This occurs when the left ventricle takes more time to empty than the right ventricle. It is seen in left bundle branch block (LBBB) and in left ventricular failure.

**Third heart sound** Third heart sound is usually not heard in many healthy individuals. Sometimes it may be heard in children and in young adults. It is usually heard in conditions in which the circulation becomes hyperkinetic. The third sound can arise from either side of the heart, but usually it arises in the left ventricle.

*Causes*

- It is caused by the vibration set up in the ventricle during the early period of rapid ventricular filling.
- Rebound fencing of the cusp of the valve and chordae of the respective valve due to vigorous elongation of the ventricle caused by rapid inflow of blood also contributes to this.

*Character* It is best heard in the mitral area. It follows the aortic component of the second sound and heard early in the diastole, that is, just after the second sound.

Duration : 0.1 second
Pitch : low-pitched

*Significance*

1. This is attributed to rapid ventricular filling. It is found in relatively hyperkinetic circulation, in young persons, and where the mitral diastolic flow is increased as in mitral regurgitation and VSD.
2. It is an important sign of heart failure due to any cause. In heart failure, the atrial pressure is increased and early filling of the ventricle is rapid.
3. It may be heard shortly after myocardial infarction or in diseases where the distensibility of the ventricular muscle is altered. The sound arises from vibration in the atrioventricular valve structures and in the ventricular muscle.

**Fourth heart sound** This is also called the atrial sound, because it is produced during atrial contraction. It is not heard in normal individuals. Presence of the fourth heart sound is always considered abnormal.

*Causes*

- It is caused by atrial contraction.
- It is produced by the vibration set up within the ventricle due to inflow of blood produced by atrial systole.

*Character* It occurs just before the first sound, that is, late in the diastole and is low-pitched.

*Significance*

1. It always indicates increased stiffnes or non-compliance of the ventricles. Therefore, when a bolus of blood is delivered into the ventricle by atrial contraction, it facilitates a sudden increase of pressure in the ventricle.
2. It is seen in left ventricular hypertrophy due to hypertension, myocardial infarction, pulmonary embolism and pulmonary hypertension.

**Triple heart sound** This consists of three heart sounds: the first and second heart sound, and the third one can be either the third or fourth heart sound. The triple rhythm associated with a normal heart may not be a serious one, but if it is present with a definite cardiac pathology, it may signify a serious condition. When the heart rate increases to more than 100 per minute, the triple rhythm is called gallop rhythm, because it produces a typical cadence of the gallop of a horse. The individual sounds cannot be identified separately. If the gallop is due to the third heart sound, it is called a protodiastolic gallop; if it is due to the fourth heart sound, it is called presystolic gallop.

**Murmurs** Murmurs occur due to turbulence in the blood flow at or near a valve, or an abnormal communication within the heart. Murmurs differ from normal heart sounds in the sense that these are of longer duration and higher frequency, whereas heart sounds have shorter duration and lower frequency. When a murmur is present, the following points are carefully noted.

1. *Site of origin* The area over which the murmur is maximally heard should be noted. The point of maximal intensity usually (but not always) indicates its site of origin.
2. *Timing and duration* Depending on the timing of the murmur, they are classified into systolic, diastolic or continuous murmurs. Depending on the duration, it may be early diastolic, mid-diastolic, early systolic, pan-systolic, and so on.
3. *Character* The murmur may be soft, blowing to harsh, rough and rumbling. Loud and rough murmurs are usually associated with organic valvular and congenital lesions, for example, murmur of mitral stenosis is always rough and rumbling in character.
4. *Radiation (conduction)* From the site of maximum intensity auscultation is done in different directions to detect whether the murmur is localised or conducted to other parts. Conduction is characteristic of some murmurs, for example, the murmur of mitral stenosis is usually localised whereas the murmur of mitral incompetence selectively propagates towards the axilla.
5. *Relation with respiration* During inspiration, the stroke volume of the right ventricle increases while that of the left decreases. Therefore, any murmur becoming louder during inspiration is considered to originate from the right ventricle, and any murmur louder during expiration is said to originate from the left side of the heart.

## VIVA

1. What are the general physical signs that are specifically looked for before commencing the clinical examination of the cardiovascular system?
2. What is the importance of detecting cyanosis in examination of the CVS?
3. What are the characteristics of edema seen in cardiac patients?
4. Why should the radial pulse be examined before the examination of the precordium?
5. What is the importance of recording blood pressure in examination of a patient of CVS?
6. Why are the neck veins usually preferred for the examination of the venous pulse?
7. How do you differentiate venous pulses from arterial pulses in the neck?
8. Why are the internal jugular veins preferred to the external jugulars for examination of the neck veins?
9. What are the waves seen in JVP and how are they produced?
10. In which conditions does an 'a' wave become more prominent?
11. What is a cannon wave and how is it produced?
12. In which pathological conditions can 'a' and 'v' waves be absent?
13. What is the significance of raised JVP and in which clinical conditions is it seen?
14. Define precordium.
15. What are the points one should look for during inspection of the precordium?
16. In what clinical conditions can precordial bulging occur?
17. Define apex beat.
18. What are the procedures to localise the apex if it is not palpable in the supine position?
19. Why should apex beat not be localised in the left lateral position?
20. Name the different conditions in which the apex beat may not be palpable.
21. What are the conditions in which the apex may become forceful and well sustained, and why?
22. What do you mean by 'tapping apex', and in which condition is it seen?
23. What is the importance of examining the position of the trachea along with the location of apex?
24. What is parasternal heave? In what conditions is this seen?

25. What are the different heart sounds normally heard?
26. What are the causes of the first heart sound, and how is it confirmed clinically?
27. What are the conditions in which the first sound becomes louder?
28. What do you mean by splitting of the second sound? Why is splitting better appreciated in inspiration?
29. What is reverse split? In which clinical condition is it seen?
30. What is gallop rhythm, and what is its significance?
31. How are murmurs produced? What are the types of murmurs?

Chapter 29

# Clinical Examination of the Sensory System

### Learning Objectives

After completing this practical, you will be able to:

- Describe the importance of performing this practical in clinical physiology.
- classify different sensations and receptors.
- draw the sensory map of the body.
- Elicit all the sensations.
- List the precautions taken during elicitation of sensations.
- Trace the pathway of all sensations.
- Name the common abnormalities of alteration in sensations.

You may also be able to:

- Explain the abnormalities of alterations of sensations.
- Correlate the clinical findings with abnormalities if present.
- Localise the diseases affecting different parts of the sensory system.
- Explain the effects of lesions at various levels in the sensory pathways.

## INTRODUCTION

### Anatomical and Physiological Considerations

The sensory information conveyed to the central nervous system by the peripheral nerves originate in the special structures that are distributed in the skin, subcutaneous tissues, muscles, tendons and joints. These special structures are known as receptors, modified nerve endings. From the peripheral nerves, the sensations enter the spinal cord through the posterior nerve roots. In the spinal cord, the sensations ascend in different sensory tracts to finally reach the sensory cortex via the thalamus. Some of the sensory inputs also reach the cerebellum, and these inputs are mainly the unconscious proprioceptive and kinesthetic sensations that are involved in the modulation of motor activities. Lesions at different levels of the sensory system produce specific sensory deficits.

### Sensory Modalities

Sensations are broadly classified into general sensations, special sensations and visceral sensations.

#### General Sensations

The different types of general sensations are:

- Touch and pressure
- Warmth
- Cold
- Pain
- Vibration
- Movement and position of joints (proprioception)

#### Special Sensations

The sensations that originate in the special sensory receptors present in the structures like the eye and ear are called special sensations. Different types of special sensations are:

- Vision
- Hearing
- Smell
- Taste
- Acceleration (rotational and linear)

#### Visceral Sensations

Sensations that originate in the visceral structures are referred to as visceral sensations. Some of the examples of visceral sensations are lung inflation, distension of the stomach and change in arterial blood pressure.

### Receptors

Receptors are transducers that convert various forms of energy in the environment into the action potentials in the neurons. They may be a part of the neuron or a specialised cell that generates action potential in the neurons. Very often, the receptors are associated with non-neural cells that surround them to form a sense organ.

## Types of Receptors

The receptors are divided into four categories:

1. **Exteroceptors** These receptors are concerned with the changes in the external environment close to the body. Exteroceptors are distributed on the surface of the body, in the skin and subcutaneous tissues. These cutaneous sense organs are broadly divided into expanded endings and encapsulated endings.

   The expanded endings are:
   - Merkel's discs and
   - Ruffini endings

   Merkel's discs and Ruffini endings are slow-adapting touch receptors.

   The encapsulated endings are:
   - Pacinian corpuscles,
   - Meissner's corpuscles and
   - Krause's end-bulbs

   Meissner's and Pacinian corpuscles are rapidly adapting touch receptors. Most of these sensory endings are present around the hair follicles, therefore, the slightest movement of hair, elicits the sensation of touch. Some of the endings especially Ruffini endings and Pacinian corpuscles are also found in deep fibrous tissues. It appears that none of these endings are needed for elicitation of sensations, because sensory modalities can be elicited from the areas that contain only free nerve endings.
2. **Interoceptors** These are concerned with the changes in the internal environment of the body, like osmoreceptors that respond to change in osmolality of body fluids.
3. **Proprioceptors** These provide information about the position of the body in space at any given time. The conscious component of proprioception comes from the receptors in the joints, and from the cutaneous touch and pressure receptors.
4. **Teleceptors** These are concerned with the events that occur at a distance from the body.

# Sensory Pathways

The sensory pathways are divided in the two systems. The pathways that ascend in the posterior column of the spinal cord are frequently called the lemniscal system and the pathways that ascend in the anterior and lateral quadrant of the spinal cord are referred to as the anterolateral system (Fig. 29.1). The neurons in the sensory pathways are placed in sequential order and accordingly they are called first, second and third order of neurons. The first order of neurons sends the encoded information from the receptors to the spinal cord and medulla. The second order of neurons transmits the impulse from the spinal cord and medulla to the thalamus from where the third order of neurons conveys the information to the cortex.

## Fine Touch

Touch receptors are present in large numbers in the skin of the fingers and lips and in fewer numbers in the skin of the trunk. The first order of neurons carrying fine touch sensation enter the spinal cord via the posterior root and then ascend up in the dorsal column of the spinal cord of the same side. They terminate in the nucleus gracilis and cuneatus of the medulla. The second order of neurons arises from these nuclei, crosses to the opposite side in the medulla and ascends in the contralateral medial leminiscus, to terminate in the ventral posterior nucleus

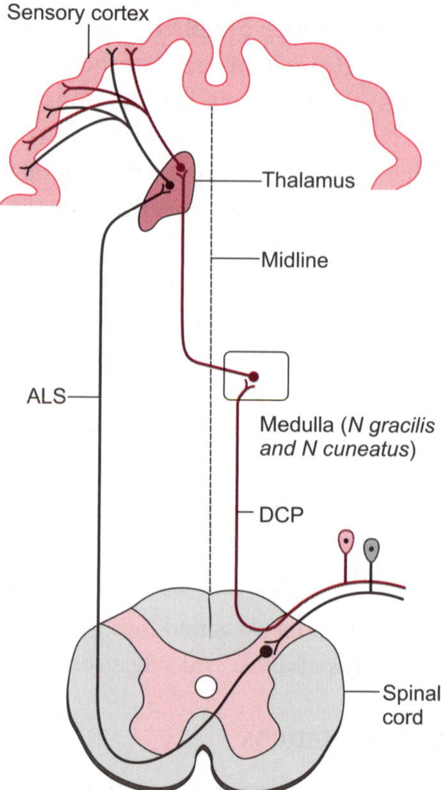


Fig. 29.1 Sensory pathways. ALS: Anterolateral system; DCP: Dorsal column pathways.

and related specific sensory nuclei of the thalamus. The third order of neurons arises from the thalamus and reaches the sensory cortex via thalamic radiation. The sensations that are carried in the posterior column of the spinal cord are:

- Fine touch
- Proprioception (joint sensation and sense of position)
- Sense of vibration
- Tactile localisation
- Two-point discrimination
- Stereognosis

### Crude Touch

The first order of neurons after entering the spinal cord synapse on the second order of neurons in the dorsal horn of the cord. The second order of neurons crosses to the opposite side at that spinal segment and ascends in the contralateral ventral spinothalamic tract to terminate in the specific sensory relay nuclei of the thalamus. The third order of neurons arises from the thalamus and terminates in the sensory cortex through thalamic radiation.

### Proprioception

The pathway for proprioceptive inputs is the same as that of fine touch. A large part of proprioceptive input goes to the cerebellum in addition to its projection to the sensory cortex, which is involved in modulation of motor activities.

### Pain

The sense organs for pain are free nerve endings. The sensation of pain is transmitted to the central nervous system by a two-fibre system. The Aδ fibres carry fast pain whereas the C fibres carry slow pain. The Aδ fibres terminate mainly on the neurons in the laminas I and V, and the C fibres terminate on the neurons in the laminas I and II. The second order of neurons crosses to the opposite side of the spinal cord, at the same segmental level and then ascends in the contralateral lateral spinothalamic tract to terminate in the specific sensory relay nuclei in the thalamus. From the thalamus, the third order of neurons arises and projects to the sensory cortex. Many fibres activated by pain terminate in the reticular system from where they project to the midline and intralaminar (non-specific projection) nuclei of the thalamus and from there to many different parts of the cortex. Many pain fibres also terminate in the periaqueductal gray in the midbrain.

### Temperature

There are two types of sense organs for temperature sensation; one type for eliciting cold and the other one for eliciting warmth. The afferents for cold are Aδ fibres and C fibres, and for warmth, only C fibres. The first order of neurons terminates in the same segmental level of the spinal cord. The second order of neurons crosses to the opposite side and ascends in the contralateral lateral spinothalamic tract to terminate in the thalamus from where the third order of neurons arises and terminates in the sensory cortex.

## Sensory Map

The spinal cord is made up of different segments. From each segment, a pair of motor and sensory nerve roots arise. The sensory fibres from each segment innervate a specific dermatome of the body. This dermatomal innervation by sensory fibres constitutes the sensory map of the body (Fig. 29.2). Sensations are elicited from the skin of different dermatomes to check the intactness of a particular segment of the spinal cord.

# METHODS

## Method of Examination of Sensory system

### Principle

Different sensory modalities are elicited from different dermatomes of both sides and compared.

### Requirements

1. Cotton
2. Von Frey's hair aesthesiometer (Fig. 29.3)
3. Compass aesthesiometer (Fig. 29.4)
4. Tuning fork (128 Hz)
5. Pin
6. Algometer
7. Test tubes containing warm and cold water
8. Ballpoint pens

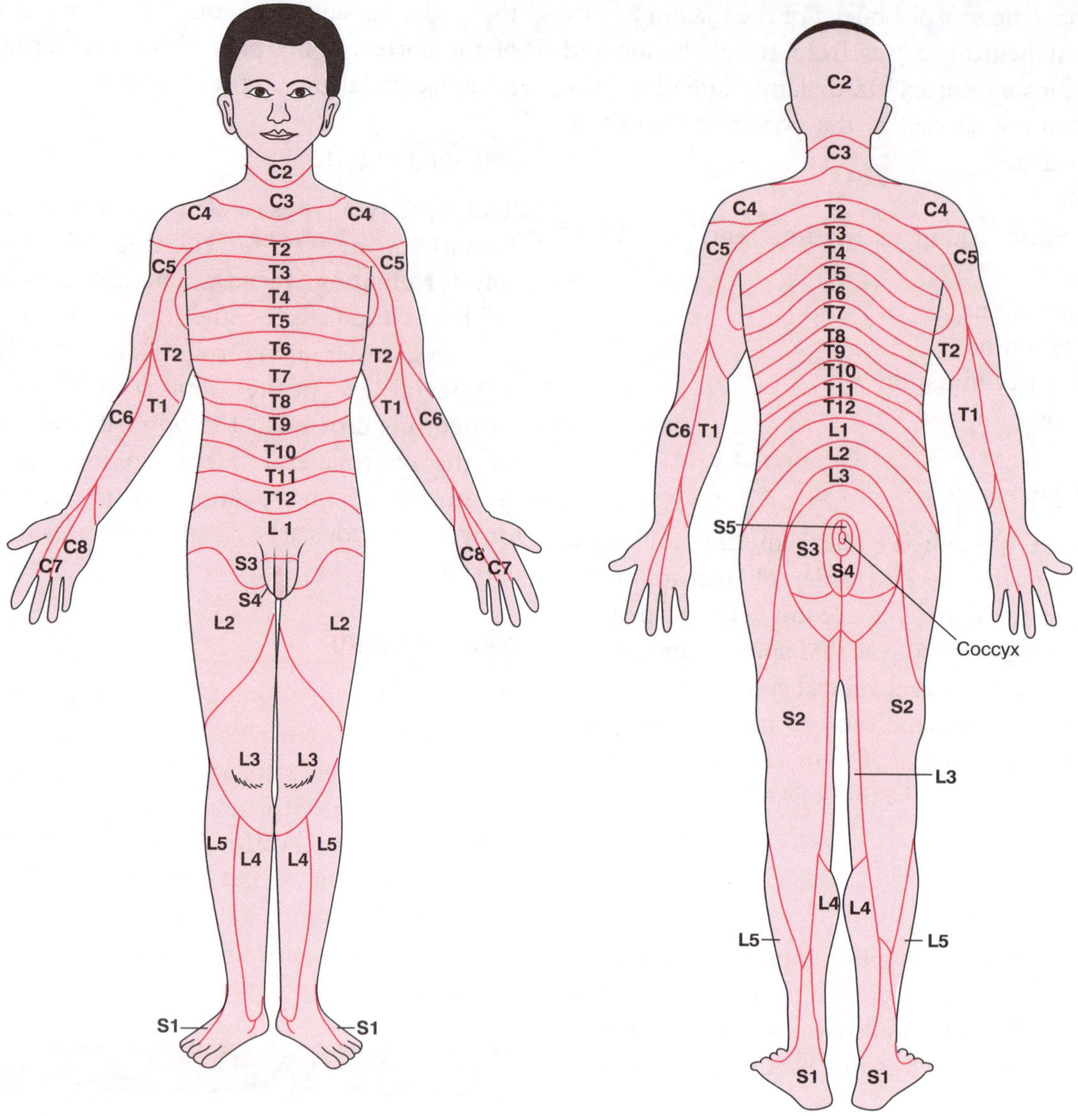


Fig. 29.2 Sensory map of the body.

## Procedure

The following different forms of sensation are tested.

1. Tactile sensibility which includes:
   - Fine touch
   - Pressure (crude touch)
   - Tactile localisation (ability to localise a point on the surface of the body being touched)
   - Two-point discrimination (ability to discriminate between two points when the two points are touched simultaneously)
   - Stereognosis (ability to feel and recognise the familiar objects by their size, shape and form)
2. Position sense, and the appreciation of passive movement (proprioception)
3 Vibration
4. Pain
5. Temperature

## Tactile Sensibility

### *Fine Touch*

**Steps**

1. Supply proper instructions to the subject (to raise his finger or say 'yes' when he feels the sensation of touch).
2. Ask the subject to close his eyes.
3. With the help of cotton wool, lightly touch the skin of the different parts of the subject.
4. If the subject raises his finger or says 'yes' enquire whether the feeling is normal or different. If the

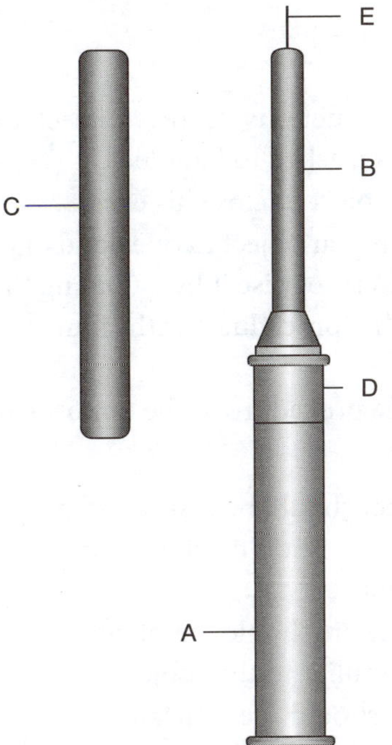


Fig. 29.3 Von Frey's hair aesthesiometer. A: Body; B: Sliding graduated tube; C: Protective cap; D: Body tube; E: Protruding horse hair.

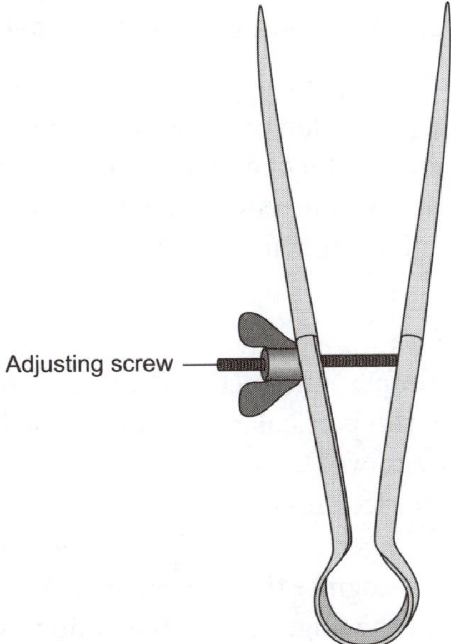


Fig. 29.4 Compass aesthesiometer.

subject does not feel the sensation, compare carefully with the corresponding area on the opposite part of the body.

5. Elicit the sensation dermatome-wise on both sides of the body.

> Note: Areas of hypoesthesia, paresthesia, or hyperesthesia, if present, should be properly delineated.

6. Note down your observation.

**Precautions**

1. Supply proper instructions to the subject to gain maximum cooperation.
2. The subject should close his eyes throughout the entire procedure.
3. Sensations should be elicited according to different dermatomes of the body.
4. Sensation of the corresponding area of the opposite side of the body should also be elicited simultaneously and compared.
5. If the sensation is altered in a particular part of the body, the area of alteration of sensation should be properly delineated.

### *Pressure (Crude Touch)*

**Steps**

1. Supply proper instructions to the subject.
2. Ask the subject to close his eyes.
3. Elicit the pressure sensation by pressing with your finger tip on the skin of different dermatomes.
4. Record your observation.

**Precautions** Same as are described for 'Fine touch'.

### *Tactile Localisation*

**Steps**

1. Supply instructions to the subject to localise (with the help of a ballpoint pen) the part of the body, which is touched by the tip of a pen.
2. Ask the subject to hold a pen and close his eyes.
3. Touch the skin of one area of the body with the help of a ball pen and ask the subject to immediately localise that point by touching with the pen that he is holding.
4. Measure the distance between the two points (this is called the localisation distance).

> Note: This distance varies greatly in different parts of the body. It corresponds with the concentration of touch spots which are numerous on the tips of the fingers and palms and fewer on the back. The localisation distance is less if the concentration of touch spots is more.

5. Likewise, determine the localisation distance on different parts of the body on both sides.

**Precautions**

1. The subject should be instructed properly regarding his role in the experiment.

2. The subject should close his eyes throughout the procedure.
3. Sensations should be elicited according to different dermatomes of the body.
4. The localisation distance of the corresponding area of the opposite side of the body should also be elicited simultaneously and compared.

### *Two-point Discrimination*

**Steps**

1. Supply instructions to the subject to say whether he feels the touch of one point or two points when he is touched by a compass aesthesiometer.
2. Ask the subject to close his eyes.
3. Separate the two limbs of the compass aesthesiometer a little and touch the skin of the subject lightly with the two points of the aesthesiometer simultaneously. Ask the subject to say whether he is being touched at one or two points.
4. If the subject says one point, increase the distance between two points a little more and repeat the test till two separate points are appreciated by the subject (the distance between two points when the subject feels it as two points is called the minimum separable distance).

> Note: This distance varies greatly in different parts of the body with the richness of touch spots. Normally, it is about 2 mm on finger tips, 5 mm on the hands and more on other parts of the body.

5. Record the minimum separable distance on different parts of the body on both the sides.

**Precautions**

1. Proper instruction should be given to the subject to gain maximum cooperation.
2. The subject should close his eyes throughout the procedure.
3. The sensation should be elicited by starting from the minimum distance between the two limbs of the aesthesiometer, and the distance should be increased little by little till the minimum separable distance is obtained.
4. The two points of the aesthesiometer should be touched simultaneously.
5. The sensation of the corresponding part of the opposite side of the body should be elicited and compared simultaneously.

### *Stereognosis*

**Steps**

1. Supply instructions to the subject to identify the object when asked to handle it.
2. Ask the subject to close his eyes.
3. Place a familiar object in one hand of the subject and ask him to recognise it by palpating the object.
4. Repeat the procedure with four to five familiar objects.
5. Repeat the procedure in the opposite hand.

**Precautions**

1. The subject should be instructed properly.
2. The subject should close his eyes during the experiment.
3. The sensation should be elicited by giving objects that are familiar to the subject.
4. The test should be repeated with at least three different objects.
5. The sensation should be elicited in one hand at a time and should be repeated in the other hand.

## Sense of Position and Joint Movement

This is tested by passively moving the limbs of the subject to a particular position with the eyes closed and asking him to recognise the position of the limb. The perception of movement is closely related to the sense of position; therefore, both the senses are tested together.

**Steps**

1. Supply proper instructions to the subject (to recognise the particular position of the limb when the limb is moved).
2. Ask him to close his eyes.
3. Move his finger or hand, up or down and ask the subject to recognise the movement by calling out the position of the finger/limb or by imitating the same movement in the other limb.
4. Repeat the procedure by changing the position of all the limbs.
5. Make movement at all the joints (all small and big joints) and ask the subject to recognise the joint movement.

> Note: Note the angle through which the limb was moved. If the sense of movement is decreased, this angle is greater than that in the normal limb. Movements of less than 10° are appreciated at all the normal joints.

6. Make a particular movement (flexion or extension at a joint) and ask the subject to recognise the direction of movement.

> Note: The patient can sometimes recognise the occurrence of a movement but not its direction.

**Precautions**

1. The subject should be properly instructed to cooperate fully in the experiment.
2. The subject should close his eyes during the experiment.
3. Movement at different joints and position of different parts of the limbs should be performed.
4. The sensation should be elicited on both the sides and compared simultaneously.

## Sense of Vibration

**Steps**

1. Supply proper instructions to the subject.
2. Make the tuning fork vibrate by hitting the blades of the fork against the hypothenar eminence of the palm or against the thigh.
3. Place the foot of the vibrating tuning fork on the surface of the body, especially on a bony prominence like the lower end of the tibia, styloid process of the radius and medial or lateral malleolus (Fig. 29.5), and ask the subject whether he feels the vibration.

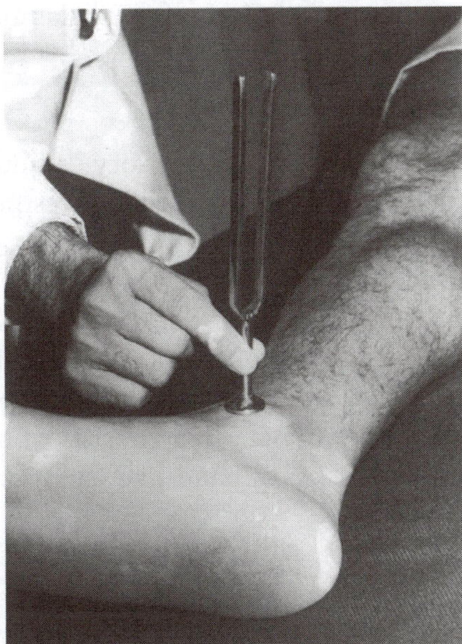

Fig. 29.5 Testing the sense of vibration. Note that the examiner places (holds the stem without touching the blade) the tuning fork on the bony prominence.

4. Ask the subject to raise his finger when he ceases to feel the vibration.
5. Immediately place the tuning fork on the corresponding bony prominence of your body and note whether you can still perceive the vibration.

> Note: If the examiner perceives the vibration after the subject ceases to perceive it, the sense of vibration is impaired in the subject.

6. Elicit vibration sense on all the bony prominences of the body.

**Precautions**

1. The subject should be instructed properly.
2. The tuning fork should be allowed to vibrate by hitting the blades of the fork against the hypothenar eminence of the palm or against the thigh, not against any hard surface.
3. The examiner should hold the tuning fork by holding the stem of the fork close to the base without touching the blades.
4. The vibrating fork should be placed only on the bony prominence.
5. After the subject ceases to feel the vibration, the examiner should place the fork immediately on the corresponding point on his own body to check if the vibration has actually ceased.
6. The sensation should be elicited on the corresponding bony prominence of the opposite side of the body.

## Pain

### *Superficial Pain*

**Steps**

1. Supply proper instructions to the subject.
2. Explain properly that you will be eliciting pain.
3. With the help of a pin (not a needle), lightly prick the skin of different parts of the body and ask the subject to indicate whether he feels pain.
4. Elicit pain from all the dermatomes of both sides of the body.
5. Delineate the area of analgesia, hypoalgesia or hyperalgesia, if present.

**Precautions** Same as described for 'Fine Touch'

### *Pressure Pain*

**Steps**

1. Supply proper instructions to the subject.

2. With an algometer, carefully press on the surface of the body and note the minimum pressure required to produce pain.
3. Repeat the procedure on the identical points of the body on the opposite side and compare the results.

> Note: Clinically pressure pain is elicited by squeezing the muscle or tendon (Achilles tendon) till pain is produced.

### Temperature

**Steps**

1. Give proper instructions to the subject (to say whether he feels cold or warm when touched with different glass tubes).
2. Take two test tubes containing warm and cold water separately.
3. Place the test tubes on the skin of the subject, each in turn or randomly and ask the subject to say whether he feels warm or cold.
4. Examine warm and cold sensation on all the dermatomes of both sides of the body and note your observation.

**Precautions** Same as described for 'Fine Touch'

## DISCUSSION

## Abnormalities of Sensation

### Tactile Sensation

*Anesthesia*

Anesthesia means loss of all sensation. Anesthesia is graded as hypoesthesia when the sensation is decreased or complete anesthesia when the sensation is totally lost.

**Causes of hypoesthesia** It is seen in lesions of the central sensory structures, like lesions of the thalamus, internal capsule or cortex. Usually it affects the distal parts of the limbs more than the proximal parts.

**Causes of complete anesthesia**

1. Usually occurs in peripheral nerve lesions. The common causes are leprosy and complicated diabetes mellitus. Lesions of peripheral nerves result in anesthesia corresponding to the distribution of sensory fibres.
2. Complete anesthesia also occurs in complete transection of the spinal cord where anesthesia is seen in the limbs and trunk below the level of the lesion.

*Dissociated Anesthesia*

When the sensation of pain and temperature is lost with the preservation of the touch sensation, the condition is known as dissociated anesthesia.

**Physiologic basis** Dissociated anaesthesia occurs in conditions where the grey matter of the spinal cord near the central canal is damaged. The fibres carrying the touch sensation ascend in the dorsal column of the spinal cord and are therefore spared. The fibres carrying pain and temperature cross to the opposite side of the spinal cord at the same segmental level of the cord. While crossing to the opposite side, the fibres travel very close to the central canal, therefore they are damaged in the disease process involving the grey matter of the spinal cord.

**Causes**

- Syringomyelia
- Intramedullary tumours
- Brainstem lesions (syringobulbia)
- Thrombosis of the posterior inferior cerebellar artery.

*Hemianesthesia*

This is loss of sensation that affects the face, arm and leg of one side (usually opposite side) of the body.

**Causes** Usually seen in lesions of the thalamus, internal capsule or cortex.

*Hyperesthesia*

When the response to a sensory stimulation is exaggerated, the condition is called hyperesthesia.

**Cause** Thalamic lesions

*Paresthesia*

When the touch sensation is perverted (touch may produce an unpleasant sensation almost amounting to pain) is called paresthesia. This consists of sensations like pricking, numbness or band-like sensations around the trunk.

**Causes**

- *Nerve compression* This is the commonest cause of paresthesia. It occurs when peripheral nerves are stretched or subjected to pressure. The commonest example is paresthesia (numbness and pricking) after sitting for a longer time with legs crossed.

- Spinal tumours
- Subacute combined degeneration of spinal cord (Vitamin $B_{12}$ deficiency)
- Disseminated sclerosis
- Thalamic lesions

## Proprioceptive Sensation

The proprioceptive sensation is that of joint movement, sense of the position of different parts of the body and the sense of vibration. The loss of proprioceptive sensation can occur without loss of other sensations. It is characteristic of the lesions of the posterior column or lesion of the fibres ascending in the posterior column to the medulla.

Loss of proprioception is seen in:

1. Tabes dorsalis
2. Subacute combined degeneration of spinal cord

## Pain

### *Analgesia*

Loss of pain sensation is called analgesia.

**Causes** Analgesia occurs with anesthesia, and usually seen in peripheral nerve lesion. Analgesia can also occur without anesthesia. A hereditary analgesia syndrome has been described, in which the pain receptors are totally absent in the body.

### *Hypoalgesia*

Partial loss of pain sensibility is called hypoalgesia.

**Cause** Nerve compression

### *Hyperalgesia*

This is a condition of exaggerated sensibility to pain. In this condition, a mild stimulus, which ordinarily does not produce pain, causes severe pain. It may occur in response to a mild cutaneous stimulus or sometimes as an intractable spontaneous activity (without stimulus).

**Causes**

- Spinal cord disease, for example, tabes dorsalis
- Thalamic lesions
- Deep-seated lesions in the parietal lobe

## Common Clinical Conditions

### *Peripheral Nerve Pain*

This occurs due to injury to the nerve, neuritis and neuropathy. It may be associated with other sensory loss with or without motor changes. Sometimes only nerve pain may occur without other sensory or motor loss. Then it is called neuralgia; for example, trigeminal neuralgia.

### *Root Pain*

Pain is seen in the area of distribution of a particular root that is affected. The most common examples are cervical and lumbar root pain distributed to the appropriate limb, as in cervical spondylosis or lumbar disc prolapse. It is characteristic of extra medullary cord compression.

### *Causalgia*

This is an abnormal type of burning sensation usually seen after limb injuries. It occurs when the nerve injury is mild.

### *Visceral Pain*

This occurs due to diseases of the viscera. For example, inflammation of abdominal viscera produces pain. Visceral pain differs from somatic pain in various ways. These are:

1. Poorly localised. The pain receptors in the viscera are relatively few, therefore, the visceral pain is poorly localised.
2. Associated with autonomic changes like hypotension, nausea, vomiting and sweating. Autonomic changes occur due to activation of visceral reflexes.
3. Associated with muscle guarding (spasm of the abdominal wall). Muscle guarding occurs due to reflex contraction of the skeletal muscle in the abdominal wall. This is a protective reflex as it prevents further injury to the viscera.
4. Often radiates or is referred to other areas. Usually visceral pain is referred to a somatic structure that is developed from the same dermatome of the visceral structure in which the pain originates. The most common example is pain of myocardial infarction radiating to the ulnar border of the left hand or the pain of cholecystitis radiating to the tip of the shoulder.

### *Brown–Sequard Syndrome*

This occurs in a hemisection of the spinal cord. It is usually seen in injury to the spinal cord or in tumours that affect one half of the cord. On the side of the lesion, the dorsal column sensations (the fine touch sensation, proprioceptive sensations and the tactile localisation and discrimination) are lost. On the opposite side of the lesion pain, temperature and crude touch sensations are lost. This occurs because the sensation for fine touch, proprioception, and two-point discrimination ascend the dorsal column of the same side, whereas the sensation for pain, temperature and crude touch ascend the anterolateral system of the opposite side of the spinal cord.

### *Syringomyelia*

In this condition there is a lesion around the central canal of the spinal cord. The lesion interrupts the pain and temperature fibres passing to the opposite side of the spinal cord. Therefore, there is loss of pain and temperature with preservation of touch and postural sensibility.

## Physiological Significance

Examination of sensory system is performed to localise disease processes that affect any part of the neuraxis of the sensory system. This is called localisation of lesion of the sensory system. Localisation of lesion partly depends on the distribution of the sensory loss and partly on the type of sensory loss. The disease may affect the nerve, the nerve root, the spinal cord, the brainstem, the thalamus or the cortex.

### *Nerve Lesion*

Lesion of a peripheral nerve results in anaesthesia corresponding to the distribution of that particular nerve (Figs. 29.6, 29.7).

### *Nerve Root Lesion*

There is segmental anesthesia in root lesions corresponding to the involvement of the segment of the spinal cord from where the nerve root arises.

### *Spinal Cord Lesion*

Complete section of spinal cord causes anesthesia in the limbs and trunks below the level of lesion. Hemisection of the spinal cord results in dissociation of anesthesia (dissociated sensory loss as seen in Brown–Sequard syndrome). A lesion around the central canal of the spinal cord results in loss of pain and temperature on both the sides below the level of the lesion with preservation of other sensations.

### *Brainstem Lesion*

Above the medulla, the spinothalamic tract (fibres of the anterolateral system) remains in close association with the trigeminothalamic tract in the tegmentum, whereas the medial lemniscus carrying the fibres of posterior column lies medial to it. A lesion of the lateral part of the tegmentum causes hemianalgesia and thermoanesthesia in the opposite side of the body without affecting other sensations (as the medial lemniscus is spared). A deep-seated lesion in the upper part of the brainstem may involve the medial lemniscus without affecting the spinothalamic fibres. This results in loss of posterior

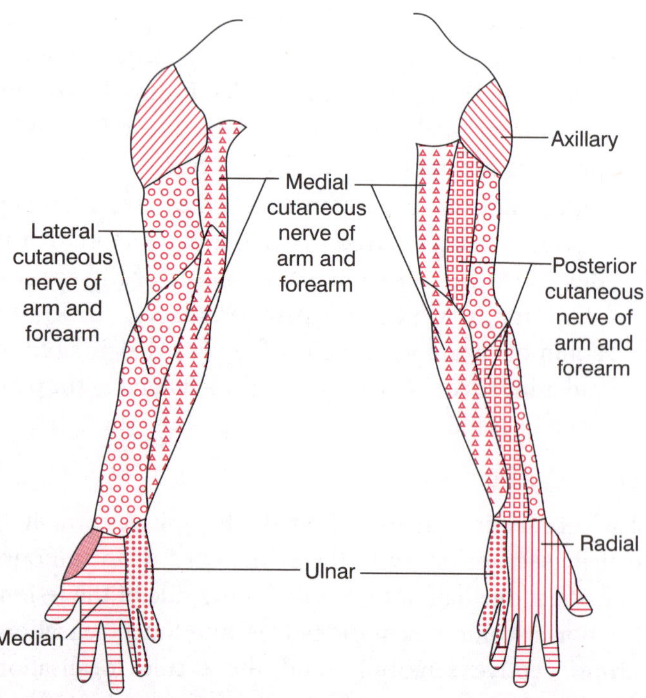


Fig. 29.6 Peripheral nerve lesions in the upper limbs.

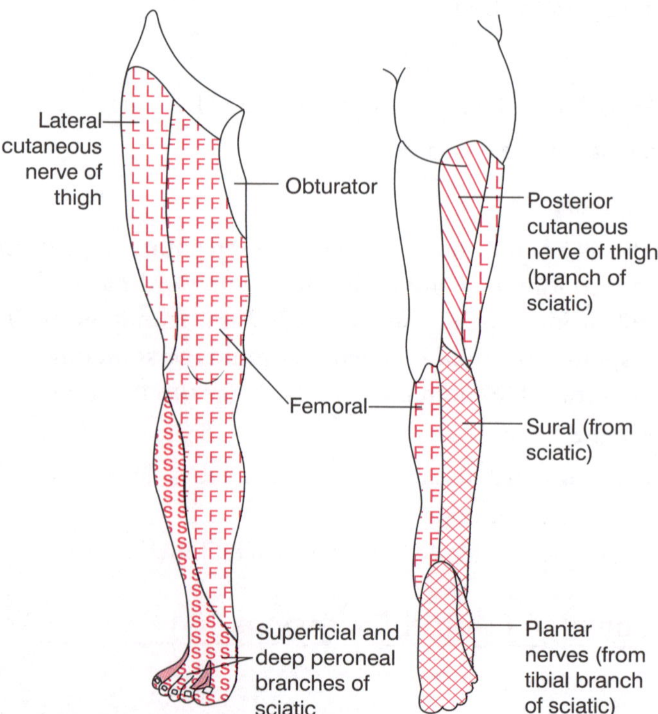


Fig. 29.7 Peripheral nerve lesions in the lower limbs.

column sensations with preservation of pain and temperature.

### *Thalamic Lesion*

Severe and extensive lesion of the thalamus results in gross impairment of sensory modalities on the opposite side of the body. The threshold for pain may be raised, but a less painful stimulus may cause an exaggerated response (hyperalgesia). The touch sensation may induce an unpleasant sensation (paresthesia). This is called the thalamic syndrome, which occurs in the lesions of the lateral and ventral nucleus.

### *Cortical Lesion*

The cortex is primarily involved in processing the finer aspect of sensations, especially the spatial and discriminatory sensibility. Tactile localisation, two-point discrimination and stereognosis are therefore called cortical sensations. The cortical lesion results in impairment of tactile localisation, two-point discrimination and stereognosis. Other sensations may remain intact.

## VIVA

1. How do you classify sensations?
2. Define a receptor.
3. What are the types of receptors?
4. What are the sensations carried in the dorsal column?
5. What are the sensations carried in the anterolateral system of the spinal cord?
6. Trace the pathway for fine touch.
7. Trace the pathway for proprioception.
8. Trace the pathway for pain and temperature.
9. What is a sensory map? What is its physiologic significance?
10. What are the precautions to be observed during elicitation of fine touch sensation?
11. What are the precautions to be observed during elicitation of tactile localisation and two-point discrimination?
12. Why is the tuning fork placed on the bony prominence for eliciting vibration sensibility?
13. What are the precautions to be taken during elicitation of vibration sensibility?
14. What is dissociated anesthesia?
15. What are the causes of dissociated anesthesia and what is the physiological basis of it?
16. What is hyperesthesia and what are its causes?
17. Define paresthesia. Give two causes of paresthesia.
18. What is hyperalgesia? What are its causes? What is causalgia?
19. How does visceral pain differ from somatic pain?
20. What is the Brown-Sequard syndrome? What are its features?
21. What are the sensory changes seen in syringomyelia?
22. What is the physiological significance of examination of the sensory system?
23. What are the sensory features of brainstem lesion?
24. What is the effect of a lesion of the thalamus on sensory functions?
25. What is the effect of a lesion of the cortex on sensory functions?

CHAPTER 30

# Clinical Examination of the Motor System

**LEARNING OBJECTIVES**

After completing this practical, you will be able to:

- Describe the importance of performing this practical in clinical physiology.
- Measure the bulk of the muscles.
- Estimate and grade the strength of various individual and groups of muscles.
- Assess the tone of flexors and extensors at various joints.
- Elicit superficial and deep reflexes.
- Test the coordination of movement in the upper and lower limbs.
- Name the descending motor pathways.
- Trace the pathway of corticospinal tracts.
- List the differences between upper and lower motor neuron paralysis.

You may also be able to:

- Trace the pathway of all descending motor tracts.
- List the functions of motor pathways, basal ganglia, cerebellum and motor cortex.
- Explain briefly the role of alpha and gamma motor neurons in regulation of muscle tone.
- Name the common conditions associated with alteration in bulk, tone and strength of the muscles and reflexes.
- Explain the changes in motor function in upper and lower motor neuron paralysis.
- List the differences in coordination of movement in cerebellar, sensory and corticospinal pathway disorders.
- Describe the different types of abnormal gaits and involuntary movement.

## INTRODUCTION

### Anatomical and Physiological Consideration

The motor system consists of motor areas in the brain, the upper motor neurons, the lower motor neurons and the muscles. The motor system deals with the body functions related to movement of different parts of the body. Movement occurs due to contraction and relaxation of the agonists and antagonists. Agonists are muscles that facilitate movement by their contraction, whereas antagonists facilitate movement by their relaxation. Movement depends on the maintenance of posture and balance. A balanced posture provides a stable background for movement.

### Muscles

Muscles can be classified in various ways. But, to understand motor physiology, the muscles can be best classified as the medial (proximal) and the lateral (distal) group.

*The Proximal Group of Muscles*

The proximal groups of muscles are the muscles of the trunk, girdles and proximal parts of the limbs. These muscles are primarily involved in the maintenance of posture and equilibrium.

*The Distal Group of Muscles*

The distal groups of muscles are the intrinsic muscles of the digits and the muscles of the distal parts of the extremities. They are not required for postural activities, but are primarily involved in the control of skilled voluntary movement, that is, manipulatory activities.

### Lower Motor Neuron

The lower motor neurons are the final common pathway for the output of the motor system. The cell bodies of the lower motor neurons are present in the anterior horn of the spinal cord. The lower motor neurons consist of the anterior horn cells and the homologous cells in the brainstem, their efferent nerve fibres that pass via the anterior spinal nerve roots and peripheral nerves to the muscles, and the terminal axonal branches that innervate the muscle fibres. In the ventral horn, the most medially situated motor neurons innervate the proximal groups of muscles (the axial muscles and the proximal limb muscles) and the most laterally situated motor neurons innervate the distal groups of muscles of the body. Therefore, the medial groups of motor neurons are involved in postural control, whereas the lateral groups of motor neurons are involved in manipulatory (skilled) activities.

## Upper Motor Neuron

The upper motor neurons originate in the motor cortex and other areas in the brain that are involved in the regulation of motor activities, and terminate on the anterior horn cells. The upper motor neurons are classically divided into two types: (i) pyramidal fibres (corticospinal tract) and (ii) extrapyramidal fibres. The pyramidal fibres are the motor neurons that pass through the pyramid in the medulla, regardless of their cells of origin. The extrapyramidal fibres are the neurons that do not pass through the pyramid of the medulla. The corticospinal tract is synonymous with the pyramidal tract for all clinical purposes. The extrapyramidal tracts are rubrospinal, vestibulospinal, reticulospinal and tectospinal tracts. Strictly speaking, some of the fibres of the pyramidal system do not pass through the pyramid and some of the fibres of the extrapyramidal system pass through the pyramids. Therefore, from the physiological point of view, the upper motor neurons are better divided into the medial system pathways and the lateral system pathways.

### The Lateral System

The upper motor neurons of the lateral system descend in the lateral funiculus of the spinal cord and terminate directly or indirectly on the laterally placed motor neurons in the anterior horns. This includes two major pathways: the lateral corticospinal tract and the rubrospinal tract. As the lateral system fibres terminate on the lateral group of motor neurons in the anterior horn that innervate the distal group of muscles of the body, they are primarily involved in regulation of skilled voluntary activities.

### The Medial System

The upper motor neurons of the medial system descend in the ventral funiculus of the spinal cord and terminate mostly indirectly on the medially placed motor neurons in the anterior horns. This includes the vestibulospinal (lateral and medial), reticulospinal (medullary and pontine), tectospinal and interstitiospinal tracts. As the medial system fibres terminate on the medial group of motor neurons in the anterior horn cells that innervate the proximal group of muscles of the body, they are primarily involved in regulation of posture and equilibrium.

#### *Corticospinal Tracts*

**Origin, course and termination** The fibres of the corticospinal tract originate in the fifth layer of the motor cortex. Fibres pass through the posterior limb of the internal capsule (Fig. 30.1) where all the fibres coming from different areas of the motor cortex converge into a narrow space (therefore a lesion in the internal capsule causes maximum motor deficit). Then the fibres descend down through the midbrain and pons into the medulla where they form the pyramid. In the medulla, 80–90 per cent of the fibres after passing through the pyramid, cross over (decussate) to the opposite side and then enter the contralateral spinal cord to form the lateral corticospinal tract. These upper motor neurons enter the anterior grey horn of the spinal cord and project directly onto the lower motor neurons. Fibres of this tract have monosynaptic connections with the motor neurons that innervate the distal groups of muscles. The remaining 10–20 per cent of the fibres in the medulla do not cross over to opposite side.

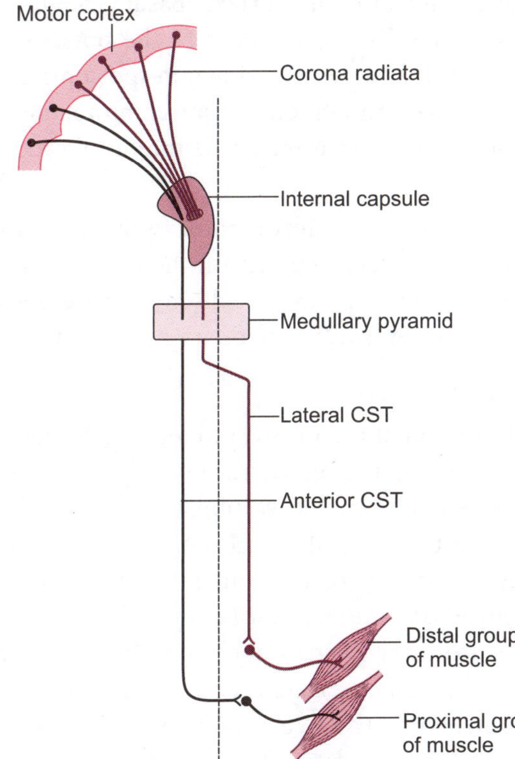


Fig. 30.1 Pyramidal (corticospinal) tract. Lateral CST: Lateral corticospinal tract; Anterior CST: Anterior corticospinal tract.

They descend down ipsilaterally in the same side of the spinal cord as the anterior corticospinal tract and cross over to the opposite side only at the segmental level (at the segments in the spinal cord where they innervate the muscles through the lower motor neurons). These fibres project onto the lower motor neurons (mostly indirectly) through interneurons that supply the proximal groups of muscles.

**Functions**

1. The lateral corticospinal tract conveys the information from the motor cortex to the distal group of skeletal muscles on the opposite side of the body that coordinates and regulates skilled voluntary movement.
2. The anterior corticospinal tract conveys the information from the motor cortex to the proximal group of skeletal muscles on the opposite side of the body that coordinates and regulates the movement of the axial skeleton (that is involved in the control of posture).

#### *Rubrospinal Tract*

**Origin, course and termination** This tract originates from the red nucleus in the midbrain, which receives input from the motor cortex, basal ganglia and cerebellum. The fibres cross over to the opposite side in the midbrain and descend down in the contralateral spinal cord to terminate on the lower motor neurons in the anterior horn that innervate the distal groups of muscles.

**Functions** This tract conveys motor impulses from the red nucleus to skeletal muscles on the opposite side of the body that governs precise, discrete movements of the hands and feet (skilled voluntary movements).

#### *Vestibulospinal Tracts*

The vestibulospinal tract conveys motor impulses from the vestibular nuclei, which receive inputs regarding head movement from the vestibular apparatus in the inner ear, to the skeletal muscles on the same side of the body that are involved in maintenance of balance and posture. The *lateral vestibulospinal tract* (LVST) originates from the Deiter's nucleus that receives input from the utricles and saccules and traverses the length of the spinal cord. The LVST is involved in adjustment of body posture in relation to linear acceleration. The *medial vestibulospinal tract* (MVST) originates from the medial and the descending vestibular nuclei that receive input from the semicircular canals and traverses up to the midthoracic level. This tract adjusts body posture (head, neck and trunk movement) in relation to angular or rotational acceleration.

#### *Reticulospinal Tracts*

The reticulospinal tracts originate from the reticular formation, traverse through the entire length of the spinal cord and convey information to the proximal group of muscles. Therefore, these tracts are involved in the regulation of posture. The *medullary reticulospinal tract* facilitates flexor reflexes, inhibits extensor reflexes and decreases muscle tone. The *pontine reticulospinal* tract inhibits flexor reflexes, facilitates extensor reflexes and increases the tone of antigravity muscles. Therefore, pontine RST is the most important tract involved in the control of posture.

#### *Tectospinal Tract*

**Origin, course and termination** The fibres in the tectospinal tract originate from superior colliculus and immediately cross over to the opposite side. This tract descends down only up to the midcervical segments in the spinal cord and innervates the muscles of the head and neck.

**Function** The tectospinal tract conveys impulses from the superior colliculus to the skeletal muscles on the opposite side of the body that are involved in movement of head and neck in response to visual stimuli. Therefore, it controls visually guided head movements.

## The Motor Areas in the Brain

The motor areas in the brain include the cortical motor areas and the other areas that are involved in regulation of motor activities. Corticospinal tracts (the pyramidal tract) arise from cortical motor areas. The other descending motor pathways, especially extrapyramidal tracts, do not directly arise from the cortical motor areas, rather they originate from the brainstem areas that receive inputs from the basal ganglia, cerebellum and motor cortex. Therefore, apart from the cortical motor areas the important motor areas in the brain are the basal ganglia and cerebellum.

### The Cortical Motor Areas

The cortical motor areas in the brain include the areas in the cortex that on stimulation produce motor activities. This includes the primary motor cortex (area

4), premotor cortex (lateral portion of the area 6), the supplementary motor cortex (medial portion of the area 6), the somatosensory cortex (areas 3, 1, 2), and the posterior parietal cortex (areas 5, 7). About 60 per cent of the fibres in the corticospinal tract come from motor areas (primary motor cortex, premotor cortex and supplementary motor cortex) whereas the remaining 40 per cent originate from the sensory areas in the cortex.

### Basal Ganglia

The basal ganglia is a subcortical structure that consists of several groups of nuclei in each cerebral hemisphere, which includes neostriatum (caudate nucleus and putamen), globus pallidus, subthalamic nucleus and substantia nigra. The basal ganglia receives inputs from the cortex and thalamus and projects back to the cortex via the thalamus. It is involved in control of posture and movement, especially in the initiation, planning, programming and smoothening of movement.

### Cerebellum

The cerebellum receives inputs from the vestibular apparatus, the spinal cord and the cortex. It influences the lower motor neuron activities indirectly via its projection to the vestibular nuclei, the brainstem areas and the cortex. The vestibulocerebellum (archicerebellum) is involved in maintenance of equilibrium and balance, the spinocerebellum (paleocerebellum) is involved in smoothening and coordination of movement, and the corticocerebellum (neocerebellum) is involved in the planning and programming of movement.

# METHODS

## Methods of Examination of Motor Functions

### Principle

The integrity of the motor system is assessed by examining the size, tone and strength of the muscles, and by evaluating the reflex response of the muscle to stretch, and coordination of movement.

### Requirements

1. Measuring tape
2. Knee hammer

### Procedure

The following aspects of motor functions are assessed while examining the motor system:

1. Bulk of muscles
2. Tone of muscles
3. Strength of muscles
4. Reflexes
5. Coordination of movement
6. Gait
7. Involuntary movement (if present)

## Bulk of Muscles

The bulk of the muscles can be easily estimated by inspection and palpation.

1. Ask the subject to sit on a stool or lie down on a couch comfortably and remove all his clothing.
2. Inspect the muscle mass of all parts of the body and note if there is any wasting (atrophy) or hypertrophy of any particular group of muscles.
3. Palpate the muscle to assess the consistency.

> Note: Wasted or atrophic muscles are not only smaller, but also softer and flabbier than normal muscles, especially when they are contracted. Hypertrophic muscles are usually firm in consistency. If muscle wasting is associated with fibrosis as is in polymyositis, the muscles are hard to palpate and inelastic.

4. Compare the bulk of the muscles of both sides of the body.
5. Measure the midarm (Fig. 30.2A) and midforearm (Fig. 30.2B) circumference in the upper limbs, and midthigh (Fig. 30.2C) and midcalf (Fig. 30.2D) circumference in the lower limbs of both sides with of a measuring tape.

> Note: Measurement of the girth of the muscles is the best way of estimating the bulk of the muscle.

## Tone of Muscles

Tone is a state of partial contraction of muscles. Clinically, tone means the resistance of the muscle to passive stretching. It is estimated by handling and passively moving the parts of the body.

1. Ask the subject to relax completely.
2. Passively move different parts of the body at various joints and try to feel the degree of resistance encountered during each passive movement (Fig. 30.3).

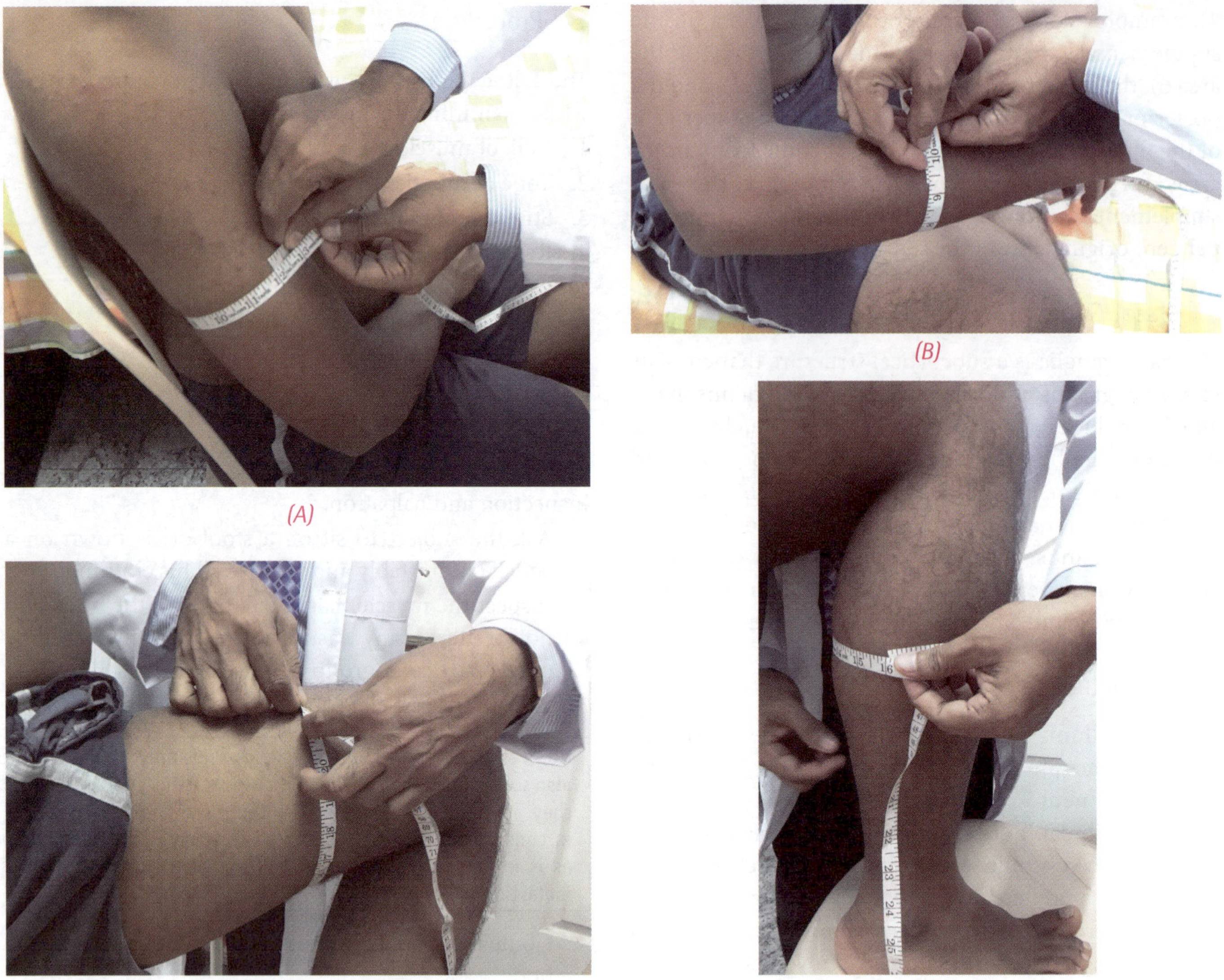

(A)

(B)

(C)

(D)

Fig. 30.2 Measurement of A: midarm, B: midforearm, C: midthigh and D: midcalf circumference.

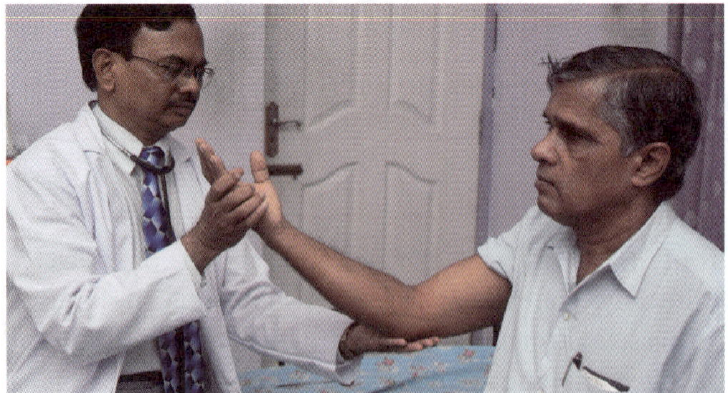

Fig. 30.3 Eliciting the tone of biceps muscle by passively extending at elbow joint. Note that the examiner appreciates the feeling of resistance offered to passive extension movement, not by actively palpating the muscle.

> Note: The degree of resistance offered by the muscle during passive movement indicates the state of tone. This is perceived by feeling the resistance to movement, not by palpating the muscle. For example, passive flexion of the forearm stretches the triceps muscle and passive extension of the forearm stretches the biceps muscle. Therefore flexion assesses the tone of the triceps and extension assesses the tone of the biceps muscle. The tone may be normal, decreased (hypotonia) or increased (hypertonia). Do not palpate muscle while making passive flexion movement for eliciting tone, as handling of muscle could stimulate muscle sensory receptors and alter muscle tone due to interference.

3. Assess and compare the tone of muscles of both sides of the body simultaneously.

## Strength of Muscles

The strength of muscles is better estimated by active movement against resistance.

1. Ask the subject to perform a movement of any part of the body (say flexion of the forearm) and you oppose the movement actively (oppose flexion of the forearm by placing your palm on his forearm and giving maximum resistance to stop flexion).

> Note: The strength of the subject is assessed by comparing with the strength of the examiner. Age, sex and build of the person should be kept in mind while comparing the strength.

2. Compare strength of the same group of muscles of the other side simultaneously.
3. Test the strength of muscles of the lower limbs, upper limbs and the trunk of the body.

### Grading of the Strength of the Muscles

Strength or weakness of muscles is graded into six degrees by the Indian Medical Research Council Scale.

Grade 0 : Complete paralysis (no contraction)

Grade 1 : A flicker of contraction only (without any resultant movement of any limb or joint)

Grade 2 : The muscle can make movement only when the opposing force of gravity is eliminated by appropriate positioning

Grade 3 : The limb can be moved against the force of gravity, but not against the examiner's resistance

Grade 4 : The muscle is able to make the full range of normal movement, but can be overcome (by resistance) to a variable extent

Grade 5 : Normal power

### Testing the Strength of Muscles of the Upper Limbs

#### *Interossei and Lumbricals*

**First dorsal interosseous** Ask the patient to abduct his index finger against resistance; while doing so, this muscle becomes prominent and the contraction of the muscle can be felt.

**Dorsal interossei** These are abductors of the fingers. Therefore, their power can be tested by asking the patient to abduct the fingers against resistance.

**Palmar interossei** These are the adductors of the fingers. These are tested by placing a paper or card between the fingers and trying to pull out the paper/card.

**Lumbricals** These are tested by asking the patient to flex his metacarpophalangeal joints and to extend his distal interphalangeal joints. This can be done by asking him to hold a pen. While the terminal phalanx of the thumb is being apposed against the terminal phalanx of any other finger, the examiner may try to dislodge the pen by force. This gives a combined test for opponens pollicis and lumbricals.

**Flexors of the fingers** Flexors of the fingers are flexor pollicis longus, flexor pollicis brevis, flexor digitorum superficialis and flexor digitorum profundus. These are tested by asking the subject to squeeze your index and middle finger.

**Flexors of the wrist** Flexors of the wrist are flexor carpi radialis, flexor pollicis brevis, and palmaris longus. Ask the subject to bring the tips of his fingers towards the front of the forearm so as to touch the crease on the front of the wrist joint.

**Extensors of the wrist** These are extensor carpi radialis and extensor carpi ulnaris. Ask the subject to flex the fingers in the form of a fist and the hand is held with the palm downwards. Then hold the wrist joint firmly and ask the subject to extend the wrist joint against resistance.

**Brachioradialis** Place the arm midway between the prone and the supine position. Then ask the subject to bend the forearm upwards. Oppose the movement by grasping the hand. The brachioradialis becomes prominent.

**Biceps** Ask the subject to lift up the forearm against resistance offered by grasping the hand or wrist with the forearm in full supination. The biceps becomes prominent as it contracts.

**Triceps** Ask the subject to straighten out his forearm while the examiner tries to keep it flexed by passive resistance.

**Supraspinatus** Ask the subject to keep his arm by the side of the body and then direct the subject to lift it straight outward at right angles to his side. The first 30° angle of movement is carried out by the supraspinatus. The remaining 60° angle is produced by the deltoid.

**Deltoid** It can be tested along with the supraspinatus. The subject is asked to make forward and backward movements of the abducted arm at a 45° angle against resistance (the anterior and posterior fibres of the deltoid help to draw the abducted arm forward and backward, respectively).

**Infraspinatus** Place the subject's elbow by his side with a forearm flexed to a right angle, then ask the subject to rotate the limb outward against the resistance applied to the middle of the outer aspect of the forearm. Contraction of the muscle can be seen and felt.

**Pectorals** Ask the subject to stretch his arm out in front of him and then to clap his hands while the examiner attempts to hold them apart.

**Serratus anterior** If the muscle is paralysed the subject will be unable to elevate his arm above a right angle when asked to do so. Paralysis of this muscle causes winging of the scapula. Therefore, look for 'winged scapula'. The deformity becomes more prominent when the patient is asked to push forward against the wall with both hands.

**Lattisimus dorsi** The subject is asked to clap his hands behind his back while the examiner (standing behind the subject), offers passive resistance to the downward and backward movement.

### Testing the Strength of Muscles of the Trunk

**Abdominal muscles** The weakness of the muscles of the abdomen is detected by observing the subject's inability to raise himself in bed without the aid of his arms. Babinski's rising-up sign is also checked. This is done by asking the subject to lie on his back with legs extended and rise without using his hands.

**Erector spinae and muscles of the back** Ask the subject to lie down on his face and try to raise his head from the bed by extending the neck and back. If the back muscles are healthy, the muscles will stand out prominently during this effort.

### Testing the Strength of Muscles of the Lower Limb

**Intrinsic muscles of the foot** It is difficult to examine the strength of intrinsic muscles of the foot (lumbricals and interossei). If the interossei are weakened or paralysed, claw-foot develops.

**Dorsiflexor and plantar flexors of the feet and toes** Dorsiflexors are peronei, and plantar flexors are tibialis posterior, gastrocnemius and soleus. These are tested by asking the patient to elevate or depress the part against resistance. The observer should try to fix the ankle or apply resistance against the patient's movement.

**Evertors and invertors of the foot** Evertors are peronei, and invertors are tibialis anterior and tibialis posterior.

**Extensors of the knee** Quadriceps are the extensors of the knee. Bend the patient's knee and then pressing with your hand on his shin, ask him to straighten his limb.

**Flexors of the knee** These are biceps femoris, semitendinosus and semimembranosus. Raise the straightened lower limb, supporting the thigh with your left hand and holding the ankle with your right hand. Then ask the subject to bend his knees.

**Extensors of the thigh** Gluteus maximus is the extensor of the thigh. Lift the subject's foot off the bed when the knee is extended and ask him to depress the limb against resistance.

**Flexors of the thigh** These are the iliopsoas and the tensor fascia lata. In the extended leg, ask the subject to raise his lower limb of the bed against resistance, without bending the limb at knee joints.

**Adductors of the thigh** These are the adductor longus, adductor brevis, adductor magnus and gracilis. Abduct the lower limb and then ask the subject to bring it back to the midline against resistance.

**Abductors of the thigh** These are the gluteus medius and gluteus minimus. Bring the lower limb to the midline and then ask the subject to move it outward against resistance.

**Rotators of the thigh or hip** These are the gluteus medius, gluteus minimus, obturator externus and obturator internus. With your lower limb extended on the bed, ask the subject to rotate the limb outwards, and inwards against resistance.

## Reflexes

Clinically, reflexes are of three types: tendon or deep reflexes, superficial reflexes, and visceral or sphincteric reflexes.

### Tendon or Deep Reflexes

The contraction of the muscle in response to a sudden stretch produced by striking the tendon (with a knee hammer) is called a tendon reflex. Tendon reflexes are stretch reflexes because they are elicited by stretching the muscle. These stretch reflexes are monosynaptic reflexes. The tendon reflexes assess the integrity of the afferent and efferent pathways and excitability of the anterior horn cells in the spinal segment of the stretched muscle.

The following precautions should be observed for eliciting tendon reflexes:

1. The subject should be completely relaxed.
2. Reassure the subject that the knee hammer is not a harmful instrument and will not cause pain while eliciting reflexes.
3. The subject's limb should be appropriately positioned.
4. Before striking the tendon, the muscle should be lightly stretched by positioning the limb.
5. The tendon should be stroked briskly by making a sudden jerky movement at the wrist joint.
6. The knee hammer should be loosely held between the thumb and the index finger, so that it swings freely in an arc, yet is controlled in its direction.
7. The homologous reflex on the opposite side should always be tested immediately for comparison.
8. If the reflexes are not elicited, the reinforcement technique (Jendrassik's maneuver) should be used.

**Grading of the tendon reflexes** Tendon reflexes can be graded into five degrees as given below.

> Note: Normal supinator jerk is less than average and normal knee jerk is brisker than average reflexes.

Grade 0 : Absent (no response)
Grade 1 : Present but diminished (as a normal supinator jerk)
Grade 2 : Brisk (as a normal knee jerk)
Grade 3 : Very brisk (hyperactive)
Grade 4 : Clonus

### *Biceps Jerk (C5,6)*

1. Ask the subject to relax.
2. Flex the elbow of the subject to a right angle and place his forearm in a semi-pronated position and support with your hand, with subject in sitting position (Fig. 30.4) or in supine position (Fig. 30.5) or by placing his elbow on his abdomen, with the subject is in the lying position on the bed (Fig. 30.6).
3. Place your thumb firmly on the biceps tendon.
4. Strike your thumb with the help of the pointed end of the knee hammer so that the biceps tendon stretches by striking the thumb.
5. Observe the contraction of the biceps muscle and the flexion at the elbow.

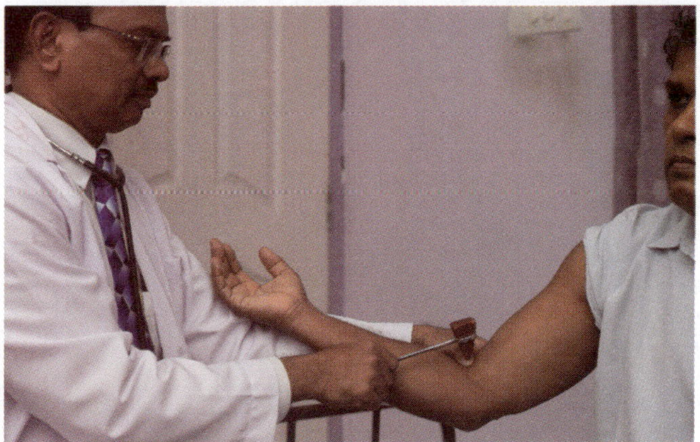

Fig. 30.4 Demonstration of elicitation of biceps jerk in sitting or standing posture. Note that the subject rests his forearm on the forearm of the examiner with elbow joint flexed. The examiner strikes the biceps tendon by striking his own thumb (placed and pressed on the tendon), using the narrow end of the knee hammer.

6. Elicit biceps jerk of the other limb and compare.

### *Triceps Jerk (C6,7)*

1. Flex the subject's arm at the elbow and allow the forearm to rest on his abdomen (Fig. 30.7) or be supported by your hand (Fig. 30.8).

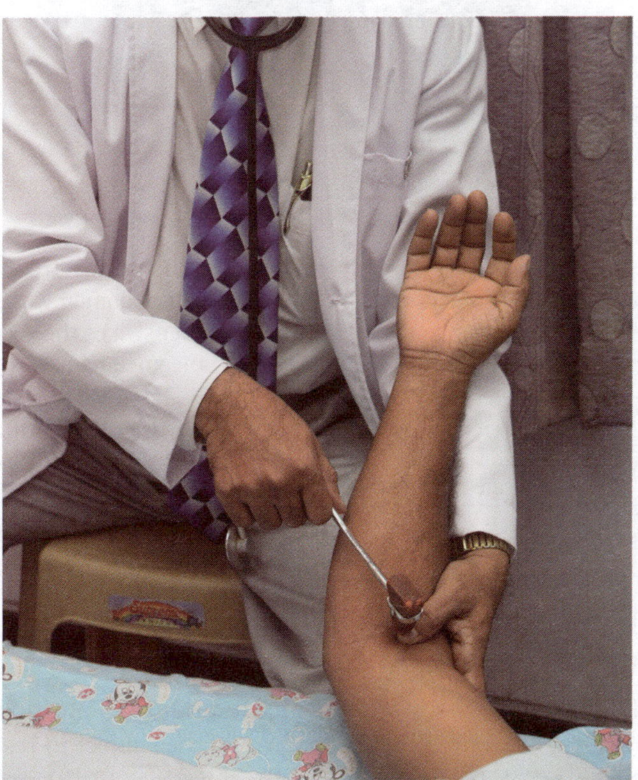

Fig. 30.5 Elicitation of biceps jerk in lying position of the subject.

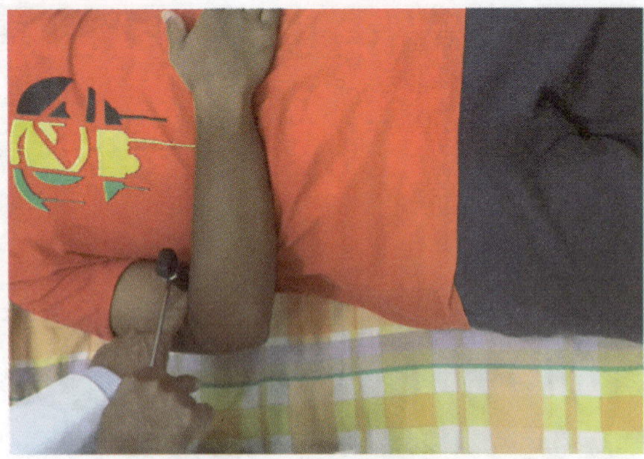

Fig. 30.6 Demonstration of elicitation of biceps jerk in supine posture. Note that the subject rests his forearm on his abdomen with elbow flexed at an angle of 90°. The examiner strikes the biceps tendon by striking his own thumb (placed and pressed on the tendon), using the narrow end of the knee hammer.

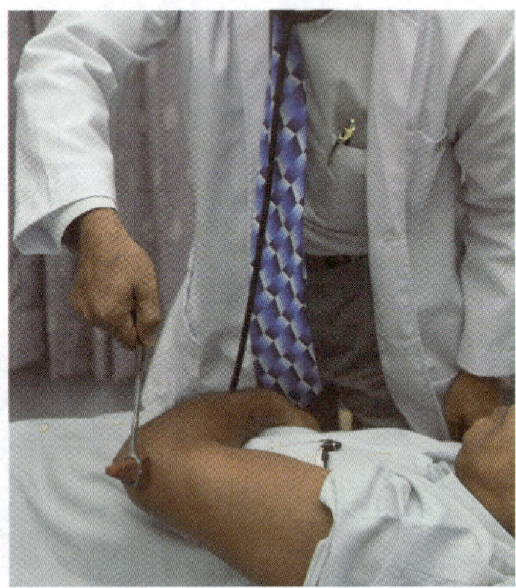

Fig. 30.7 Demonstration of triceps jerk in supine posture. Note that the subject rests his forearm on his abdomen with elbow flexed at an angle of 90°. The examiner strikes the triceps tendon by using the broad end of the knee hammer.

2. Tap the triceps tendon directly above the olecranon.

Note: Take care not to strike the belly of the triceps muscle.

3. Observe the contraction of the triceps muscle and extension at the elbow.
4. Elicit the triceps jerk of the other side and compare.

*Supinator or Brachioradialis Jerk (C5,6)*

1. Hold the hand of the subject in sitting position (Fig. 30.9) or allow the forearm of the subject to rest on his abdomen in supine position (Fig. 30.10) and slightly stretch the brachioradialis muscle by laterally bending the hand in the opposite direction.

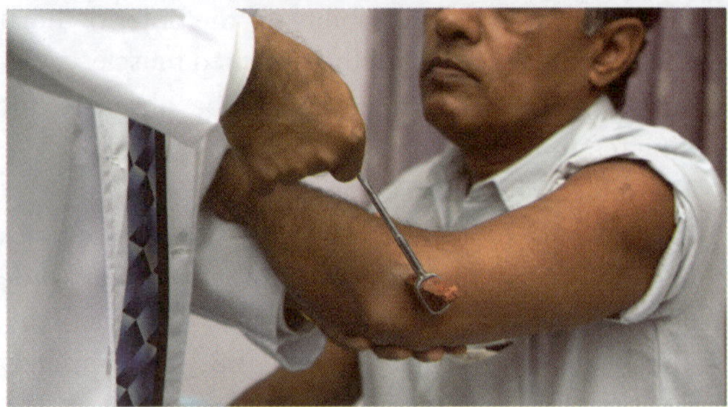

Fig. 30.8 Demonstration of triceps jerk in sitting or standing posture. Note that the forearm of the subject rests on the forearm of the examiner with his elbow joint flexed at 90°. The examiner strikes the triceps tendon by using the broad end of the knee hammer.

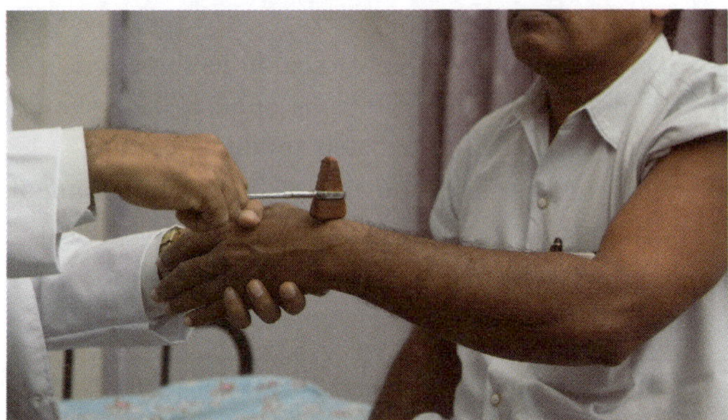

Fig. 30.9 Demonstration of supinator jerk in sitting or standing posture. Note that the examiner holds the hand of the subject and slightly dorsiflexes it and then strikes the brachioradialis tendon at the wrist by using the broad end of the knee hammer.

2. With the help of a knee hammer strike the radius 1–2 inches above the wrist over its styloid process.
3. Observe the flexion at the elbow and supination of the forearm.
4. Elicit the supinator jerk of the other side and compare.

*Knee Jerk (L2,3,4)*

It can be tested with the subject either in the supine or the sitting position.

**In the supine position** (Figs. 30.11, 30.12 and 30.13)

1. Expose the part (up to the upper thigh)
2. Pass your forearm under the knee to be tested and place your hand on the opposite knee (the knee to be tested should rest on the dorsum of your wrist and forearm).

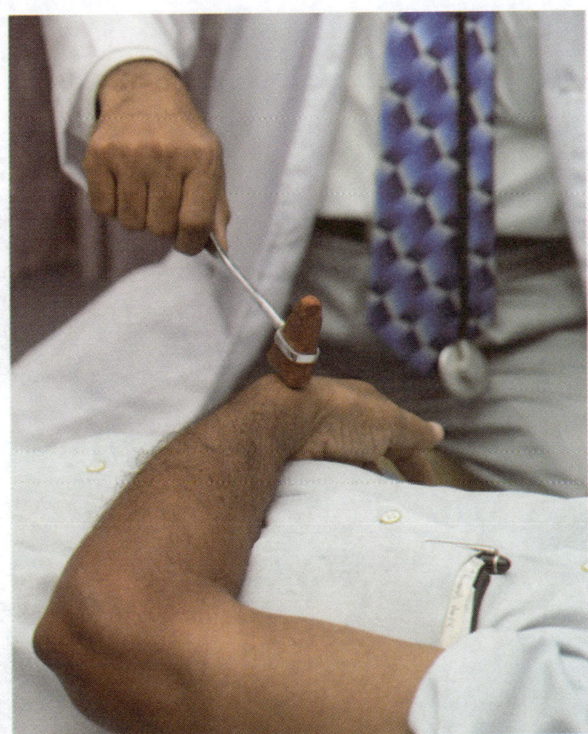

Fig. 30.10 Demonstration of supinator jerk in supine posture. Note that the subject rests his forearm on his abdomen and the examiner strikes the brachioradialis tendon at the wrist by using the broad end of the knee hammer.

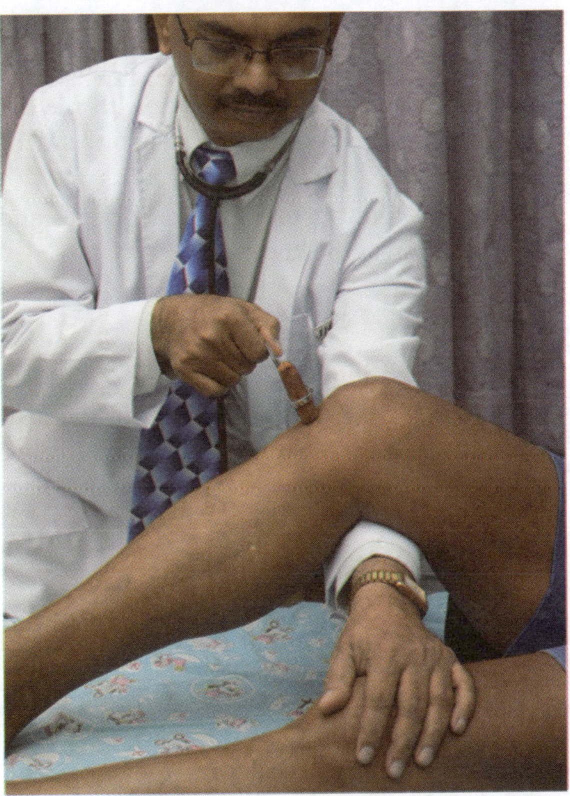

Fig. 30.11 Demonstration of knee jerk in supine position. Note that the examiner supports the leg to be examined by placing his hand below the leg in such a way that he lifts it with the help of the other leg.

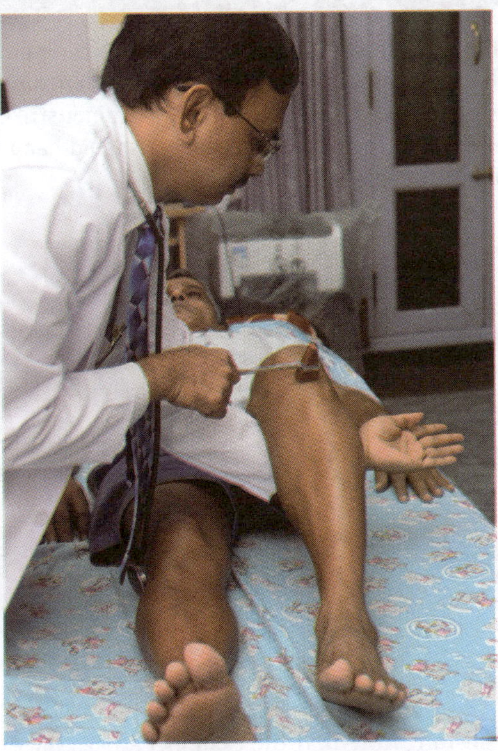

Fig. 30.12 Elicitation of knee jerk of left side, in supine position, lifting the leg by forearm of examiner as shown.

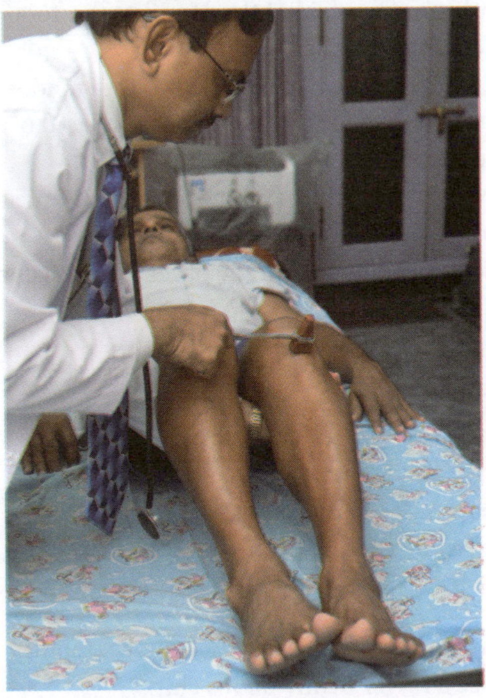

Fig. 30.13 Elicitation of knee jerk of both the sides in one lifting, in supine position.

3. Semiflex the knee and lift your hand slightly so that the weight of the knee rests on your hand.
4. Strike the patellar tendon directly with the help of a knee hammer (by using the narrow end of the hammer).
5. Observe the contraction of the quadriceps and the brief extension at the knee.
6. Elicit the knee jerk of the opposite side and compare.

**In the sitting position** (Fig. 30.14)

1. Ask the subject to sit over the edge of the bed or a stool in such a way that his legs dangle freely from the edge, or ask the subject to keep one knee (the knee to be tested) on the other knee.
2. Ask him to relax completely.
3. Strike the patellar tendon.
4. Observe the contraction of the quadriceps and the extension at the knee joint.

### *Ankle Jerk (S1,2)*

The ankle jerk can be tested with the subject in the supine or kneeling position.

**In the supine position** (Fig. 30.15)

1. Place the lower limb (to be examined) of the subject on the bed in such a way that it is everted and slightly flexed.
2. With one hand, slightly dorsiflex the foot so as to stretch the Achilles tendon.
3. With the other hand, strike the tendon on its posterior surface (by using the broad end of the knee hammer).
4. Observe for any contraction of calf muscles and plantar flexion of the foot.
5. Elicit the ankle jerk of the other side and compare.

**In the kneeling position** (Fig. 30.16)

1. Ask the subject to kneel on a chair or on a bed with feet projecting out.
2. Slightly dorsiflex the foot.
3. Strike the Achilles tendon.
4. Observe for contraction of calf muscles and plantar flexion of the foot.

### *Jaw Jerk (Fig. 30.17)*

1. Ask the subject to partially open his mouth.
2. Place a finger firmly on his chin.
3. Strike the finger with the help of a knee hammer (using the narrow end of the hammer).

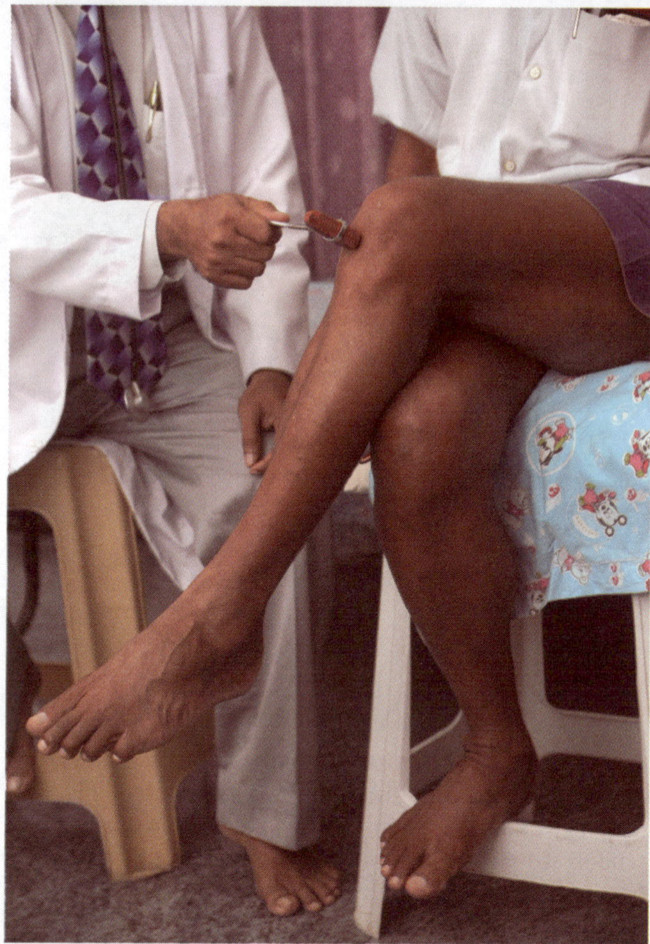

Fig. 30.14 Demonstration of knee jerk in sitting position. Note that the subject sits on a stool or chair crossing the leg to be examined on the other leg. The examiner strikes the patellar tendon. The legs of the subject should hang freely (should not touch the ground).

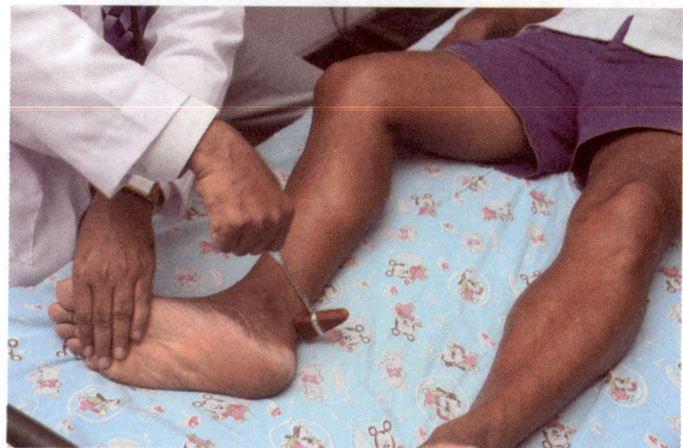

Fig. 30.15 Demonstration of elicitation of ankle jerk in supine posture. Note that the examiner strikes the Achilles tendon after slightly dorsiflexing the foot. Also note that the knee of the examined leg is flexed to an angle of 120°.

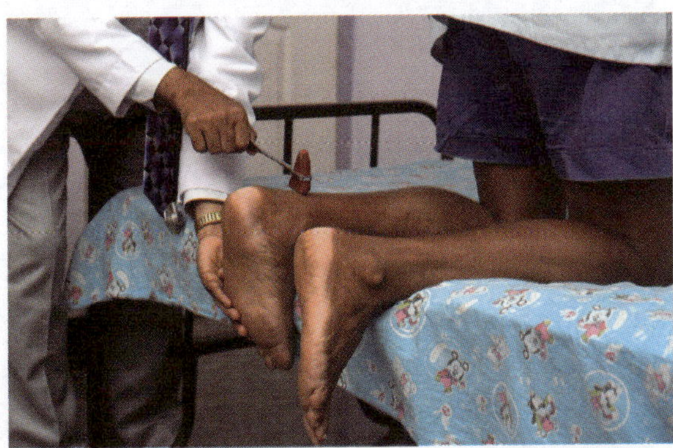

Fig. 30.16 Demonstration of ankle jerk in kneeling posture. Note that the subject kneels on a chair or on the bed and the examiner strikes the Achilles tendon after slightly dorsiflexing the foot.

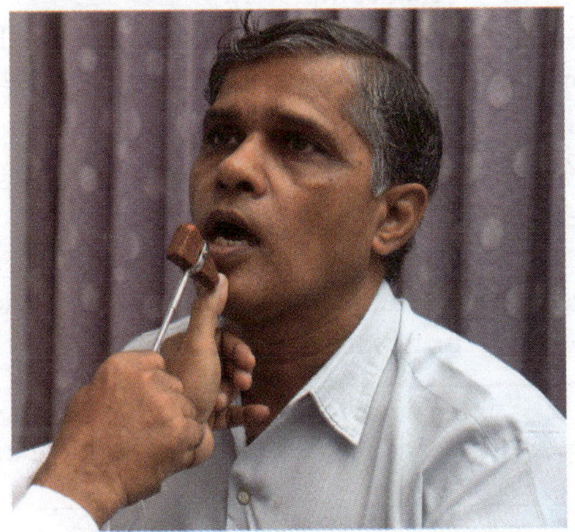

Fig. 30.17 Demonstration of jaw jerk. Note that the examiner strikes the thumb placed on the chin of the subject (subject partially opens his mouth).

4. Observe for immediate closure of the mouth (due to contraction of the elevators of the jaw).

*Jendrassik's Maneuver*

This is performed by asking the subject to make a strong voluntary muscular effort using following methods:

1. While testing the reflexes of the lower limb, ask the subject to hook the fingers of two hands together and then pull them apart (against one another) as hard as possible (Fig. 30.18).
2. While testing the reflexes of the upper limb, ask the subject to clench his teeth or to make a fist in the other hand (Fig. 30.19).

> Note: Jendrassik's maneuver works by increasing the excitability of the anterior horn cells and by increasing the sensitivity of the muscle spindle primary sensory endings to stretch by increasing the gamma fusimotor discharge.

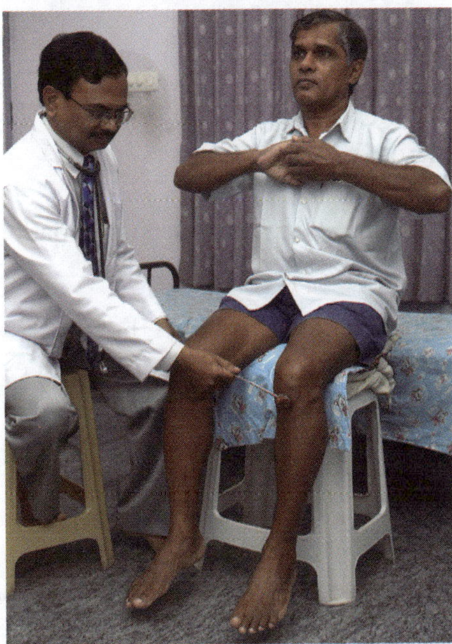

Fig. 30.18 Demonstration of Jendrassik's maneuver. Note that the subject pulls apart the fingers of both the hands hooked against each other, during which the examiner elicits the jerk.

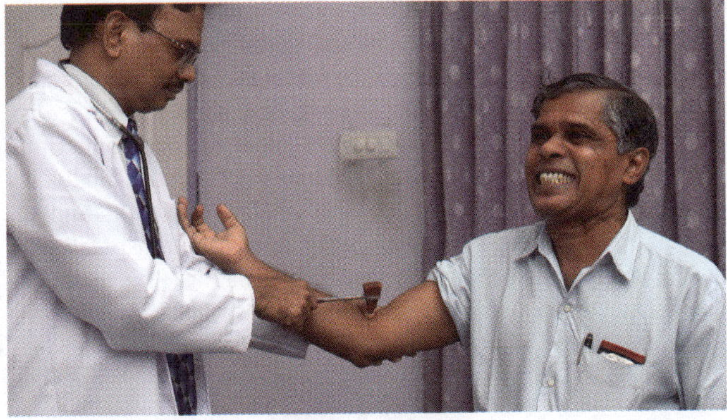

Fig. 30.19 Jendrassik's maneuver for upper limbs. Note that subject clenches his teeth while examiner elicits the reflex.

## Superficial Reflexes

The superficial reflexes are elicited by stimulating the cutaneous receptors. The stimulation of an area of the skin by scratching results in contraction of certain muscles supplied by the same spinal segment. These reflexes are polysynaptic reflexes. Superficial reflexes are of two types, spinally mediated and cranially mediated.

Chief superficial reflexes of the spinal origin are:

- Plantar reflex
- Cremasteric reflex
- Bulbocavernosus reflex
- Anal reflex

- Abdominal reflex
- Scapular reflex

Superficial reflexes of cranial origin are:

- Conjunctival reflex
- Corneal reflex
- Pupillary reflexes (light and accommodation reflex)

### *Plantar Reflex (L5 S1)*

1. Ask the subject to lie down on the couch.
2. Partially flex the lower limb and rotate it externally.
3. With one (left) hand, grasp the leg just above the ankle joint.
4. Ask the subject to relax completely.
5. In the other hand, with the help of a pointed object (pointed metallic portion of the knee hammer or a pointed key) gently scratch the outer edge of the sole of the foot from the heel towards the little toe and then medially across the metatarsus towards the ball of the great toe (Fig. 30.20).
6. Observe for the plantar response.

> Note: The plantar response may be a flexor plantar response or an extensor plantar response. The flexor plantar response is characterised by inversion and dorsiflexion of the ankle with flexion of all the toes at the metatarsus. This is normally present in healthy subjects. The extensor plantar response is characterised by dorsiflexion of the great toe and abduction or fanning of other toes with dorsiflexion of the ankle. It is found in patients with corticospinal tract lesions and is a pathognomonic feature of upper motor neuron paralysis. This abnormal response is also called Babinski's sign as it was first described by Babinski. It is also normally seen in newborns and infants.

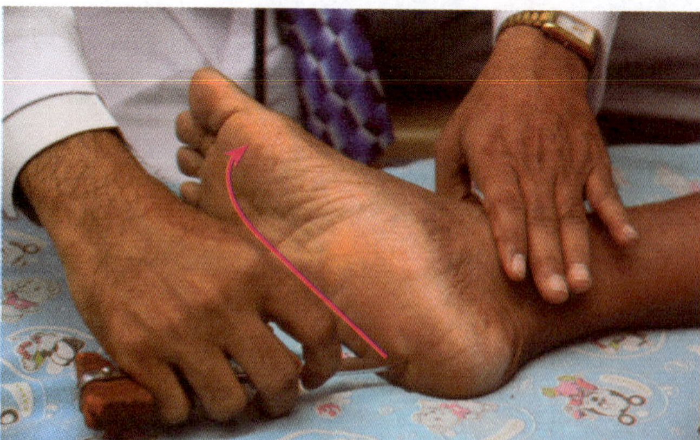

Fig. 30.20 Demonstration of elicitation of plantar reflex. Note that a pointed object is used to stroke or scratch on the lateral aspect of the sole in the direction of the arrow depicted in the figure.

### *Cremasteric Reflex (L1,2)*

This is elicited only in male subjects.

1. Expose the part (genitalia and upper thigh).
2. Lightly scratch the inner aspect of the upper part of the thigh.
3. Observe the elevation of the testicle on that side and the contraction of the dartos muscle as evidenced by increase in wrinkling of the skin of the scrotum.
4. Elicit the cremasteric reflex of the opposite side.

### *Abdominal Reflex (T7–12)*

1. Ask the subject to lie down in the supine position.
2. Expose the abdomen fully.
3. Ask him to relax completely.
4. Stroke lightly but briskly each side of the abdomen above and below the umbilicus, with a key or a pencil or the pointed metallic end of the knee hammer (Fig. 30.21), from the outer aspect towards the midline (Fig. 30.22).
5. Observe the contraction of the abdominal muscles after every stroke as evidenced by the deviation of the umbilicus towards the stimulus.

> Note: It is often impossible to elicit abdominal reflexes in obese, elderly and anxious patients and in multiparous women.

### *Bulbocavernosus Reflex (S3,4)*

This is elicited only in male subjects.

1. Expose the part (external genitalia).
2. Pinch the dorsum of glans penis.
3. Observe the contraction of the bulbocavernosus muscle.

### *Anal Reflex (S3,4)*

1. Expose the anal region.
2. Ask the subject to relax completely.
3. Stroke or scratch the skin near the anus.
4. Observe the contraction of the anal sphincter.

### *Scapular Reflex (C5–8, T1)*

1. Expose the upper portion of the back.
2. Stroke the skin in the interscapular region.
3. Observe the contraction of the scapular muscles.

## Sphincteric Reflexes

These reflexes are concerned with swallowing, defecation and micturition. They depend upon complex muscular

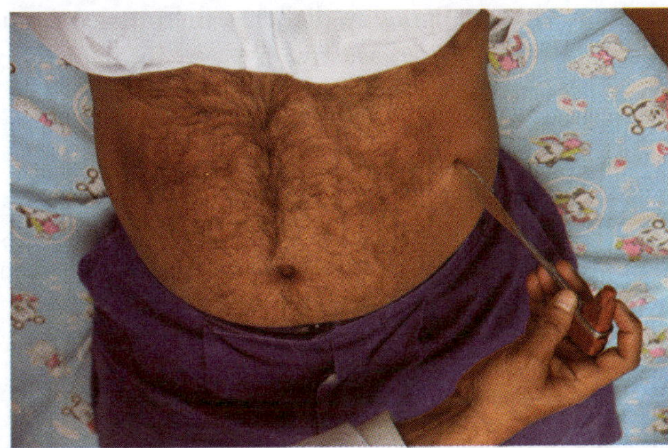

Fig. 30.21 Note that with the pointed metallic end of the knee hammer, surface of abdomen is scratched from the outer aspect towards the midline.

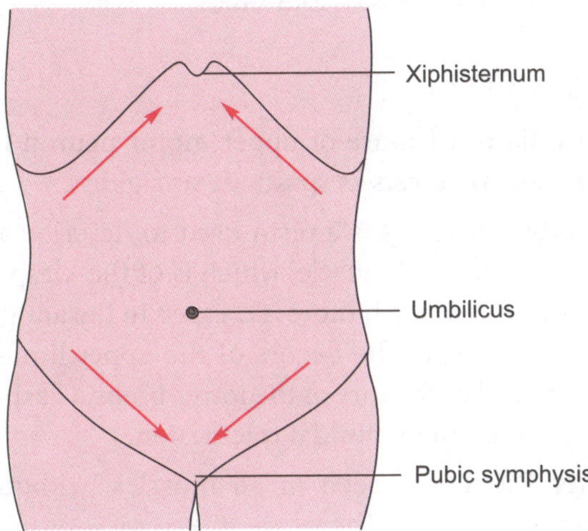


Fig. 30.22 Site and direction of stimulation for elicitation of abdominal reflex.

movement excited by increased tension in the wall of the viscera concerned.

**Swallowing** Ask the subject whether he has any difficulty in swallowing (dysphagia). Also ask whether there is any regurgitation of food through the nose. If dysphagia is present, ascertain whether it is predominantly for liquids or solids or both.

**Defecation** Ask the subject if he has any problem in passing stools. The subject should also be questioned regarding the presence of normal or abnormal anorectal sensation.

**Micturition** The subject should always be asked regarding his bladder habits, and whether he has any problem in controlling or initiating micturition. Retention of urine, incontinence or urgency of micturition should be noted.

## Coordination of Movement

Coordination of movement means smooth recruitment, interaction and cooperation of muscles or groups of muscles to carry out a precise and definite motor act. Coordination of movement should be tested both in the upper and the lower limbs.

### In the Upper Limbs

#### *Finger-Nose Test*

1. Supply proper instructions to the subject regarding the test.
2. Ask the subject to touch the tip of his nose with the tip of his index finger rapidly and repeatedly, first with the eyes open, and then with the eyes closed.
3. Observe whether the subject is able to touch his nose every time.
4. Ask him to repeat the test with the other hand.

#### *Making a Circle*

1. Supply proper instructions to the subject regarding the test.
2. Ask the subject to draw a circle in the air with his forefinger.
3. Observe whether the subject is able to draw a circle.
4. Ask him to repeat with the other hand.

#### *Dysdiadokokinesis*

Dysdiadokokinesia is the inability to execute rapidly repeated alternate movements. Diadokokinesis can be tested in different ways.

1. Ask the subject to flex his elbow to a right angle and then ask him to perform supination and pronation of his forearm as rapidly as possible, or
2. Ask him to tap the palm with the tips of his fingers as fast as possible in an arhythmic manner, or
3. Ask the subject to clap over the dorsum of one hand with the palm of another hand as quickly as possible. He may be asked to perform this movement alternately on either hand.

### In the Lower Limbs

#### *Knee-Heel Test*

1. Ask the subject to lie down in the supine position.
2. With the eyes open, ask him to place one heel on the opposite knee and then to slide the heel down the shin of his leg towards the ankle.

3. Ask him to repeat the procedure in quick succession.
4. Observe whether he performs the action properly.
5. Ask him to repeat the procedure with the other limb.

*Making a Circle*

1. Ask the subject to draw a circle in the air with his toes.
2. Observe whether he is able to draw a circle.

*Walking*

1. Ask the subject to walk on a straight line.
2. Observe whether he is able to walk on a straight line.

## Gait

Gait is defined as the attitude of walking. It is tested by asking the subject to walk with bare feet on a straight line. Ask him to walk a distance and then to turn round and come back. While the subject is walking observe the following points:

1. Whether he walks at all.
2. If he walks, does he walk in a straight line or does he tend to deviate to one side.
3. If he tends to fall, in what direction?

## Involuntary Movement

Involuntary movements are not seen normally. In some diseases of the nervous system there are involuntary, unintended movements. Observe whether there is any involuntary movement of any part of the body. If involuntary movements are present, note the type of movement.

# DISCUSSION

## Bulk of the Muscle

The bulk of the muscle may be normal, decreased (atrophy) or increased (hypertrophy).

### Muscle Atrophy

Muscle atrophy is seen in neurological disorders, especially in lower motor neuron disease. Generalised wasting of the muscle occurs in non-neurological conditions like malignancy, diabetes, thyrotoxicosis and tuberculosis. Localised wasting is seen in arthritis or myopathy.

### Muscle Hypertrophy

Hypertrophy occurs due to excessive use of muscles as in athletes and gymnasts. It can also occur in some myotonic disorders.

## Tone of the Muscle

The tone of the muscle is the state of partial contraction of the muscle. Healthy muscles always exhibit certain degrees of tone. In some diseases, the tone of the muscles increases (hypertonia) and in others the tone of the muscles decreases (hypotonia).

### Hypertonia

Hypertonia is a feature of upper motor neuron lesion. Hypertonia manifests as spasticity or rigidity.

**Spasticity** Spasticity is a term used to describe a state of increased tone of muscle, which is of the 'clasp-knife' type. The tone is much more increased in the antigravity muscles, that is, in the flexors of the upper limbs, and extensors and adductors of the lower limbs. Clasp-knife rigidity is seen in pyramidal tract lesion.

**Rigidity** Rigidity is seen in all muscles, without any relation to gravity. There are two types of rigidity: lead pipe and cogwheel. This is seen in lesions of extrapyramidal tracts.

**Lead pipe rigidity** The resistance to passive movement is uniform throughout the range of movement. It is seen in catatonic states, dementia and Parkinsonism.

**Cogwheel rigidity** The resistance to passive movement is seen alternately, that is, there is alternate resistance and relaxation. This is typically seen in diseases of the basal ganglia, particularly in the involvement of the substantia nigra.

## Strength of Muscles

If muscle strength is decreased, there is paresis and if there is no strength, there is paralysis.

**Hemiplegia** means paralysis of one side of the body, especially of the arms and legs, paraplegia means paralysis of both legs, monoplegia means paralysis of one limb and quadriplegia means paralysis of all four limbs.

Hemiplegia is usually seen in lesions of the corticospinal tract at the level of the internal capsule. Paraplegia is seen in spinal cord lesions below the midthoracic level and quadruplegia is seen in spinal cord lesion above the upper throacic level. Monoplegia usually occurs due to lesions of a nerve plexus. Crossed paralysis refers to paralysis of the ipsilateral cranial musculature with contralateral hemiplegia. It is usually seen in brainstem disease.

Weakness of the muscle may occur in the absence of paralysis. It occurs due to myasthenia gravis, myopathies and myotonic dystrophy.

## Reflexes

### Tendon Reflexes

Tendon reflexes are stretch reflexes that are activated in response to a sudden stretch of the muscle. These are monosynaptic reflexes that are activated by stretching of the muscle spindle that conveys information via Ia fibres directly to the motor neurons in the spinal cord (Fig. 30.23). Stimulation of the α motor neuron causes contraction of the muscle that was stretched. The presence of the tendon reflexes indicates the integrity of the afferent and efferent pathways, and of the excitability of the anterior horn cells in the spinal segment of the stretched muscles. The tendon reflexes are continuously affected by the activities in the descending (from supraspinal centres) pathways. The higher centres usually inhibit the spinal reflexes. Therefore, the tendon reflexes are exaggerated in upper motor neuron lesions.

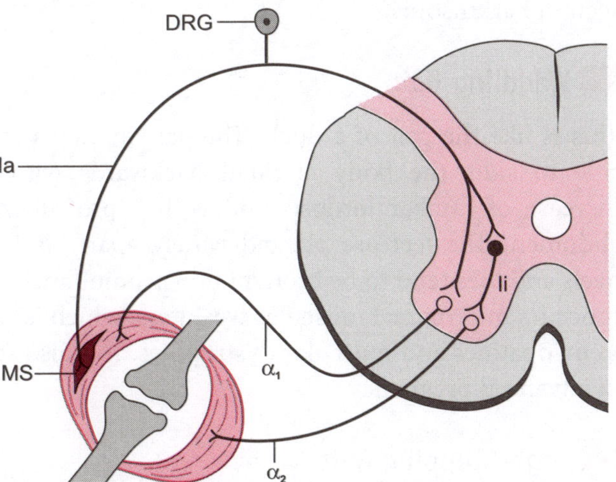


Fig. 30.23 The stretch reflex. DRG: Dorsal root ganglion; MS: Muscle spindle; Ii: Inhibitory interneuron; $\alpha_1$ and $\alpha_2$: Motor neurons; Ia: Ia afferents.

The tendon reflexes are diminished or absent in lower motor neuron lesions as there is disruption in the final common pathway.

Gamma motor neurons increase the sensitivity of the muscle spindle to stretch. Therefore, increased γ motor neuron discharge increases the reflex activity. The γ motor neurons are usually under the inhibitory influence of supraspinal inputs. Therefore, a lesion of the upper motor neuron results in exaggeration of deep reflexes.

### Superficial Reflexes

The superficial reflexes are polysynaptic and involve many centres in the neuraxis. These are elicited by stimulating the cutaneous receptors that carry information to higher centres by sensory pathways. The higher centres then convey information to the concerned muscles by motor pathways. Therefore, superficial reflexes are lost in both upper and lower motor neuron paralysis.

## Coordination of Movement

Normal movement is dependent on the ability of the agonist muscles to contract to the degree needed and the simultaneous relaxation of the antagonist muscles. Impairment in these abilities produces incoordination of movement. This incoordination may be due to a disease of the cerebellum, the corticospinal tract or the sensory system. Lack of proper coordination is known as ataxia.

### Cerebellar Disease

In cerebellar ataxia, the errors of movement tend to occur at right angles to the intended direction of movement. A useful sign of cerebellar ataxia is dysdiadokokinesia which is the impaired ability to execute rapidly repeated alternate movements. All the aspects of movement (initiation, rate, range, direction and termination) are affected.

### Corticospinal Tract Disease

The incoordination is characterised by slowness and clumsiness in finger movements. This is tested by asking the patient to rapidly approximate each finger to the thumb. Corticospinal tract disease does not cause incoordination of movement at the more proximal joints, that is, knee, hip, elbow and so on; it also does not cause incoordination of movement in the leg. However, if it is associated with muscle weakness, impairment in walking occurs.

### Sensory System Disease

Incoordination of movement can be produced in the arms or legs by impaired sensation. This is called sensory ataxia. It is tested by the Romberg sign. The patient is asked to stand with his feet close together and if he can do so, he is asked to close his eyes. If the subject sways or falls, the Romberg sign is positive. It is an important physical sign of impaired position and joint sense in the lower limb.

## Gait

Gait is the posture of the subject while walking. The character of the gait is often important in the diagnosis of neurological diseases. Normally, when a person walks, he partially flexes the hip and knee joint of one lower limb and dorsiflexes his foot. As he does so, his foot is lifted above the ground and the other lower limb supports the whole weight of the body. As the first lower limb is moved forward and takes up his weight, the other lower limb is flexed and the whole cycle is repeated. If the smooth manner in which the whole movement is performed is disturbed, the gait becomes abnormal. The common abnormal gaits are:

- Spastic gait
- Ataxic gait
- Festinant gait
- Waddling gait
- High-stepping gait
- Limping gait

### Spastic Gait

The spastic gait is probably the commonest abnormal type. The patient walks on a narrow base, has difficulty in bending his knees and drags his feet along as if they are glued to the ground. The movement is slow and the flexion of the knee and hip joints is either absent or imperfectly performed. The affected leg tends to remain adducted. The foot is raised from the ground by tilting the pelvis and the leg is then swung forwards so that the foot tends to describe an arc (circumduction), the toe scraping along the floor. It is characteristically seen in corticospinal tract lesions. There are two types of spastic gaits: (i) hemiplegic and (ii) scissor.

**Hemiplegic gait** In this type of gait only one leg is affected. It is seen in hemiplegia.

**Scissor gait** The spasticity is present on both sides. The patient walks in a typical criss-cross fashion. It is typically seen in congenital spastic paraplegia.

### Ataxic Gait

This occurs due to ataxia. Ataxic gaits are of two types, stamping and drunken.

**Stamping gait** It is a high-stepping ataxic gait in which the movements in the lower limbs are not coordinated. The patient raises his feet suddenly and often abnormally to a higher level and then jerks them forward, bringing them to the ground again with a stamp, and often heel first. Ataxia increases in darkness or if the eyes are closed. It is best seen in tabes dorsalis and severe peripheral neuritis.

**Drunken gait** The patient walks on a broad and irregular base, the feet being planted widely apart. The ataxia is equally severe whether the eyes are opened or closed. It is typically seen in cerebellar disorders.

### Festinant Gait

The patient walks with an attitude of generalised flexion (bent forward) so that the centre of gravity of the body lies outside in front of him. To bring the centre of gravity to its proper place, the patient takes rapid, short and shuffling steps. But, the centre of gravity moves forward and continues to elude him. Thus, he attempts to catch the centre of gravity. His arms do not swing. It is typically seen in Parkinsonism.

### Waddling Gait

This is like the gait of a duck. The patient sways from side to side, the body is tilted backwards with an increase of lumbar lordosis and with a protruberant abdomen. The feet are planted widely apart, and the heels and toes tend to be brought down simultaneously. It occurs in proximal muscular weakness, which is seen in myopathies and muscular dystrophies. It is also seen in advanced pregnancy.

### High-Stepping Gait

The patient walks taking high steps. It is typically seen in foot drop, as in peripheral neuritis or peroneal muscular dystrophy.

### Limping Gait

The patient limps with short steps, keeping the painful limb semiflexed and dropping the pelvis towards the painful side. It is seen in tuberculosis of the knee and hip joints and in sciatica.

## Involuntary Movement

Involuntary movements can occur either at rest or during voluntary movement. Involuntary movements are classified into two types, localised and generalised.

### Localised Involuntary Movement

1. Fibrillation
2. Fasciculation
3. Myoclonus
4. Tremor

### Generalised Involuntary Movement

A. Extrapyramidal abnormalities
   Athetosis
   Chorea
   Choreoathetosis
   Hemiballism
   Torsion dystonia

B. Spasms
   Tonic spasm
   Clonic spasm

**Fibrillation** This occurs due to contraction of a single muscle fibre. Usually it cannot be seen. Clinically, fibrillation, if present, can be observed in the tongue but it can be recorded electromyographically.

**Fasciculation** This occurs due to contraction of a bundle of muscle fibre. It can be seen as well as recorded electromyographically. It occurs due to irritation of the anterior horn cells or nerve roots during inflammation or degeneration.

*Causes*

- Motor neuron disease
- Cervical spondylosis
- Syringomyelia
- Peroneal muscular dystrophy

**Myoclonus** Sudden shock-like contraction of a single muscle or group of muscles is called myoclonus. It is involuntary and arrhythmic. There are different varieties of myoclonus. When myoclonus occurs in the face, it is called facial myoclonus, when it occurs during muscular activity it is called action myoclonus, and when it occurs in different parts of the body and disappears during sleep it is called myoclonus simplex.

**Tremor** Tremor is a regular, rhythmic, purpose-less, to and fro movement of a part of the body (usually limbs) due to contraction of a group of muscles and their antagonists. It usually involves the distal parts of the limbs, tongue, and rarely the trunk. It is divided into resting or static tremor (when it occurs at rest) and intention or kinetic tremor (when it occurs during a purposeful movement of limbs). Resting tremor is typically seen in Parkinsonism and intention tremor in cerebellar disorder. Tremor is also divided into fine and coarse tremors. Fine tremor is seen in anxiety, hyperthyroidism and so on. coarse tremor is seen in Parkinsonism (pin-rolling tremor).

*Causes of tremor*

I. Physiological
   1. Anxiety
   2. Exposure to cold
   3. Old age (senile tremor)
   4. Congenital

II. Pathological
   A. Neurological
      1. Parkinsonism
      2. Cerebellar disorder
      3. Disseminated sclerosis
      4. Benign essential tremor
   B. Metabolic
      1. Thyrotoxicosis
      2. Hypoglycemia
      3. Hepatic coma
      4. Uremia
   C. Toxic
      1. Alcoholism
      2. Barbiturate poisoning
      3. Opium poisoning
      4. Heavy metal poisoning

**Chorea** This is a rapid involuntary dancing type of movement. It occurs in lesions of the caudate nucleus. It is seen in Huntington's disease (Huntington's chorea) and chronic rheumatic disease (Sydenham's chorea).

**Athetosis** This is characterised by continuous, slow or writhing movements. It occurs due to a lesion in the globus pallidus.

**Choreoathetosis** When chorea and athetosis are present together, the condition is called choreoathetosis.

**Ballism** This is an involuntary movement, which is sudden, flailing, intense and violent. It occurs in the lesion of the subthalamic nucleus. When it occurs in one side of the body, it is called hemiballism.

**Torsion dystonia** The torsion of the limbs and vertebral column causes distorted posture of the limbs and trunk. Persistent increase in muscle tone occurs. The dystonia disappears during sleep.

**Tonic spasm** Tonic spasm of the muscle is seen in tetanus and strychnine poisoning.

**Clonic spasm** Clonic spasm of the muscle is seen in epilepsy.

**Tics** These are sudden rapid, repeated, coordinated and purposeless movements that occur usually in the same region intermittently. Usually tics occur in the form of blinking of the eyes or wriggling of the shoulders.

## Upper Motor Neuron (UMN) Paralysis

### *Features*

- Muscles are affected in groups (individual muscles are never affected)
- No muscle atrophy (disuse atrophy may occur in chronic patients)
- Spasticity (hypertonia)
- Exaggeration of tendon reflexes
- Loss of superficial reflexes
- Positive Babinski sign (extensor plantar response)
- No fascicular twitches
- No denervation potential in EMG
- Normal nerve conduction studies

### *Causes*

The corticospinal pathways can be interrupted by lesions at any level, starting from the cerebral cortex, subcortical white matter, internal capsule, brainstem, to the spinal cord. The most common site of lesion of the corticospinal tract is the internal capsule that is usually involved in cerebral hemorrhage due to damage to Charcot's artery (the artery of cereberal hemorrhage), a branch of the middle cerebral artery. Corticothalamic, corticostriate, corticorubral, corticopontaine, cortico-olivary, and corticoreticular fibres also pass through the internal capsule. Therefore, a lesion in the internal capsule not only affects the pyramidal (corticospinal) tract but also the extrapyramidal and other fibres. Therefore, the paralysis is called upper motor neuron paralysis, instead of pyramidal paralysis.

The extrapyramidal motor system includes the basal ganglia and the cerebellum. These two structures influence the extrapyramidal tracts by projecting directly or indirectly to the brainstem. Extrapyramidal lesions do not cause paralysis (Table 30.1).

### *Physiological Basis*

In upper motor neuron (UMN) paralysis there occurs not only lesions of the corticospinal tract (the so-called pyramidal tract), but a few extrapyramidal fibres (especially corticoreticular fibres that project onto the reticulospinal tract) are also disrupted. This occurs in UMN paralysis due to a lesion at the internal capsule (the commonest site of UMN lesion). The pontine reticulospinal tract is excitatory to the muscles involved in postural control, that is, the antigravity muscle, and this reticulospinal tract is under the inhibitory control of corticoreticular fibres. In UMN lesions, disruption of corticoreticular fibres facilitates the excitatory output of the pontine reticulospinal pathway. Therefore, hypertonia and spasticity occur in a UMN lesion. Deep reflexes are exaggerated because of the increased discharge and sensitivity of the gamma motor neurons.

Table 30.1 Differences between pyramidal (corticospinal) and extrapyramidal lesions.

| | Pyramidal | Extrapyramidal |
|---|---|---|
| 1. Muscle tone | Spasticity (clasp-knife rigidity) | Plastic (cogwheel rigidity) |
| 2. Distribution of hypertonus | Flexors of arm and extensors of leg | Generalised |
| 3. Shortening and lengthening reaction | Present | Absent |
| 4. Involuntary movement | Absent | Present |
| 5. Tendon reflexes | Exaggerated | Normal |
| 6. Babinski's sign | Positive | Negative |
| 7. Paralysis | Of voluntary movement | No paralysis |

Excitability of the gamma motor neurons regulates spinal reflex activity. gamma motor neurons are usually inhibited by many supraspinal influences. In UMN lesions, loss of inhibitory influence increases gamma motor neuron discharge and therefore increases the reflex activity.

The corticospinal tract excites flexor motor neurons and inhibits the extensor motor neurons of the digits of the limbs. Therefore, normally stroking of the sole elicits plantar flexion. In UMN paralysis, disruption of corticospinal influence on the lumbosacral motor neurons causes dorsiflexion of the big toe and fanning of other toes (Babinski's sign or extensor plantar response).

## Lower Motor Neuron (LMN) Paralysis

Lower motor neurons may be injured or diseased in the cranial nerve nuclei or spinal anterior horn cells, in the anterior nerve roots, or in the nerves themselves. The most common acute lesion of the anterior horn cell is poliomyelitis. The chronic degeneration of anterior horn cells occurs in motor neuron disease (progressive muscular atrophy). The anterior nerve roots may be damaged by trauma, especially in association with cervical spondylosis or by an inflammatory or neoplastic lesion. The peripheral nerves are mainly affected by injury, inflammation and toxic or metabolic disorders (neuropathies). As the nerves carry both motor and sensory information, pure motor deficit rarely occurs. Usually muscular paralysis is associated with sensory changes.

### *Features*

- Usually individual muscles are affected
- Muscle atrophy is pronounced (Table 30.2)
- Flaccidity
- Hypotonia is seen in the affected muscles
- Tendon reflexes and superficial reflexes are diminished or absent
- Babinski's sign is negative (plantar flexion)
- Fascicular twitches may be present
- Denervation potentials (fibrillation, fasciculation, positive sharp waves) are observed in the EMG
- Nerve conduction studies reveal abnormalities

Table 30.2 Comparison of upper motor neuron and lower motor neuron paralysis.

| | UMN paralysis | LMN paralysis |
|---|---|---|
| 1. Muscles affected | Muscles are affected in groups | Individual muscles are affected |
| 2. Size of the muscles | Atrophy not seen (slight atrophy may occur due to disuse) | Pronounced atrophy (may be up to 80 per cent of the total bulk) of muscles |
| 3. Type of paralysis | Spastic paralysis | Flaccid paralysis |
| 4. Tone of the muscles | Hypertonia | Hypotonia |
| 5. Power of the muscles | Paralysis occurs (no voluntary movement) | Paralysis occurs |
| 6. Tendon reflexes | Exaggerated | Diminished or absent |
| 7. Superficial reflexes | Absent | Absent |
| 8. Babinski's sign | Positive (extensor plantar reflex) | Negative (flexor plantar reflex) |
| 9. Involuntary movement | Absent | Fascicular twitches may be present |
| 10. EMG changes | No denervation potentials seen in EMG | Denervation potentials (fibrillations, fasciculations, and sharp waves) are seen in EMG |
| 11. Nerve conduction | No abnormalities in nerve conduction | Abnormal nerve conduction (decreased studies conduction) |

## VIVA

1. What are the different aspects of motor functions that are assessed while examining the motor system?
2. How do you measure the bulk of the muscles in the upper and lower limbs?
3. What is the tone of the muscle and how is it assessed?
4. How do you grade the strength of muscles?
5. How do you estimate the strength of intrinsic muscles of the hands?

6. How do you assess the strength of the flexors and extensors of the wrist?
7. How do you assess the strength of the biceps, triceps and brachioradialis?
8. How do you assess the strength of the abdominal muscles?
9. How do you assess the strength of the intrinsic muscles of the foot?
10. How do you assess the strength of extensors and flexors of the knee and those of the thigh?
11. What are the precautions observed for eliciting deep reflexes?
12. How do you grade tendon reflexes?
13. What is the root value of different tendon jerks?
14. Name the superficial reflexes.
15. What are the tests for coordination of movement in the upper and lower limbs?
16. What is dysdiadokokinesis?
17. Define gait.
18. In what conditions are atrophy and hypertrophy of muscles observed? Why?
19. What is the cause of spasticity in upper motor neuron paralysis?
20. What is the cause of flaccidity in lower motor neuron paralysis?
21. What are the differences between pyramidal and extrapyramidal tract lesions?
22. What are the differences between upper motor neuron and lower motor neuron paralysis?
23. How do you classify muscles clinically?
24. What do you mean by lower and upper motor neurons?
25. What are the descending motor tracts?
26. Name the extrapyramidal systems.
27. Trace the pathway of corticospinal tracts.
28. What are the functions of corticospinal tracts?
29. What are the functions of extrapyramidal systems?
30. What are the areas in the brain involved in regulation of motor activities?
31. What are the functions of the motor cortex?
32. What are the functions of the basal ganglia?
33. What are the functions of the cerebellum?

Chapter 31

# Clinical Examination of the Cranial Nerves

## Learning Objectives

After completing this practical, you will be able to:

- Describe the importance of performing this practical in clinical physiology.
- List the functions of all the cranial nerves.
- Perform clinical examination of all the cranial nerves.
- List the precautions observed while examining each of the cranial nerves.
- List the common effects of lesions of the cranial nerves.

You may also be able to:

- Trace the pathway of all the cranial nerves.
- Explain the abnormalities observed following lesions of the cranial nerves.
- List the differences between supra- and infranuclear palsy of the 7$^{th}$ and 12$^{th}$ cranial nerves.

## INTRODUCTION

There are twelve pairs of cranial nerves. Some of them contain only sensory fibres and are thus known as *sensory cranial nerves*. Few cranial nerves are predominantly motor in function and are therefore called *motor cranial nerves*. The remaining cranial nerves contain both sensory and motor fibres and are thus called *mixed cranial nerves*. A systematic and thorough examination of cranial nerves is part of the clinical evaluation of a patient with neurological deficit. The cranial nerves may be affected by a primary disease of the cranial nerve or by a disease of the brain or the meninges, or sometimes secondary to other systemic disorders.

### Anatomical and Physiological Considerations

#### Olfactory or First Cranial Nerve

**Anatomy** This nerve arises from the olfactory mucosa. The nasal mucous membrane contains bipolar sensory cells that constitute the first order of neurons. Their central processes pass through the olfactory foramina in the cribiform plate of the ethmoid bone and terminate in the olfactory bulb. From the olfactory bulb, the second order of neurons arises and projects to the olfactory cortex, which consists of the periamygdaloid and prepiriform areas of the piriform lobe.

**Function** The olfactory nerve carries the sensation of smell from the nasal mucosa to the olfactory cortex of the brain.

#### Optic or Second Cranial Nerve

**Anatomy** This is one of the important cranial nerves as it subserves vision. The fibres of the optic nerve arise in the retina and pass through the optic foramen to form the optic chiasma and then the optic tract. At the chiasma, the fibres from the inner half of each retina decussate while those from the outer half remain on the same side. Thus each optic tract consists of fibres from the outer half of the retina of the same side and from the inner half of the retina of the opposite side (Fig. 32.1). Most of the fibres of the optic tract pass onto the lateral geniculate body of the thalamus, and some fibres from the optic tract reach the pretectal area, which is involved in regulation of pupillary reflexes and movement of the orbital muscles. The fibres from the lateral geniculate body travel in the optic radiation to reach the visual (calcarine) cortex. The calcarine cortex constitutes the main visual centre and represents the opposite half of the field of vision. The area of central or macular vision has extensive cortical representation and has dual blood supply from the middle and posterior cerebral artery.

**Function** The optic nerve serves the most important special sensation, vision. Normal vision is dependent on the integrity of the visual pathway, that is, receptors in

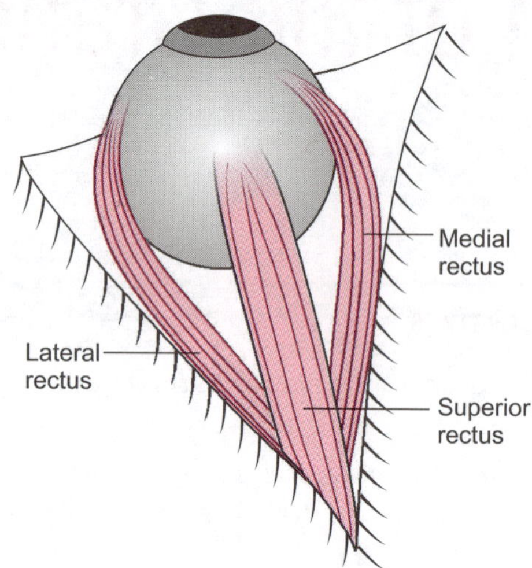


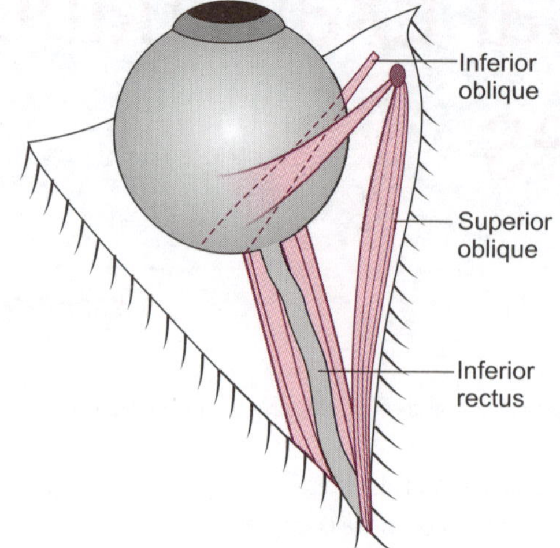


Fig. 31.1 Muscles attached to the left eye.

the retina, optic nerve, optic chiasma, optic tract, lateral geniculate body and visual cortex.

## Oculomotor or Third Cranial Nerve

**Anatomy** This is predominantly a motor nerve. The third cranial nerve nuclei lie in the midbrain, just anterior to the cerebral aqueduct, at the level of the superior and inferior colliculi. The nerve fibres emerge at the upper border of the pons, pass through the cavernous sinus and superior orbital fissure, and supply the four extrinsic muscles of the eyeball (superior rectus, medial rectus, inferior rectus and inferior oblique) (Fig. 31.1). It also supplies the levator palpebrae superioris of the upper eyelid. It carries parasympathetic innervation to the sphincter muscles of the iris (sphincter pupillae) and ciliary muscles (involved in control of accommodation).

**Functions**

1. It controls all the movements of the eyeball except lateral deviation of the eye and depression of the medially deviated eye.
2. It controls the size of the pupil.
3. It is involved in accommodation of vision.

## Trochlear or Fourth Cranial Nerve

**Anatomy** This is primarily a motor cranial nerve. The nucleus of the fourth cranial nerve is present in the midbrain. The fibres decussate before emerging from the brain and enter the orbit through the superior orbital fissure to supply the superior oblique muscle. It supplies the superior oblique muscle of the opposite side of the eyeball. This is a peculiar nerve in the sense that it is the only cranial nerve that decussates between its nuclei of origin and the point of emergence.

**Function** It causes depression of the medially deviated eye.

## Trigeminal or Fifth Cranial Nerve

**Anatomy** This consists of both motor and sensory fibres. It has three subdivisions: ophthalmic, maxillary and mandibular. The ophthalmic and maxillary divisions are sensory whereas the mandibular division is both motor and sensory.

***Motor component of the fifth nerve*** The motor fibres originate in the pons and come out of the brain through the foramen ovale to innervate the muscles of mastication (masseters and temporalis). Motor fibres of the fifth nerve are present only in the mandibular division of the nerve.

***Sensory component of the fifth nerve*** Sensory fibres of the fifth nerve are present in all the three divisions of the nerve (Fig. 31.2).

*Ophthalmic division* The ophthalmic division carries fibres that receive sensation from the skin over the upper eyelid, eyeball, lacrimal glands, nasal cavity, side of the nose, the conjunctival surface of the upper but not the lower lid, forehead and the scalp as far as the vertex. These fibres pass through the superior orbital fissure.

*Maxillary division* The maxillary division carries sensations from the upper part of the cheek, the lower eyelid and its conjunctival surface, skin and mucus membrane of the nose, the upper lip, the upper teeth, the upper part of the pharynx, the roof of the mouth

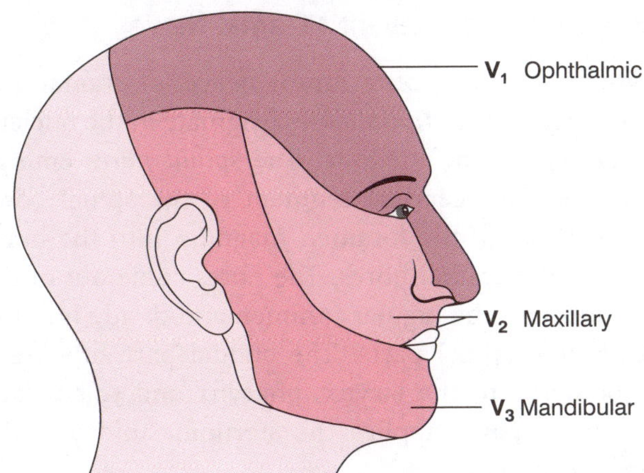


Fig. 31.2 Areas supplied by the three peripheral sensory branches of the trigeminal nerve.

and soft palate and the medial inferior quadrant of the cornea. The fibres in the maxillary division enter the brain through the foramen rotundum.

*Mandibular division* The sensory fibres in the mandibular division carry sensations from the lower part of the face, the lower lip, the ear, anterior two-thirds of tongue (not taste) and the lower teeth. These fibres pass through the foramen ovale. The sensory fibres from all the three divisions of the trigeminal nerve end in the pons.

**Functions** The trigeminal nerve carries general sensation from different parts of the face, and a part of the head and neck. Through its motor functions, it is involved in mastication (chewing).

## Abducent or Sixth Cranial Nerve

**Anatomy** This is primarily a motor nerve. The fibres originate in the nucleus, that is, in the lower part of the pons near the internal genu of the facial canal. After emerging from the pons, it traverses a long intracranial course to enter the orbital cavity through the medial end of the superior orbital fissure to supply the lateral rectus muscle. The long intracranial course of this nerve makes it liable to the effects of raised intracranial pressure.

**Function** It helps in lateral deviation of the eye.

## Facial or Seventh Cranial Nerve

**Anatomy** The seventh cranial nerve is a mixed nerve. It has motor and sensory components.

*Motor component* The motor fibres originate in the pons, pass through the stylomastoid foramen and innervate the muscles of facial expression, scalp and platysma (neck muscle).

*Sensory component* Fibres arise from the taste buds present in the anterior two-thirds of the tongue, pass through the stylomastoid foramen and end in the geniculate ganglion, a nucleus in the pons from where fibres go to the gustatory area in the parietal lobe of the cerebral cortex through the thalamus.

During its course, the facial nerve travels through the facial canal in the temporal bone. The chorda tympani nerve carrying the taste sensation from the anterior two-thirds of the tongue, and joins the facial nerve in the facial canal. This part of the nerve is vulnerable to injury and edema as it is enclosed in a bony tube.

**Functions**

1. It supplies all the muscles of the face and scalp, (except the levator palpebrae superioris) and platysma. Therefore, it carries out all facial expressions.
2. It carries the taste sensation from the anterior two-thirds of the tongue.

## Vestibulocochlear or Eighth Cranial Nerve

**Anatomy** It has two components, the cochlear and the vestibular.

*The cochlear nerve* The auditory (cochlear) fibres arise in the spiral organ (organ of Corti) and form the spiral ganglion. Fibres from the spiral ganglion pass through the internal auditory meatus to reach the nuclei in the medulla, from where the fibres project to the thalamus and from there to the auditory cortex.

*The vestibular nerve* The vestibular fibres originate in the semicircular canals, saccule and utricle and form the vestibular ganglion. The fibres from the vestibular ganglion terminate in the vestibular nuclei present in the pons and medulla. A good deal of projection also reaches the cerebellum.

**Functions**

1. The cochlear fibres convey impulses associated with hearing.
2. The vestibular fibres convey impulses associated with equilibrium.

## Glossopharyngeal or Ninth Cranial Nerve

**Anatomy** The glossopharyngeal nerve is a mixed nerve. It has motor and sensory components.

***The motor fibres*** The fibres originate in the nucleus ambiguous in the medulla. It accompanies the tenth and eleventh cranial nerve and comes out of the skull through the jugular foramen to supply the middle constrictor of the pharynx and stylopharyngeous muscle. It also supplies parasympathetic fibres to the parotid gland.

***The sensory fibres*** These fibres arise from the taste buds in the posterior third of the tongue and from baroreceptors in the carotid sinus. They carry general sensation from the nasopharynx and posterior aspect of the soft palate. The fibres terminate in the nucleus tractus solitarius (NTS).

**Functions**

1. It is involved in activation of the pharyngeal reflex.
2. It carries the taste sensation from the posterior third of the tongue.
3. It helps in the secretion of saliva.
4. It is involved in regulation of blood pressure (baroreceptor reflex).

### Vagus or Tenth Cranial Nerve

**Anatomy** The vagus nerve is a mixed nerve. It has motor and sensory components.

***The motor fibres*** The motor fibres originate in the nucleus ambiguous in the medulla. The nerve comes out of the skull through the jugular foramen to supply the structures in the neck, thorax and abdomen. Its function is motor to the soft palate (with the exception of tensor palati), pharynx, larynx, the respiratory passages, esophagus, stomach, small intestine, most parts of the large intestine, gall bladder and heart. Its function is secretomotor to most of these organs.

***The sensory fibres*** It carries sensation from the aortic arch and aortic bodies that mediate baroreceptor and chemoreceptor reflexes. It also carries the sensation from the structures that it innervates. The fibres pass through the jugular foramen and terminate in the medulla and pons.

**Functions**

1. It regulates the functions of the cardiovascular system, gastrointestinal tract, respiratory system, urogenital tract and other thoracic and abdominal viscera.
2. It is involved in the elicitation of the palatal reflex.
3. It subserves laryngeal and pharyngeal functions.

### Accessory or Eleventh Cranial Nerve

**Anatomy** This is a pure motor nerve, of cranial and spinal origin. The *cranial fibres* originate in the nucleus ambiguous in the medulla. The *spinal fibres* emerge from the sixth cervical segment of the spinal cord, ascend through the foramen magnum into the brain and join the cranial fibres. The fibres come out of the skull through the jugular foramen and divide into the cranial and spinal parts. The cranial part supplies a motor nerve to the larynx, pharynx and soft palate. The spinal part supplies the sternomastoid and the trapezius muscle.

**Functions**

1. The cranial portion mediates swallowing movements.
2. The spinal portion mediates head and shoulder movements.

### Hypoglossal or Twelfth Cranial Nerve

**Anatomy** The twelfth cranial nerve is a pure motor nerve. The fibres originate from its nucleus, which is present in the medulla. It leaves the skull via the hypoglossal canal (anterior condyloid foramen) and joins the ansa hypoglossi in the cervical region. It supplies the muscles of the tongue of the same side. It also supplies the hypoglossus, styloglossus and genioglossus muscles.

**Functions**

1. It helps in the movement of the tongue and therefore assists in speech and swallowing.
2. It assists in depressing the hyoid bone.

## METHODS

## Method to Test Olfactory Nerve

### Principle

The olfactory nerve carries the sensation of smell. Therefore, this nerve is tested by various olfactory stimuli.

### Requirements

One small bottle each of clove oil and peppermint oil.

### Procedure

1. Ask the subject to sit comfortably on a stool.

2. Make sure that both the nostrils are patent and there is no inflammation of the nasal mucosa (no nasal obstruction due to common cold).
3. Ask the subject to close his eyes and one of his nostrils.
4. Remove the cap of the bottle containing clove oil and take the bottle close to the open nostril.
5. Ask the subject if he correctly perceives the smell.
6. Repeat the procedure with peppermint oil.
7. Ask the subject to close this nostril and open the other nostril, and repeat the procedure.
8. Compare the results of both the nostrils.
9. Ask the subject if he has any hallucination of smell.
10. Note your result. Express the result as smell normal, reduced, absent or perverted, separately for each nostril.

### Precautions

1. The subject should close his eyes.
2. The subject must be familiar with the odour.
3. Both the nostrils should be examined separately.
4. One nostril should be closed when the other is examined.

## Method to Test Optic Nerve

### Principle

The optic nerve carries the sensation of vision. Examination of this nerve reveals intactness of the visual pathway, field of vision and acuity of vision.

### Requirements

1. Snellen's chart
2. Lister's or Goldmann's perimeter
3. Ishihara chart

### Procedure

The optic nerve is tested for acuity of vision, field of vision and colour vision. Tests for acuity of vision, colour vision and field of vision are described in detail in Chapters 33, 34 and 32, respectively. The field of vision is detected by 'confrontation test' at the bedside of the patient.

#### *Confrontation Test*

1. Ask the subject to sit on a stool comfortably in an erect position.
2. Sit on a stool in front of the subject in such a way that your eyes and the subject's eyes remain at the same level and at a distance of about 3 feet (Fig. 31.3).
3. Ask the subject to fix his gaze at the tip of your nose.
4. Ask the subject to close one of his eyes and close your opposite eye.
5. Move your finger midway between you and the subject to test the field of vision of four quadrants (upper, lower, nasal and temporal). Bring your finger from the periphery of the four quadrants to the centre of the visual field and ask the subject to say 'yes' when he sees the finger.

> **Note:** If the subject's vision is normal, at the point at which the examiner catches sight of the moving finger, the subject can also see it.

6. Compare the patient's field of vision with yours and note your observation.
7. Repeat the procedure with the other eye.

### Precautions

1. The distance between the examiner and the subject should be 3 feet.
2. The eye of the examiner should remain level with that of the subject's.
3. The field of vision of the examiner should be normal.

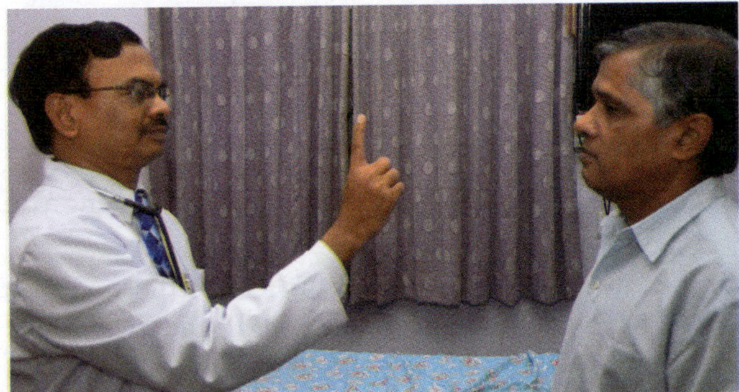

Fig. 31.3 Procedure for testing eye ball movements for assessment of oculomotor nerve function. Note that the eye level of examiner and subject is approximately same. Subject fixes his gaze at the tip of examiner's index finger (with a distance of approximately 25 cm) and follows the movement of examiner's finger.

4. The subject should fix his gaze at the centre.
5. The examiner should move his finger midway between him and the subject.
6. One eye should be closed while the other eye is being examined.
7. The subject should wear glasses during the procedure if he uses them constantly for refractive errors. Restriction of the field of vision due to glasses should be kept in mind.

## Method to Test Oculomotor, Trochlear and Abducent Nerves

### Principle

The third, fourth and sixth cranial nerves are tested together as they innervate all the external ocular muscles. The eyeball moves in different directions and the movements are named accordingly. Horizontal movement in an outward direction is called *abduction* and in an inward direction is called *adduction*, vertical movement in the upward direction is called *elevation* and in the downward direction is called *depression*. The eye is also capable of rotatory movements. The rolling movement of the eye towards the nose is called *internal rotation* and movement away from the nose is called *external rotation*. The superior and inferior rectus elevate and depress the eye when the eye is in abduction, and the inferior and superior oblique elevate and depress the eye when the eye is in adduction.

### Requirements

1. Torch
2. Cardboard

### Procedure

1. Ask the subject to sit comfortably on a stool and you sit in front of the subject.
2. Examine the eyes of the subject for the presence of ptosis (drooping of the eyelid) and nystagmus (rhythmic, involuntary and jerky movement of the eyeball) if any.
3. Give instructions to the subject to follow the direction of the movement of your finger.
4. Bring your index finger to the front of the subject's eyes, keeping a distance of around 25 cm (the normal visual distance) from the subject.
5. Ask the subject to look at and follow the movements of your index finger, and observe the movement of the eyeball of the subject while moving your finger (Fig. 31.3).
6. First, move your finger laterally to the right of the subject (this tests the function of the lateral rectus of the right eye and the medial rectus of the left eye simultaneously). From there move your finger vertically upwards (this tests the superior rectus of the right eye and the inferior oblique of the left eye) and downwards (this tests the inferior rectus of the right eye and superior oblique of the left eye).
7. Then move your finger laterally to the left (this tests the lateral rectus of the left eye and the medial rectus of the right eye). From there, move your finger vertically upward (this tests the superior rectus of the left and inferior oblique of the right eye) and downward (this tests the inferior rectus of the left and superior oblique of the right eye).
8. Examine the pupillary reaction to light (*light reflex*). Put a piece of cardboard between the two eyes or place your hand between the eyes (Fig. 31.4). Switch on the torch and bring the torch from the side of the subject and immediately focus the light onto one of his eyes and look for the reaction of the pupil of that eye (direct light reflex) as well the pupil of the other eye (indirect or consensual light reflex).
9. Examine the pupillary reaction to accommodation (*accommodation reflex*). Ask the subject to look at a distant object. Bring the index finger of your hand to a point midway between the two eyes and very close to the eyes of the subject. Ask the subject to look at the tip of your index finger (Fig. 31.5). Examine for

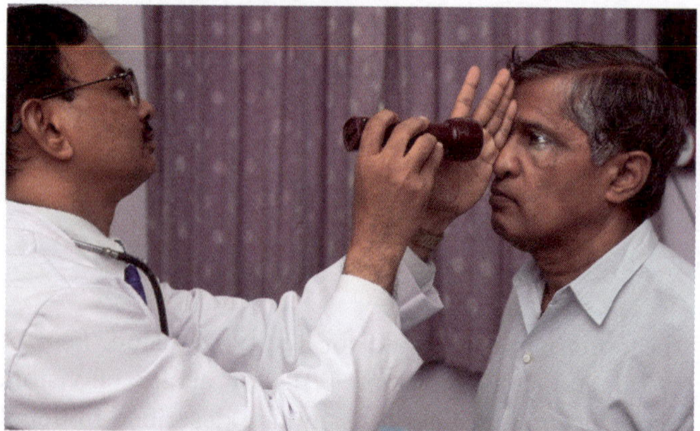

Fig. 31.4 Procedure for assessing light reflex. The examiner, while placing the hand between eyes, focuses light on the eye and looks for pupillary constriction.

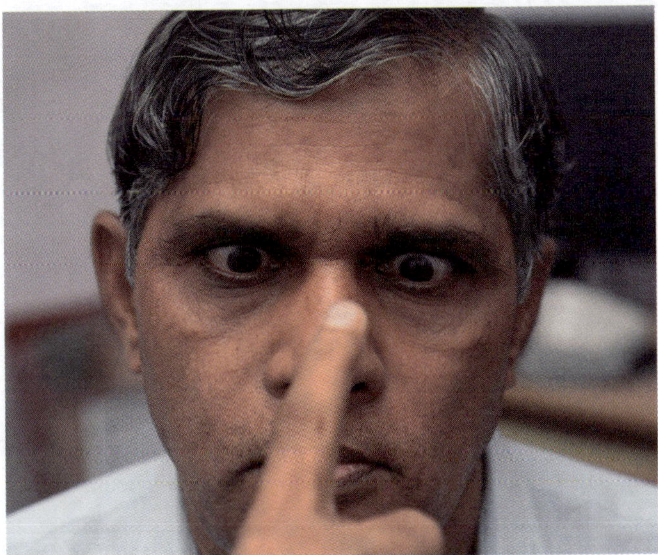

Fig. 31.5 Procedure for assessing accommodation reflex. Note the medial deviation of the eye of the subject and constriction of pupil when he looks at the tip of the examiner's finger kept close to his eyes.

medial deviation and pupillary constriction of both the eyes.

### Precautions

1. The examiner's finger should remain about 25 cm (the normal visual distance) from the subject's eyes while testing for eye movement.
2. The light reflexes of both the eyes should be elicited separately by placing a cardboard between both the eyes.
3. For eliciting light reflex, the light should not be projected to the eyes from the front; rather it should be brought from the side of the eye and then immediately focussed on the pupil.
4. For eliciting accommodation, the subject should shift his gaze immediately from a distant object to an object very close to his eyes.

## Method to Test Trigeminal Nerve

### Principle

The trigeminal nerve supplies the muscle of mastication and carries sensations from the face. Examination of the different sensations on the face and the ability of the subject to chew tests the intactness of the trigeminal nerve.

### Requirements

1. Cotton wool
2. Pin
3. Tuning fork (128 Hz)
4. Glass tubes containing warm and cold water
5. Knee hammer

### Procedure

1. Supply proper instructions to the subject and explain to him the nature of the examination.
2. Ask the subject to sit comfortably on a stool.
3. Examine all the sensations (as described in Chapter 29) of the face keeping the area supplied by the ophthalmic, maxillary and mandibular division in mind (Fig. 31.2).
4. Examine the motor function. Ask the subject to clench his teeth and palpate the prominence of the temporal and masseter on both sides by palpating the temple and the upper part of the cheek. Ask the subject to open his mouth and look for deviation of the jaw, if present.

> Note: If there is paralysis of one side, the muscle on that side will fail to become prominent and on opening the mouth, the jaw deviates towards the paralysed side because it is pushed over by the lateral pterygoid muscle of the healthy side. Normally, the lateral pterygoid muscle pushes the jaw towards the midline.

5. Test the conjunctival reflex. Bring a piece of cotton wool from the side of the subject (the subject should not know that you are going to touch his conjunctiva) and immediately touch the conjunctiva. Look for the response (the subject blinks his eyes).
6. Test the corneal reflex. Touch the limbus, that is, the sclerocorneal junction of the eye with cotton wool and look for the response (blinking of the eyes).
7. Elicit *jaw jerk* (Fig. 30.17, Chapter 30). Ask the patient to partially open his mouth. Place your left index finger in the groove under the lower lip and lightly tap on the nail of the finger with the help of the knee hammer. Observe the response (if the jerk is present, the mouth snaps shut).

### Precautions

1. The subject should be instructed properly.

2. All the sensations should be elicited from the face according to the distribution of the three subdivisions of the fifth nerve.
3. The masseter and temporalis should be examined on both the sides and compared simultaneously.
4. While eliciting the corneal and conjunctival reflex, the subject should not be aware of the procedure, otherwise he will close his eyes before the conjunctiva is touched.

## Method to Test Facial Nerve

### Principle

The facial nerve carries the taste sensation from the anterior two-thirds of the tongue and supplies the muscles of facial expression. Therefore, the examination of the taste sensation of the anterior two-thirds of the tongue and the ability of the subject to perform all facial expressions test the intactness of the facial nerve.

### Requirements

1. Four small vials containing strong solutions that are sweet (sugar), salty (common salt), bitter (solution of quinine or chloroquine) and sour (lime juice or weak solutions of citric acid) separately.
2. Four glass rods.

### Procedure

1. Ask the subject to frown or open his eyes wide. Look for the wrinkling of the forehead (to test the frontal belly of the occipitofrontalis).
2. Ask the subject to shut his eyes as tightly as he can. Try to open the eyes while he tries to keep them closed (Fig. 31.6). This is the test for orbicularis oculi.

> Note: If one side of the nerve is paralysed, the affected eye is either not closed at all, in which case the eyeball rolls upward to make up for the failure of the lid to descend (Bell's phenomenon), or if the eye is closed, the eyelashes are not buried. Bell's phenomenon is a normal phenomenon preserved in facial palsies of the lower motor neuron type.

3. Ask the subject to show his teeth. Look for deviation of the angle of the mouth if present (to test for orbicularis oris).

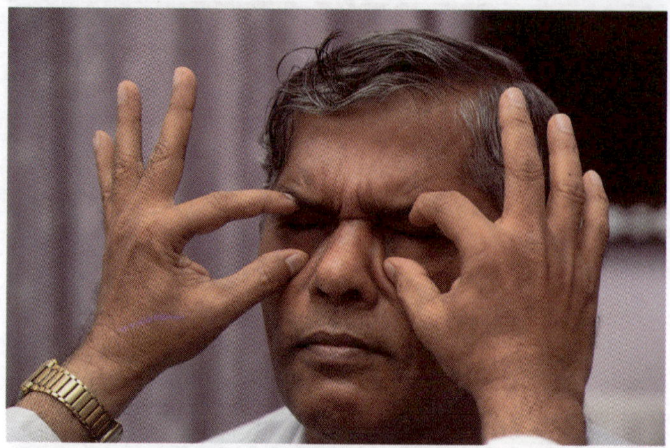

Fig. 31.6 Procedure for testing the orbicularis oculi.

> Note: If the seventh nerve is paralysed, the angle of the mouth on the affected side becomes less prominent and instead of being elevated upwards and laterally, is drawn towards the midline by the unopposed action of the orbicularis oris of the healthy side.

4. Ask the subject to inflate his mouth with air and blow out his cheeks. Tap with the finger on each inflated cheek (test for the buccinator muscle) (Fig. 31.7).

> Note: Air escapes from the mouth more easily from the paralysed side.

5. Ask the subject to whistle (test for both orbicularis oris and buccinator).
6. Ask the subject to clench his teeth and observe the prominence of the platysma muscle in the neck (Fig. 31.8).
7. Test the taste sensations from the anterior two-thirds of the tongue. Ask him to protrude his tongue. Dip one glass rod in the sweet solution and

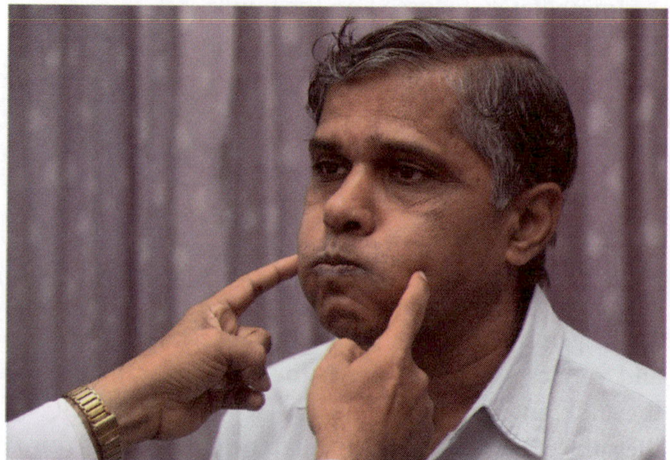

Fig. 31.7 Procedure for testing of buccinator muscle.

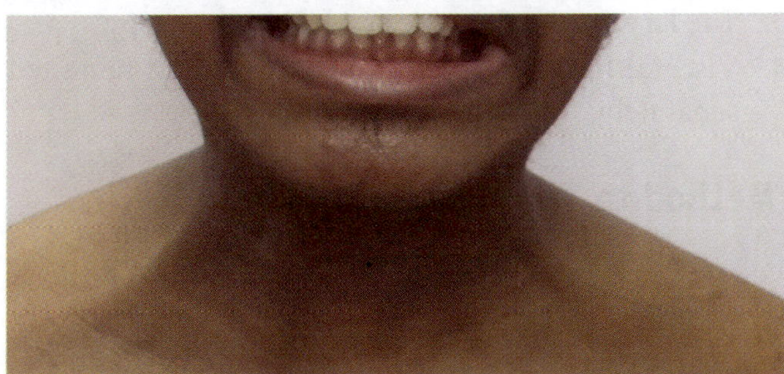

Fig. 31.8 Procedure for testing the platysma. Note the prominence of platysma in the neck, while subject clenches his teeth.

touch different parts of the tongue of the subject with the tip of the rod. Ask him what taste he senses. Similarly repeat the procedure with the salty, sour and bitter solutions by using separate glass rods for each solution.

> Note: While testing for different taste sensations, the relative distribution of taste buds in the tongue for different modalities of taste should be kept in mind. The taste buds for sweet are more concentrated at the tip, bitter at the back and salt and sour on the sides of the tongue.

### Precautions

1. The subject should be properly instructed.
2. Functions of both sides of facial muscles should be tested simultaneously and compared.
3. Separate rods should be used for testing different taste solutions.
4. Sensation for bitterness should be tested last.
5. Rinse the mouth after testing with each solution.

## Method to Test Vestibulocochlear Nerve

### Principle

The eighth nerve has two components, vestibular and cochlear. The cochlear nerve is involved in hearing and the vestibular in balance and equilibrium. Therefore, eighth nerve functions are tested by performing hearing and vestibular tests. The tests of hearing are described in Chapter 35.

### Requirements

No special requirement.

### Procedure

1. Ask the subject whether he has giddiness, dizziness and vertigo (external objects seem to move around him).
2. Examine the subject's eye for the presence of nystagmus (involuntary rhythmic jerky movement of the eyeball).

> Note: Nystagmus is observed by asking the subject to look in a different direction, if not found. Nystagmus can be elicited clinically by hyperextending the neck and rapidly moving the head from side to side.

3. Elicit nystagmus by performing caloric test or rotation test (not usually done in physiology).

#### *Caloric Test*

Irrigate the ear with warm water or with cold water. This produces nystagmus. Irrigation with warm or cold water sets up convection currents in the endolymph of the semicircular canals and produces nystagmus.

#### *Rotation Test*

Rotate the subject in a special rotating chair. Rotation induces nystagmus.

## Method to Test Glossopharyngeal Nerve

### Principle

The ninth cranial nerve carries general as well as taste sensations from the posterior third of the tongue and mucous membrane of the pharynx, and supplies motor fibres to the middle constrictor of the pharynx and the stylopharyngeous muscle. It also carries sensation from the carotid sinus. Therefore, functions of the ninth nerve are tested by eliciting taste sensations from the posterior third of the tongue, pharyngeal reflex, and by testing the heart rate and blood pressure response to standing.

### Requirements

1. Different taste solutions, as described for the seventh nerve
2. Swab stick
3. Sphygmomanometer

## Procedure

1. Ask the subject to sit comfortably on a stool and elicit all the taste sensations in the posterior third of the tongue as described for the seventh nerve.
2. Ask the subject to open his mouth wide. Tickle the back of the pharynx with the help of a swab stick, and observe the contraction of the posterior pharyngeal wall.
3. Ask the subject to lie down and record his blood pressure. Then ask him to stand up and immediately record his blood pressure.

> Note: A fall in blood pressure of more than 20 mm Hg is considered as orthostatic hypotension, and may indicate dysfunction of the ninth nerve.

## Precautions

1. Similar precautions should be followed as for testing the taste sensations of the seventh nerve.
2. Swab sticks should not be placed for a longer duration in the pharynx to elicit pharyngeal reflex.
3. The blood pressure should be recorded immediately (preferably within 15 seconds) after standing.

# Method to Test Vagus Nerve

## Principle

The vagus nerve supplies motor fibres to the soft palate, pharynx and larynx. It also innervates the respiratory passage and most of the thoracic and abdominal viscera. Therefore, this nerve is tested by eliciting palatal, pharyngeal and laryngeal reflexes, and by assessing visceral function.

## Requirement

1. Swab stick

## Procedure

1. Ask the subject to open his mouth wide and say 'aaah'. Observe the arch of the palate and whether the arch is formed equally on both the sides or is flat on one side or both sides.
2. Elicit the pharyngeal reflex as described for the ninth nerve.
3. The laryngeal reflex is tested by laryngoscopy.
4. Visceral functions of the tenth nerve can be tested separately.

# Method to Test Accessory Nerve

## Principle

The accessory nerve supplies the sternomastoid and trapezius muscles. Therefore, its functions are tested by testing the actions of these muscles.

## Requirements

No special requirements.

## Procedure

1. Stand behind the subject and press his shoulder. Ask the subject to shrug his shoulders against the passive resistance (Fig. 31.9).

> Note: This test is done to assess the function of the trapezius.

2. Ask the subject to move his chin to one side. Try to prevent it by opposing the movement (Fig. 31.10). Note the prominence of the sternomastoid muscle of the opposite side. Repeat the procedure by asking the subject to move his chin against resistance to the opposite side. Ask the subject to depress his chin against the resistance of your hand (Fig. 31.11).

> Note: Movement of chin to one side against resistance assesses the power of the sternomastoid of the opposite side. Depressing the chin against resistance assesses the power of the sternomastoid of both sides simultaneously.

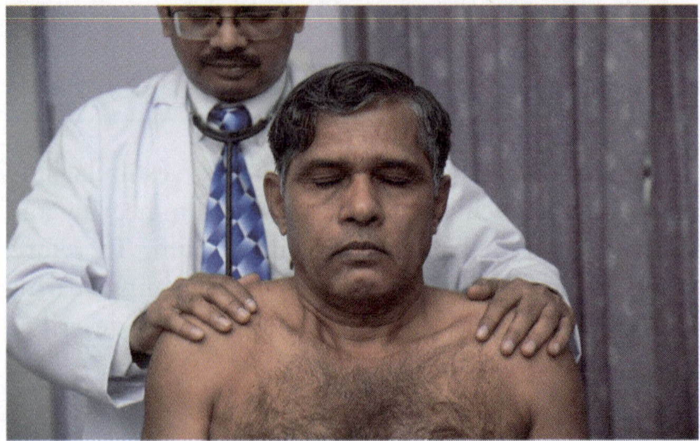

Fig. 31.9 Testing the function of the 11th cranial nerve (Trapezius muscle)

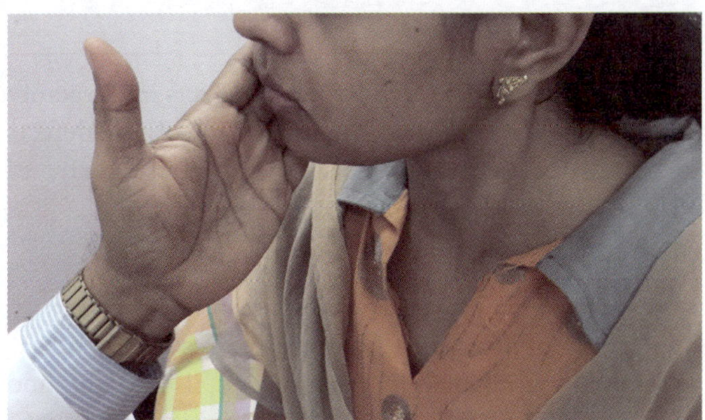

Fig. 31.10 Testing the function of the 11th cranial nerve (sternocleidomastoid muscle of one side)

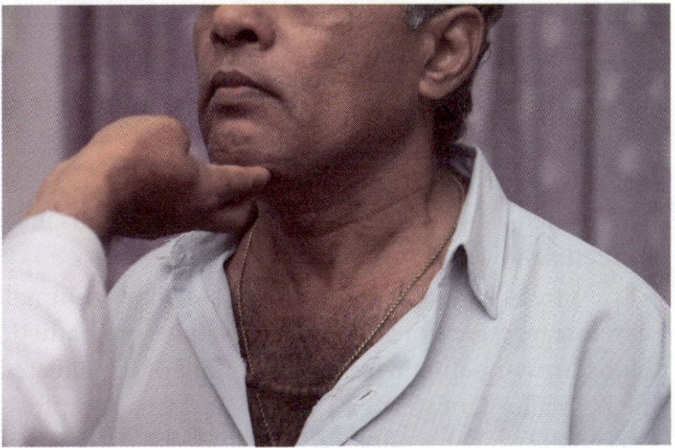

Fig. 31.11 Testing the function of the 11$^{th}$ cranial nerve (sternocleidomastoid muscle of both the sides). Note the prominence of both sternocleidomastoid muscles, while the subject depresses his chin against resistance.

### Precautions

1. The examiner should stand behind the subject for testing the trapezius.
2. While testing for trapezius, press moderately on the shoulders.
3. While testing for the sternomastoid, offer gentle resistance against the movement of the chin.

## Method to Test Hypoglossal Nerve

### Principle

The hypoglossal nerve is a pure motor nerve that supplies the muscles of the tongue and the depressors of the hyoid bone. Therefore, this nerve is tested by testing the movement of the tongue and hyoid bone.

### Requirements

No special requirements.

### Procedure

1. Ask the subject to protrude his tongue and note if the median raphe of the tongue is concave towards one side. Also observe atrophy, fasciculation or tremor if present.
2. Ask the subject to move his tongue from side to side and push his cheek laterally from inside. Resist the tongue movements by pressing it from the outside of the cheek (Fig. 31.12).

## DISCUSSION

The cranial nerves are examined thoroughly to detect the abnormalities of these nerves and to localise the lesions at various levels of the brainstem. The lesions of the cranial nerve may occur either in the supranuclear pathway (in the corticonuclear fibres), in the nucleus, or in the infranuclear pathway, that is, in the nerves. The nuclear and infranuclear palsies of the cranial nerves, whether unilateral or bilateral, manifest with definite clinical features, but the unilateral supranuclear palsies of most of the cranial nerves do not manifest with physical signs because of their bilateral cortical representation.

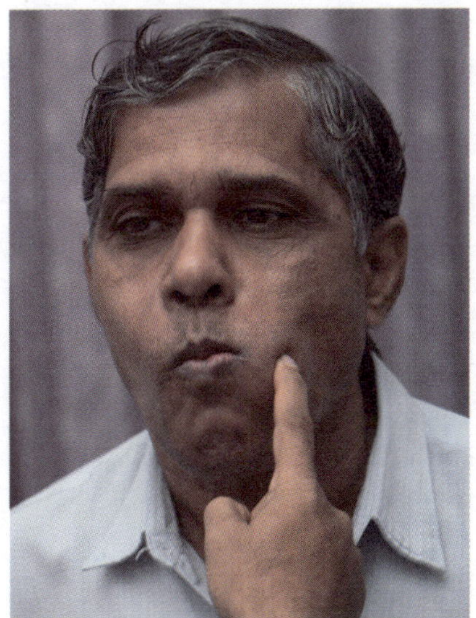

Fig. 31.12 Testing the function of hypoglossal nerve (strength of tongue muscle). Subject pushes his cheek with the tongue from inside and the examiner resists it from outside.

The bilateral supranuclear lesions of the cranial nerves manifest with specific features, especially the lesions of facial and hypoglossal nerves.

## Olfactory Nerve

A lesion of the olfactory nerve manifests as various disorders of smell like anosmia, parosmia and olfactory hallucinations.

### Anosmia

**Definition** Complete abolition of sense of smell is called as anosmia.

**Causes** Unilateral and bilateral anosmia could have different causes.

***Unilateral anosmia***

- Tumour of olfactory bulb
- Tumour of frontal lobe
- Meningiomas pressing on the olfactory bulb or olfactory tract

***Bilateral anosmia***

- Common cold
- Head injuries in which the cribiform plate of the ethmoid bone is fractured
- Atrophic rhinitis

### Hyposmia

**Definition** Decreased sensation of smell is called hyposmia.

**Causes** Same as anosmia.

### Parosmia

**Definition** When the sensation of smell is perverted, it is known as parosmia. The offensive smell may seem like a pleasant odour or vice versa. This is also called *cacosmia.*

**Causes** It could be due to

- Mental disorders
- Can occur as an aura in epilepsy
- Sometimes in head injury

### Olfactory Hallucination

**Definition** When the sensation of smell is perceived without actual presence of any odour.

**Cause** It is typically seen as an aura of temporal lobe epilepsy.

## Optic Nerve

A lesion of the optic nerve results in defects in the acuity of vision, field of vision and colour vision. These defects are discussed separately under 'Perimetry', 'Acuity of Vision' and 'Colour Vision'.

## Oculomotor Nerve

The lesion of the oculomotor nerve results in ptosis, nystagmus, abnormal reaction of pupil to light and accommodation, diplopia and defects in eye movement.

### Ptosis

**Definition** Drooping of the eyelid is called ptosis.

**Causes**

- Impairment of the functions of the third cranial nerve
- Horner syndrome (sympathetic lesion)
- Myasthenia gravis (disorder of neuromuscular junction)

The ptosis of Horner syndrome is always minimal. Therefore, presence of gross ptosis excludes sympathetic lesions. In sympathetic lesions, the pupil of the affected side is smaller (constricted). In third nerve palsy, ptosis is complete and the pupil of the affected side is larger (dilated). In myasthenia, ptosis is usually bilateral and the pupil remains unaffected.

### Nystagmus

**Definition** This is the involuntary, rhythmic and jerky movement of the eyeball. The nystagmus may be horizontal, vertical or rotatory.

**Causes**

- Vestibular lesion
- Cerebellar lesion
- Lesion of third cranial nerve
- Congenital

Nystagmus of visual origin is mostly pendular and often rotatory on central fixation of the eyes.

### Pupillary Reactions

The pupils constrict in response to the light (light reflex). In accommodation reflex, there is convergence of the eyeballs, constriction of pupils and increased convexity of the lens. There are different abnormalities in which pupillary reactions are altered.

*1. Argyll Robertson Pupil*

**Definition** Absence of the reaction of pupils to light with preservation of the reaction to accommodation is called Argyll Robertson pupil (ARP, mnemonic for accommodation reflex present).

**Causes** It is usually seen in neurosyphilis. Neurosyphilis is very rare in recent times after the advent of modern antibiotics.

*2. Adie's Pupil*

**Definition** The extremely decreased reaction of the pupil to light and darkness is called Adie's pupil. In light, the pupil constricts very slowly, and in darkness, it dilates very slowly. It also reacts sluggishly to accommodation.

**Causes**

- Holmes-Adie syndrome (decreased tendon reflexes)
- Sometimes seen in young girls

*3. Unilateral Dilated and Fixed Pupil*

**Cause** Unilateral third nerve palsy. It is associated with ptosis and laterally deviated eye.

*4. Hippus*

**Definition** Alternate rhythmic dilatation and constriction of pupil in response to light is called hippus.

**Cause** Usually seen in retrobulbar neuritis.

### Abnormalities of Ocular Movement

Normally the movements of the two eyes are symmetrical, so that the visual axes meets at the point at which the eyes are directed. This is called conjugate movement of the eyes. In third nerve palsy, the ability of the eye to move medially, to move upward in the adducted position and to move upward and downward in the abducted position is lost. The eye deviates laterally due to unopposed action of the lateral rectus, which is supplied by the sixth cranial nerve.

### Strabismus

**Definition** Deviation of the eyeball is called strabismus or *squint*. The visual axes do not meet at the point of fixation.

There are two types of strabismus: paralytic and non-paralytic. *Paralytic strabismus* occurs due to weakness of extraocular muscles. Paralytic strabismus causes diplopia (double vision) because defective movement of one eye results in images formed by the two eyes falling upon non-identical points of two retinas. Therefore, binocular fusion cannot occur in the visual cortex and two separate images are perceived.

### Diplopia

**Definition** The occurrence of double vision is called diplopia.

**Physiologic basis** Diplopia occurs only over that part of the field of vision towards which the affected muscles move the eye. If both the eyes are functional, and one deviates, *binocular diplopia* results. *Monocular diplopia* results from lens opacities and astigmatism.

**Causes** Diplopia can occur in third, fourth and sixth nerve palsy.

## Trochlear Nerve

The trochlear nerve innervates the superior oblique muscle. Therefore, a lesion of the trochlear nerve results in impaired downward movement of the eye. The eyeball rotates outward by the unopposed action of the inferior rectus when the subject attempts to look downward. Usually there is no squint, but diplopia may occur below the horizontal plane.

## Abducent Nerve

The abducent nerve innervates the lateral rectus muscle. Therefore, lesions of the sixth nerve result in the inability to move the eye outwards and diplopia occurs when the subject looks in that direction. A convergent squint may occur because of unopposed action of the medial rectus.

## Trigeminal Nerve

A lesion of the trigeminal nerve results in sensory and motor deficits.

**Sensory deficits**

1. There is loss of general sensation from different parts of the face depending on the division of the fifth nerve affected.
2. Though the fifth nerve does not carry the taste sensation, in the suspected lesion of the fifth nerve the sensation of taste should be examined as the seventh nerve runs in close association with the fifth nerve in the brain.

**Motor deficits**

1. Paralysis of the fifth nerve of one side the muscles of mastication on that side will fail to become prominent. On opening the mouth, the jaw deviates towards the paralysed side, being pushed over by the healthy lateral pterygoid muscle.
2. Jaw jerk is diminished in infranuclear fifth nerve palsy. The jaw jerk is exaggerated in supranuclear fifth nerve palsy (upper motor neuron lesion above the nucleus of the fifth nerve).

**Reflex deficits** Corneal and conjunctival reflexes are abolished in fifth nerve lesions.

*Trigeminal neuralgia* Neuralgia (nerve pain) of one or more branches of the trigeminal nerve is called the trigeminal neuralgia (tic douloureux). It may be associated with sensory loss and muscle weakness in the area of its distribution.

## Facial Nerve

A lesion of the facial nerve is the commonest of the cranial nerve lesions. **Bell's palsy** is the most common cranial nerve disorder.

**Effects of paralysis**

1. The affected side of the face loses its expression.
2. The nasolabial fold is less pronounced.
3. The eye on the affected side is more widely open than on the other side, and does not close totally even during sleep.
4. The mouth is drawn to the healthy side.
5. The food is collected between the lips and gum on the affected side.
6. The fluid and saliva escape from the affected angle of the mouth.
7. There is loss of taste sensation from the anterior two-thirds of the tongue. However, if the lesion is below the joining of the chorda tympani nerve that is distal to the stylomastoid foramen, taste will not be affected.

**Types of paralysis** Facial nerve lesion may be infranuclear or supranuclear.

*Infranuclear facial palsy* This is the commonest of all lesions of cranial nerves. The idiopathic infranuclear facial palsy is called Bell's palsy. It usually occurs due to viral infection, or may be idiopathic. common features are:

1. Both upper and lower parts of the face are equally affected.
2. Taste sensation may be lost depending on the site of lesion.
3. No involvement of emotional components of facial expression.

*Supranuclear facial palsy* Facial palsy due to a lesion above the nucleus involving the corticonuclear fibres is called supranuclear facial palsy. common features are:

1. The lower part of the face is mainly affected whereas the upper part of the face is either totally spared or affected minimally. This is because the frontal belly of occipitofrontalis has bilateral cortical innervation.
2. Taste sensation may not be altered.
3. Muscles of the voluntary movement of the face are paralysed, but muscles involved in emotional expressions of the face, for example, crying, remain intact or exaggerated (mimic paralysis). This occurs because the emotional movements are not dependent on the same cortical innervation as voluntary movements.

## Vestibulocochlear Nerve

Functional aspects of cochlear nerve have been described in Chapter 35 (Hearing Tests).

**Effect of lesion of vestibular nerve**

1. Patient complains of vertigo, dizziness and giddiness. Vertigo is the sensation of rotation in the absence of actual rotation (hallucination of movement).
2. Patient may vomit and nystagmus may be present.
3. Orientation in space may be lost.

## Glossopharyngeal Nerve

**Effects of paralysis**

1. Loss of taste and general sensation from the posterior third of the tongue.
2. Absence of pharyngeal reflex and difficulty during swallowing.
3. Decreased secretion of saliva.
4. Orthostatic hypotension may occur.

## Vagus Nerve

**Effects of paralysis**

1. Loss of the pharyngeal and palatal reflex. Swallowing becomes difficult.
2. Nasal regurgitation of fluid may occur.
3. Uvula deviates to the healthy side.

4. Paralysis of vocal cord causes aphonia.
5. Paralysis of larynx (all the muscles of the larynx except the cricothyroid are supplied by the recurrent laryngeal nerve, a branch of the vagus nerve) results in hoarseness of voice.
6. Impairment of sensation from many organs.
7. Increase in heart rate and impairment in regulation of blood pressure.

## Accessory Nerve

A lesion of the accessory nerve causes inability to raise the shoulders and difficulty in turning the head. There may be drooping of shoulders.

## Hypoglossal Nerve

The features of hypoglossal nerve lesion depend on the type of paralysis.

### *Lower Motor Neuron Paralysis*

**Unilateral paralysis** Common features are:

1. Tongue is pushed to the paralysed side.
2. Median raphe becomes concave towards paralysed side.
3. Atrophy (with flaccidity) of tongue occurs on the affected side.
4. Fasciculation may be seen on the affected side.

**Bilateral paralysis** Common features are:

1. Marked wasting with fasciculation on both sides.
2. Protrusion of tongue becomes impossible.
3. Dysarthria and difficulty in pronouncing 'T' and 'D' may be seen.

### *Upper Motor Neuron Paralysis*

**Unilateral paralysis** Common features are:

1. Usually asymptomatic.
2. Tongue may be pushed to the opposite side.

**Bilateral paralysis** Common features are:

1. Tongue is spastic.
2. Dysarthria may be associated with emotional disturbances.
3. Dysphagia may be present. This is due to the inability to swallow because the tongue cannot manipulate food properly.

## VIVA

1. Which cranial nerves are sensory in function, motor in function, or mixed?
2. What is the pathway for olfactory nerves?
3. What is anosmia? What are its causes?
4. What is parosmia?
5. Why should a distance of 3 feet be maintained between the subject and the examiner for performing confrontation test and for detecting acuity of vision?
6. What are the functions of the third cranial nerve?
7. Why should a distance of 25 cm be maintained between the eye of the subject and the finger of the examiner for assessing eye movements?
8. What are the effects of a lesion of the third cranial nerve?
9. What is diplopia and what are its causes?
10. What is ptosis and what are its causes?
11. What is nystagmus?
12. What are the causes of unilateral and bilateral dilated pupils?
13. What are the divisions of the fifth cranial nerve and what are their functions?
14. How do you test for the motor function of the fifth cranial nerve?
15. Why is the fourth cranial nerve more liable to be affected by raised intracranial pressure?
16. What is the course of the seventh cranial nerve?
17. How do you test for the motor functions of the seventh cranial nerve?
18. Why is the facial nerve more prone to injury in the facial canal?
19. What is Bell's palsy?

20. Differentiate between supranuclear and infranuclear palsy of the seventh nerve?
21. Why does the upper part of the face escape in supranuclear seventh nerve palsy?
22. How do you assess the functions of the vestibular division of the eight nerve?
23. What are the functions of the ninth cranial nerve?
24. What are the effects of a lesion of the ninth cranial nerve?
25. What are the functions of the vagus nerve?
26. What are the effects of a lesion of the vagus nerve?
27. How do you assess the functions of the eleventh cranial nerve?
28. What are the effects of a lesion of the eleventh cranial nerve?
29. How do you assess the functions of the twelfth cranial nerve?
30. What are the effects of a lesion of the twelfth cranial nerve?
31. What are the differences between upper motor and lower motor neuron paralysis of the twelfth cranial nerve?

# Chapter 32

# Perimetry

## Learning Objectives

After completing this practical, you will be able to:

- Describe the importance of perimetry in clinical physiology.
- Define field of vision, visual axis, isopters, meridians and blind spot (scotoma).
- Read the perimeter chart.
- State the principle of perimetry.
- Chart the field of vision by using a perimeter.
- List the precautions for perimetry.
- Explain the extent of visual field in different quadrants.
- List the factors that affect field of vision.
- Trace the visual pathway.
- Name the visual field defects with lesions at various levels of the visual pathway.

You may also be able to:

- Name and describe different perimeters.
- Describe a perimeter chart.
- Explain physiological and pathological blind spots.
- Explain the effect of lesions of visual pathway.

## INTRODUCTION

Perimetry is the method of accurate charting of peripheral field of vision, using a perimeter. A perimeter is the instrument used to determine the field of vision. Clinically, the field of vision is determined at the bedside of the patient by the confrontation method (as described in Chapter 31). The confrontation method gives a rough idea of the field of vision. Perimetry is performed to detect the exact nature and extent of defects in the field of vision. The defects in the field of vision occur due to lesions at various levels of the visual pathway.

### The Visual Pathway

Visual fibres originate in the nerve cell layer in the retina (from bipolar and ganglion cells). The neurons travel as optic nerves to the optic chiasma where partial decussation of the fibres takes place. The fibre coming from the temporal side of the retina (that receives information from the nasal half of the visual field), remain uncrossed and the fibre emerging from the nasal hemiretina (that receives information from the temporal half of the visual field) cross to the opposite side at the optic chiasma. Thus, the optic tract contains fibres from the temporal hemiretina of the same side and nasal hemiretina of the opposite side. This means that the left optic tracts carry the fibres from the left halves of both retina and the right optic tract from the right halves of both the retina. In the optic tract, the fibres before crossing ascend in the optic chiasma for a short distance, which is known as von Willebrand's knee. Most fibres in the optic tract terminate in the lateral geniculate body of the thalamus, from where the second order of neurons originates and ascend the geniculocalcarine pathway to reach the visual cortex. Few fibres from the optic tract enter the superior colliculus, from where the fibres project to the pretectal area that mediates visual reflexes (Fig. 32.1). The fibres originating from the lateral geniculate body form a loop at their origin called Meyer's loop.

### Field of Vision

The portion of the external world visible to the eye when the gaze is fixed at a particular point is called the field of vision. The visual field depends mainly on the size and colour of the object used for mapping the field. In the temporal side of the fixation point at about 12°–15° a scotoma (blind spot) is located where perception of light does not occur. This is called physiological scotoma and it corresponds to the optic disc in the retina, which does not contain rods and cones. It measures approximately 7.5° in height and 5.5° in width. The visual fields of both the eyes overlap in their medial part to form the area of binocular vision, in which objects are seen by both the eyes. The extent of visual field is described under the discussion section.

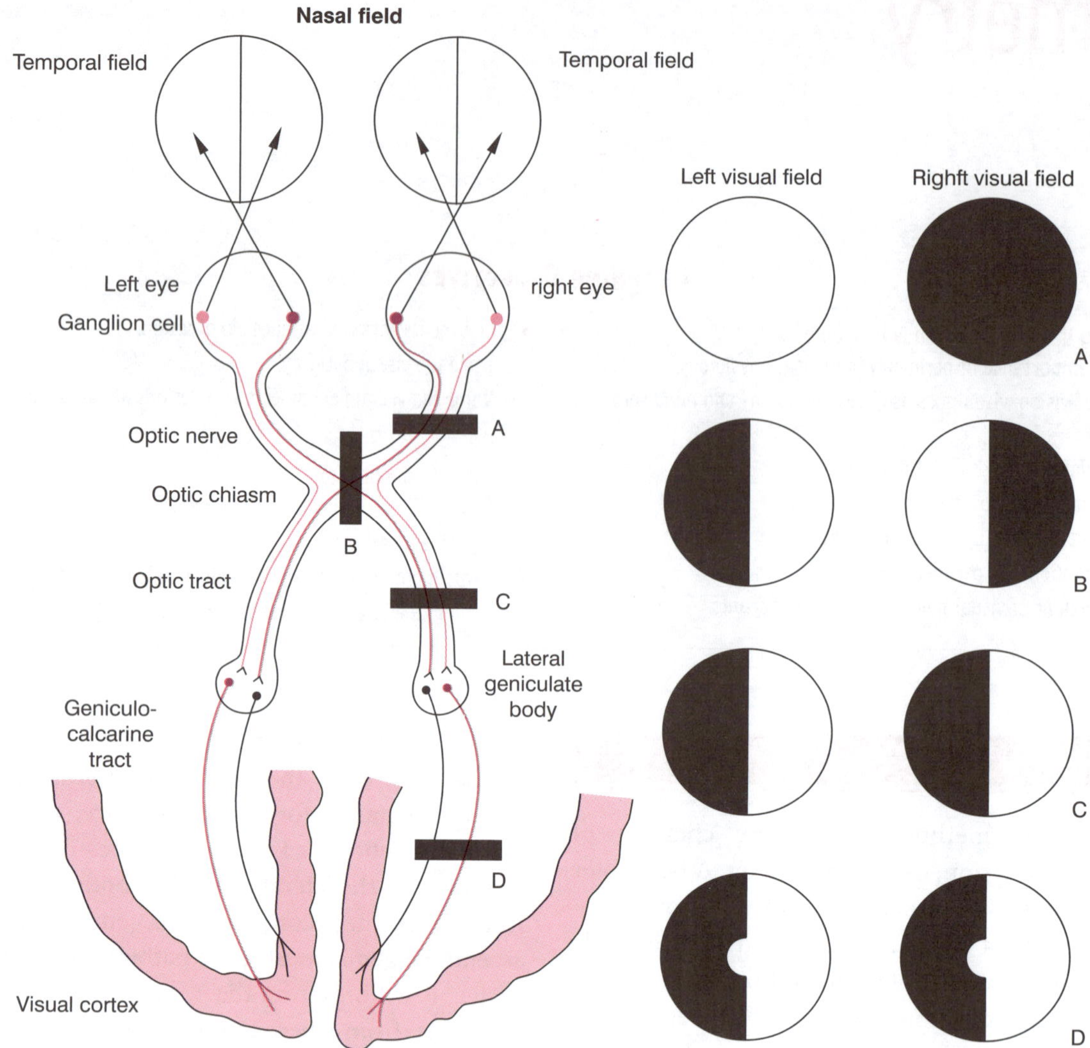


Fig. 32.1 Effects of lesions at various levels of visual pathway. A: lesion of right optic nerve produces blindness in right eye; B: lesion of optic chiasm produces bitemporal hemianopia; C: lesion of right optic tract produces left homonymous hemianopia; D: lesion of right geniculocalcarine tract produces left homonymous hemianopia with macular sparing.

## METHODS

### Method of Determining Perimetry

#### Principle

The part of the external world visible to a person when he fixes his gaze on an object is called the **field of vision**. The method of charting the field of vision is called perimetry. The field of vision charted with one eye (the other eye closed) gives the field of vision for that eye. One eye is covered while the other is fixed on a central point. A small target is moved towards this central point along the selected meridians. Along each meridian, the location where the object becomes first visible is plotted in degrees, and is repeated in all meridians. Determination of the visual field by the *confrontation method* is described in Chapter 31 (2$^{nd}$ cranial nerve).

#### Requirements

1. **Perimeter** Perimeter is the instrument that accurately maps the field of vision. There are different types of perimeters available. The commonly used perimeters are Priestley–Smith's perimeter, Lister's perimeter and student's perimeter (a simple hand perimeter). The most commonly used perimeter in physiology laboratories is Lister's perimeter.

*Lister's perimeter* This consists of a broad concave metal arc which can be rotated around its centre, clockwise or anticlockwise (Fig. 32.2). The metallic arc is graduated in degrees. There is a groove in one limb of the metallic arc, into which a test object is fitted. The concavity of the arc faces the subject. The arc rotates through various angles on a pivot in any direction along with the test object. There are two metallic chin rests. At the back of the perimeter, there is an arrangement for fixing the perimeter chart.

2. **Perimeter chart** The centre of the chart (Fig. 32.3) corresponds to the visual axis. The concentric circle around the centre denotes the point of equal visual acuity called isopters and is marked in degrees (at 10° intervals) from the central fixation points. Perimeter charts contain lines through the centre of the circle denoting various meridians in degrees. These radii (meridians) are marked at 15° intervals. A black oval dot present on the horizontal meridian (15° on either side of the central fixation point) corresponds to the normal blind spot. For comparison with the normal field of vision, right and left visual fields are marked on the chart as dotted lines. For mapping the visual field, the chart is fixed to the back of the perimeter.

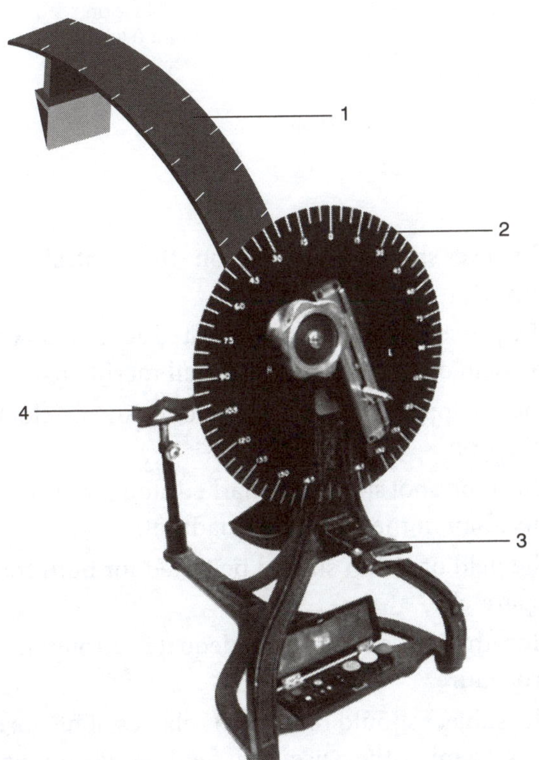


Fig. 32.2 Lister's perimeter. 1: Metallic arc; 2: Removable shield; 3: Chart plate; 4: Chin rest.

3. **Test objects** Test objects of different colours and diameters are used. Usually, the size of the test objects is 3, 5, 10, 15 and 20 mm. The test object is fitted into a carrier, which moves in a groove in one limb of the metal arc. The test object moves with a knob, which causes movement of a pin on the back of the metal arc. The most commonly used object is white and 5 mm in size.

## Procedure

1. Read the perimeter chart.
2. Supply proper instructions to the subject.
3. Ask the subject to sit on a stool comfortably in front of the perimeter.
4. Arrange the perimeter in such a way that the concavity of the arc faces the subject.
5. Ask the subject to sit straight and rest his chin on one of the chin rests.

> Note: When the field of vision of the right eye is to be tested, the subject should rest his chin on the left chin rest. This brings his right eye in line with the fixation point.

6. Focus the eye to be examined on the fixed object which is a white object of 5 mm size placed at the centre of the metallic arc.

> Note: It should be emphasised that the subject's gaze should be fixed at the object throughout the maneuver.

7. Fix the metallic arc in one meridian.
8. Move the test object (which is fixed to the carrier along the arc) gradually from the periphery (90°) towards the central fixation point and ask the subject to indicate when he first sees the object, and note the point.
9. Note this reading in degrees on the arc by marking on the chart for that meridian.
10. Repeat the procedure at 15° intervals till the field of vision is plotted in all meridians of the four quadrants.

> Note: The blind spot is marked along the horizontal meridian in the temporal quadrant.

11. Mark the point of disappearance by bringing the test object towards the centre after initial appearance in the field and point of reappearance with further movement of the object in the same line. This gives an idea of the size of the blind spot.

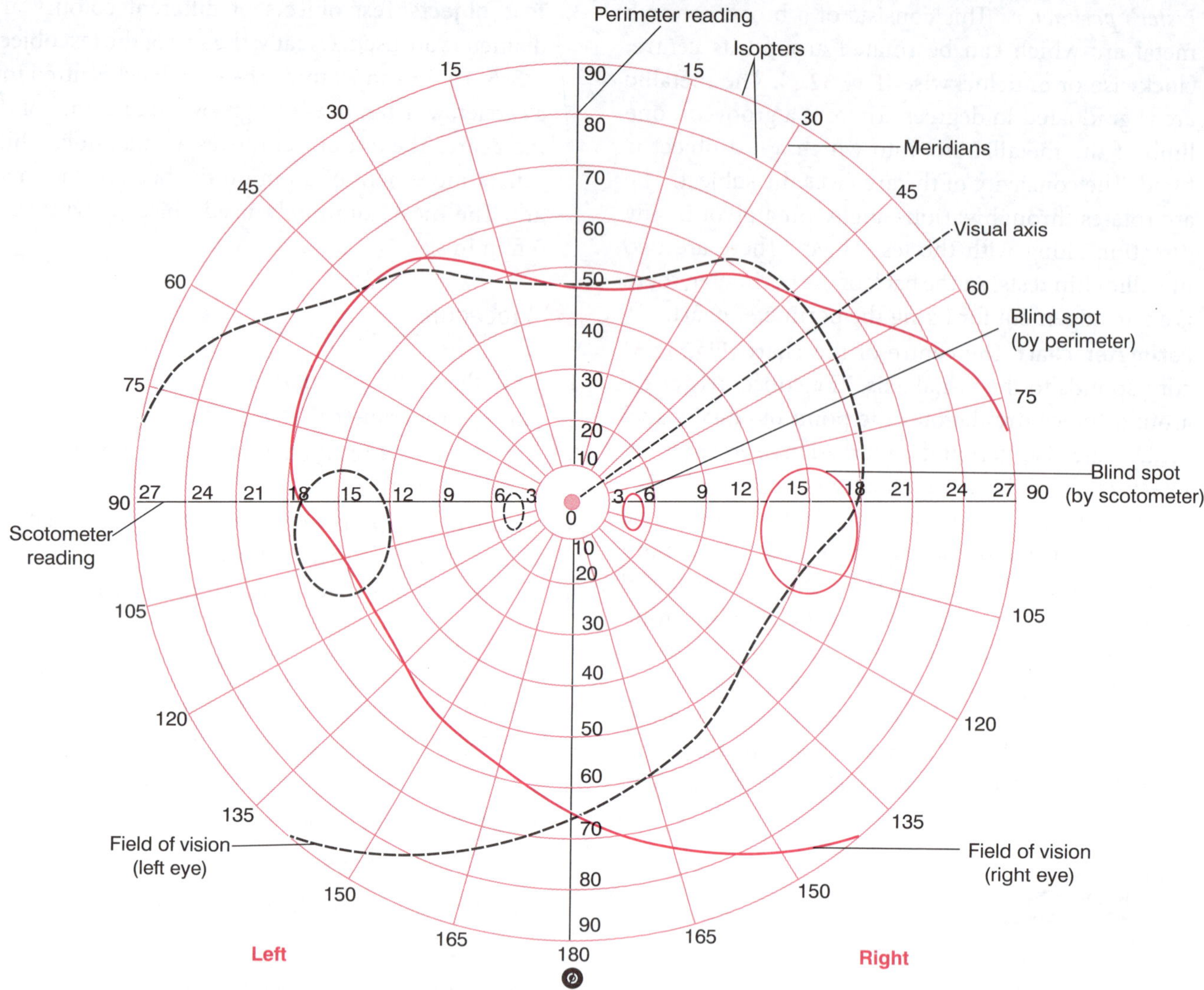


Fig. 32.3 Lister's perimeter chart.

12. Repeat the whole procedure in the opposite eye on the same chart.

## Observation

Observe the obtained field of vision and compare it with the normal visual field depicted in the chart. Note the site and size of blind spot.

## Precautions

1. The subject must be instructed properly.
2. Before mapping the field of vision, the perimetry chart should be studied thoroughly.
3. While testing for one eye, the other eye should be closed.
4. The eye should be fixed on the central fixation point.
5. The procedure should be repeated at 15° intervals till the field of vision is plotted in all meridians.
6. The mapping should be done in a clockwise direction.
7. The blind spot should be marked along the horizontal meridian in the temporal quadrant.
8. The field of vision should be tested for both the eyes separately.
9. Illumination should be adequate throughout the procedure.
10. The subject should remove his glasses, if he normally uses them, otherwise the field of vision will be restricted.

## DISCUSSION

The visual field of each eye is the portion of the external world visible in that eye. The visual field theoretically should be circular, but actually is restricted by the nose medially and roof of the orbit superiorly. Mapping of visual fields is one of the important tests in clinical neurology to detect different diseases of the brain, especially of those that affect the visual pathway.

The visual field is divided into the peripheral and central field of vision. The peripheral field of vision is mapped by perimetry whereas the central field of vision is mapped with the help of a *tangent screen (Bjerrum's screen)* in which a white target is moved across a black screen.

### Factors that Affect Field of Vision

The field of vision depends on:

1. **Colour of the object** Visual acuity is better for a white object than coloured objects. Thus the field of vision is better delineated with a white object. Roughly, the field of vision obtained by using blue and yellow objects is less by 10° and that by using red and green objects is less by 20° from the visual field obtained by a white object.
2. **Size of the object** The larger the size of the object the better is the visual acuity. However, a standard size object is used in perimetry.
3. **Brightness of the object** Brightness, contrast and illumination affect visual acuity and therefore, field of vision.
4. **Illumination** Poor illumination decreases the visual field.

### Normal Field of Vision

The normal field of vision with a white object of 5 mm size is:

Temporal : 100° (since there is no anatomical obstruction on the temporal side of the eyes, the extent of the field of vision in this quadrant is more).

Inferior : 75° (maxilla of the cheek provides anatomical obstruction and reduces the extent of the field in this quadrant.)

Superior : 60° (supraorbital margin provides anatomical obstruction and reduces the extent of the field in this quadrant.)

Nasal : 60° (nasal bridge provides anatomical obstruction and reduces the extent of the field in this quadrant.)

### Visual Field Defects

A defect in the same side of both visual fields is called a **homonymous defect** and a defect in half of the visual field is called **hemianopia**. A defect in the opposite sides of the visual field is called **heteronymous defect** (Fig. 32.1).

*Complete blindness* This occurs due to lesion of the optic nerves. If the lesion is on one side, it causes blindness of that eye.

*Heteronymous hemianopia* The lesions that affect optic chiasma, for example, tumours of pituitary gland expanding the sella turcica causes this defect. Bitemporal hemianopia is seen commonly whereas binasal hemianopia occurs rarely.

*Homonymous hemianopia* The lesion of the optic tract causes this defect. Lesion of the right side of the optic tract produces left homonymous hemianopia and lesion of the left optic tract produces right homonymous hemianopia.

*Homonymous hemianopia with macular sparing* The lesion in the geniculocalcarine tract causes this defect. The macular sparing (loss of peripheral vision with intact macular vision) occurs because the macular representation is separate from that of the peripheral field and is large relative to that of the peripheral fields. Therefore, the lesion in the occipital cortex must extend to large areas to affect peripheral as well as macular vision.

## VIVA

1. What is perimetry?
2. What is the use of perimetry in ophthalmology and neurology?
3. What are the different types of perimeters?

4. What are the precautions taken for doing perimetry?
5. Why is the visual field not circular?
6. What are the factors that affect field of vision?
7. Trace the visual pathway.
8. What are the visual field defects produced by lesions at various levels in the visual pathway?
9. How is central field of vision determined?
10. What is blind spot? How is it detected?
11. What is scotoma?

# CHAPTER 33

# Visual Acuity

## LEARNING OBJECTIVES

After completing this practical, you will be able to:

- Explain the importance of determining visual acuity in clinical medicine.
- Define visual acuity.
- List the factors that affect visual acuity.
- Determine the visual acuity for distant and near vision.
- List the precautions taken for determining visual acuity.
- Define myopia and hypermetropia.
- Name the type of lens used to correct the defects of visual acuity for distant and near vision.

## INTRODUCTION

Visual acuity is defined as the resolving power of the eyes, that is, the extent to which the eye can perceive the details and contours of an object. It can be explained in terms of minimum separable distance, that is, the smallest gap by which two lines can be separated and still be seen as two separate lines. Visual acuity is the function of cones. It is tested separately for distant vision and near vision.

### Factors Affecting Visual Acuity

Visual acuity is mainly affected by three factors: optical factors, retinal factors and stimulus factors.

#### Optical Factors

The image forming mechanism is the primary factor that determines visual acuity. Optical aberrations and defects of the image forming mechanism decrease the visual acuity.

#### Retinal Factors

Visual acuity is the function of the cones. Cones are more in number at the centre (densely packed in the fovea centralis) than in the periphery of the retina. Therefore, visual acuity is maximal at the fovea and less in the periphery of the retina.

#### Stimulus Factors

The main stimulus factors are the size and colour of the object.

**Size of the object** Size of the object and its distance from the eye affect visual acuity. Visual acuity is directly proportional to the visual angle (VA).

$$\text{VA} = \frac{\text{Size of the object}}{\text{Distance of the object from the eye}}$$

**Colour of the object** Visual acuity is better for white objects than for coloured objects. Visual acuity also depends on the brightness of the stimulus, contrast between the stimulus and the background, and the length of time the subject is exposed to the stimulus.

## METHODS

### Test for Distant Vision

#### Principle

A series of letters of varying sizes are constructed in such a way that the top letter is visible to normal eyes at 60 metres, and the subsequent lines at 36, 24, 18, 12, 9, 6, and 5 metres respectively. Visual acuity is recorded according to the formula $V = d / D$, where $V$ is the visual acuity, $d$ is the distance at which the letters are read, and $D$ is the distance at which the letters should be read.

#### Requirement

**Snellen's chart** Snellen's letters are depicted on a cardboard (Fig. 33.1) with eight rows of black letters of different fonts. The topmost line can be read by a normal subject at a distance of 60 metres and subsequent lines at 36, 24, 18, 12, 9, 6, and 5 metres respectively.

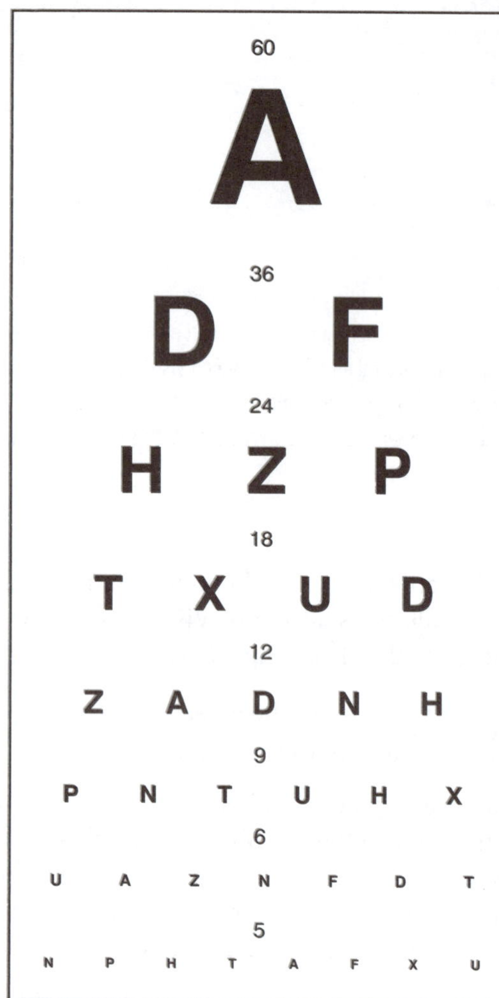


Fig. 33.1 Snellen's chart.

## Procedure

1. Supply proper instructions to the subject.
2. Ask the subject to sit at a distance of 6 metres from the chart ($d = 6$).
3. Ask him to close one of his eyes and read the chart with the other eye.
4. Note up to which line the subject is able to read comfortably.
5. Ask him to repeat the procedure with the opposite eye.

## Precautions

1. The subject should be instructed properly.
2. It should be ascertained that the subject knows the letters (language) written on the Snellen's chart.
3. The Snellen's chart should be well-lit.
4. The patient should sit exactly at a distance of 6 metres from the chart.
5. Each eye should be tested separately.
6. If the subject wears glasses, visual acuity should be tested with and without them.

## Observation

If only the top letter of the chart is visible, the visual acuity is 6/60. If the subject can read the lowest line the visual acuity is 6/5, that is, he has better than normal vision. Normal visual acuity is 6/6. Accordingly visual acuity is expressed as 6/6, 6/9, 6/12, 6/18, 6/24, and 6/36, respectively, depending on the line up to which the subject can read. If his visual acuity is less than 6/60, that is, the subject cannot read the top line from a distance of 6 metres, he should move closer until he can read the top letter. If the top letter is visible at 2 metres, the visual acuity is expressed as 2/60. If the acuity of vision is less than 1/60, the subject is asked to count fingers held up (*finger counting method*) or to perceive hand movement (*hand movement method*). If the subject cannot count the finger or perceive hand movement, a light is focused in front of his eyes and he is asked whether he perceives the light (*light perception method*).

# Test for Near Vision

## Principle

The visual acuity for near vision is tested by reading Jaeger's chart at ordinary reading distance. This consists of letters of various sizes based on the principle of *Printer's point system.*

## Requirement

**Jaeger's chart** This chart (Fig. 33.2) consists of letters of various sizes on the Printer's point system. The smallest point is N5 and the largest point is N36.

## Procedure

1. Supply proper instructions to the subject.
2. The room should be well-lit and the subject should sit comfortably.
3. Hold Jaeger's chart at a distance of 10–12 inches from the subject's eyes.

N5

When I was ten years old, my father had a small estate near Satara where he used to take us during the holidays. It was situated in rough and uncultivated country side where wild animals were often seen. Once we heard that there was a panther in the surroundings who was killing the cattle and attacking the villagers. Father had warned me not to wander for from home in the evenings. I had made friends with a your villager called Ramu.

N6

Ramu used to drive the cattle to graze and bring them back to shelter at the end of the day. He was lean and of a short build and was barely fifteen. He used to be my companion whenever I meet him winding his way home. One afternoon, just about five o'clock, early in the month of March, chance brought us together.

N8

As there had been considerable variation in the series of Jaeger's test types produced by different printers, a new series of standard graduated test types for near vision has been recommended by the Faculty of Opthalmologist of England in which Times Roman types are used with standard spacing.

N10

The eye to be examined is anaesthetised with 1% solution in anaethine and the instrument is lightly pressed against the eye in the suspected area. If there is a solid tumour, the pupil remains dark. Then the instrument is placed on another region when the pupil is found to be read.

Fig. 33.2 Jaeger's chart.

4. Ask the subject to read the letters of the different sizes.
5. Note the smallest type of the letters that the subject can read comfortably.
6. Repeat the test separately for each eye with the other eye closed.

## Precautions

1. It should be ascertained that the subject knows the language in which the letters are written.
2. The room should be adequately lighted.
3. The Jaeger's chart should be kept at a distance of about 25 cm from the subject.
4. The test should be performed with both eyes open. It should also be performed separately for each eye with the other eye closed.

## Observation

Express the result by noting the smallest size of letters that the subject can read.

# DISCUSSION

The visual acuity of a normal person is 6/6, that is, the subject should be able to read up to the seventh line. If his visual acuity is less than 6/6, it is considered to be reduced. For correction of the acuity of vision, concave lenses are prescribed after doing a thorough postmydriatic examination of the eye.

If the subject wears glasses, the type of lens used should be mentioned. The examiner can detect the type of lens by holding the lens in front of the eye and looking at an object through it. By moving the lens side to side if the object moves in the opposite direction, the lens is convex; and if the object moves in the same direction, the lens is concave. Concave lenses are used for myopia and convex lenses for hypermetropia.

For young children, simple pictures constructed on a chart on the basis of Snellen's principle can be used. Another test used for children is the *Sheridan–Gardiner* test in which Snellen's letters are matched with different types of objects. For illiterate persons the 'E' test is effective.

## Myopia

Myopia or shortsightedness is an error of refraction in which parallel rays of light coming from a distant object are focused in front of the retina. The person cannot see distant objects. It is corrected by using concave lenses.

## Hypermetropia

Hypermetropia or longsightedness is an error of refraction in which parallel rays of light coming from distant object are focused behind the retina. Thus the person cannot see near objects. It is corrected by using convex lenses.

## VIVA

1. Define visual acuity.
2. What are the factors that affect visual acuity?
3. What is visual angle? How does it affect visual acuity?
4. How do you test visual acuity for distant vision?
5. How do you test visual acuity for near vision?
6. What are the precautions for the tests of visual acuity?
7. What is the Sheridan–Gardiner test? What is its significance?
8. What is myopia? How do you correct it?
9. What is hypermetropia? How do you correct it?

# Chapter 34

# Colour Vision

## Learning Objectives

After completing this practical, you will be able to:

- Explain the clinical importance of performing the test of colour vision.
- Test the colour vision by using Ishihara chart.
- Give the function of cone systems.
- Trace the pathway of colour vision.
- Classify and define different types of colour blindness.

You may also be able to:

- Name the theories of colour vision.
- Explain different types of and the mode of transmission of colour blindness.
- Describe other methods of detecting colour vision.

## INTRODUCTION

The human eye has the ability to respond to all wavelengths of light from 400 to 700 nm. This is called the visible part of the spectrum. The sense of colour is perceived by cones. There are three types of **cone systems**: red, green and blue. There are also three types of cone pigments: cyanolabe, chlorolabe and erythrolabe showing highest response to specific parts of the spectrum. Each cone shows maximum absorption of light at a particular wavelength. Due to differential stimulation of the three types of cones by different wavelengths of light, the human eye perceives all the colours. For example, the wavelength of 580 nm stimulates red cones maximally and we perceive the colour red. It also stimulates the green cones to some extent and therefore we see the colour orange. Likewise, the wavelength of 535 nm stimulates green cones and the wavelength 445 nm stimulates blue cones maximally, therefore, we perceive the colours green and blue.

There are three primary colours: red, green and blue, each responding maximally to the light of certain wavelengths. When colours are mixed in appropriate amounts, the object looks white. Therefore, for any colour, there is a complementary colour which, when properly mixed with a specific colour, produces white.

### Pathway of Colour Vision

Neurons carrying colour vision in the optic nerve pass through the optic tract to reach the parvocellular part of the lateral geniculate body (LGB) of the thalamus. From parvocellular laminas of the LGB, fibres project to blob regions in layer four of the visual cortex. Blobs are the clusters of cells arranged in a mosaic in the visual cortex and are concerned with colour vision.

### Mechanism of Colour Vision

There are two mechanisms of colour vision, the retinal and the cortical.

#### The Retinal Mechanism

The retinal mechanism of colour vision is based on **Young and Helmholtz's theory**. According to this theory, the perception of the three primary colours is possible due to the presence of three types of cone systems in the retina, each containing a specific pigment which is maximally sensitive to one type of primary colour.

#### The Cortical Mechanism

The colour-sensitive ganglion cells project to the cells of the lateral geniculate body (single opponent cells), which in turn project to the cells of the primary visual cortex (double opponent cells). The cortical cells in turn project to area 18. It is believed that different colours are perceived by the activities in the primary visual cortex and the cortical association areas.

## METHODS

### Ishihara's Chart Method

There are different methods of detecting colour vision. However, the Ishihara chart is routinely used for this purpose.

## Principle

Colour vision is tested by using Ishihara's chart which consists of lithographic plates where numericals are drawn in coloured spots amidst other parts of different colours and sizes. The subject reads the number and traces the pathway by appreciating the colour. The colour of these plates is such that they are liable to be confused with spots in the background by people with defective colour vision.

## Requirements

**Ishihara's chart** This consists of lithographic plates in which numerals are written in different colour spots (Fig. 34.1). The colour of these spots is such that they are liable to be confused with spots in the background by people with defective colour vision. These plates are so constructed that a person with colour vision defect will read a different number from a normal person.

## Procedure

1. Give proper instructions to the subject.
2. Ask the subject to sit comfortably in a well-it room.
3. Instruct the subject to read the numbers or trace the lines in each plate of the book.
4. Note if he reads the number or traces the pathway properly.

## Precautions

1. The room should be adequately lit.
2. All the plates of the book should be read.
3. While reading the plates, a maximum of 5–10 seconds should be allowed per plate.

# Other Methods

There are other two methods of testing colour vision: Edridge–Green lantern test and Holmgren's wool-matching test.

## Edridge–Green Lantern Test

In this test, different colours are shown by a lantern and the subject is asked to name the colours. The lantern contains the following colours: pure red, red of different intensities, yellow, green, signal green, blue and purple. The subject sits in a dimly illuminated room 6 metres from the lantern. He names the colour of the light,

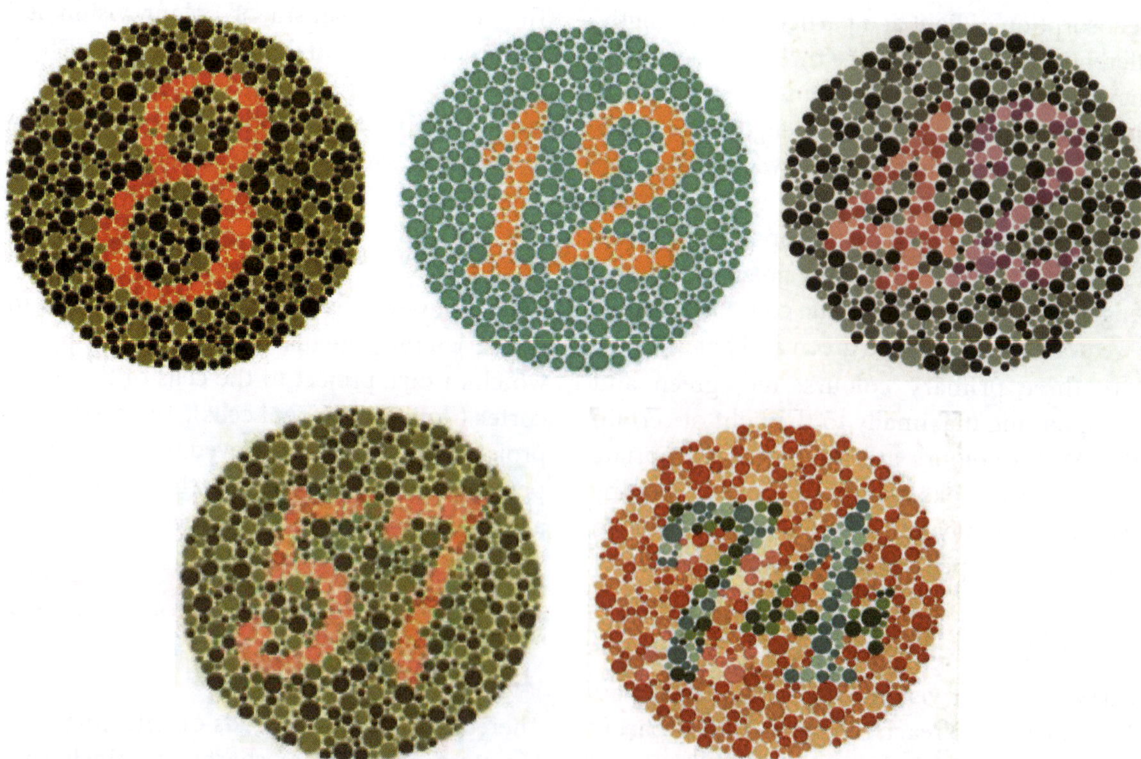

Fig. 34.1 Lithographic plates of Ishihara's chart.

focused through the glass fixed on a rotating disc in the lantern. This test is usually employed for railway recruitment.

### Holmgren's Wool-Matching Test

In this test, the subject is asked to perform a series of colour-matching from a collection of wools of different colours. There are three sets of coloured wools: test colours, match colours and confusing colours. The subject matches different colours of all the three groups.

## DISCUSSION

### Clinical Significance

Test for intactness of colour vision is performed routinely as part of the health check for recruitment to a government job or admission to any professional courses. Intact colour vision is mandatory for selection for posts related to driving, traffic services, railways and armed forces. Defect in the perception of colour is called **colour blindness**.

### Types of Colour Blindness

Colour blindness is classified into three types:

1. **Trichromats** Trichromats are of two types: protanomaly and deuteranomaly. The person is less sensitive to one of the primary colours.
2. **Dichromats** Dichromats are of three types: protanopia, deuteranopia, and tritanopia. The person perceives two primary colours.
3. **Monochromats** The person perceives only one primary colour.

The suffix "anomaly" represents colour weakness and the suffix "anopia" represents colour blindness. The prefixes "prot", "deuter" and "trit" represent red, green and blue colour defects. For example, protanomaly means weakness of perception of red and protanopia means blindness for red. A trichromat has all the three cone systems but one system may be weak (protanomaly or deuteranomaly). A dichromat is an individual having only two cone systems, with one cone system absent. Depending on the absence of a cone system, a subject can be protanopic, deuteranopic or tritanopic. A monochromat is a person having only one cone system, with two systems absent.

Colour blindness is inherited as an X-linked recessive. This occurs due to an abnormal gene on the X chromosome. Women are the carriers but suffer from the disease only when both X chromosomes carry the defective gene.

## VIVA

1. What is the clinical significance of the test of colour vision?
2. What is the chart used for detecting colour blindness? What is its principle?
3. What do you mean by colour blindness? How do you classify it?
4. What is the mode of transmission of colour blindness?
5. What are the theories of colour vision?
6. What is the pathway for colour vision?
7. What are the other methods of detecting colour vision? What is the principle behind each of these methods?

CHAPTER 35

# Hearing Tests

## LEARNING OBJECTIVES

After completing this practical, you will be able to:
- Explain the importance of performing this practical in clinical physiology.
- Name the hearing tests.
- State the principles of the tuning fork test.
- Perform and interpret the tuning fork tests.
- List the precautions to be taken for tuning fork tests.
- Differentiate conductive deafness from neural deafness.

You may also be able to:
- Trace the auditory pathway.
- State the attributes of sounds.
- State the principles of audiometry and BAEP.
- Explain the abnormalities of hearing tests.

## INTRODUCTION

Hearing tests are commonly performed by audiologists to detect the type and degree of hearing loss for prescribing hearing aids. Hearing tests also help neurologists establish the extent of lesions, especially if the brainstem is involved in the pathological process.

## Anatomical and Physiological Considerations

### Physiological Basis

**Characteristics of sound** Perception and interpretation of speech is a complex phenomenon. There are four attributes of sound: frequency, intensity, direction and pattern. The sound waves are sensed by the hair cells of the cochlea and the impulses are transmitted to the auditory cortex by a very complex pathway. The actual perception and interpretation of most aspects of sound take place in the auditory cortex.

**Frequency** The frequency of the sound stimuli is detected by the basilar membrane. Sharpening of frequency occurs in the hair cells and auditory neurons. The cells in the auditory cortex respond only to a narrow range of sound frequency. The frequency of the nerve impulses is related to the intensity of the stimulus.

**Intensity** Intensity of the sound is coded as early as with the receptors. The outer hair cells respond to weaker stimuli because of the lower threshold of the cilia of the outer hair cells that are embedded in the tectorial membrane. In the auditory cortex, there are neurons that are maximally sensitive to a specific intensity of the stimulus.

**Direction** The direction of sound is judged by the difference in time and intensity at which it arrives at the two ears. Though the direction of sound is detected by the superior olivary nucleus, the auditory cortex is essential for perception of the direction of sound.

**Pattern** The pattern of a sound is the sequence in which different components of the sound appear. This property of sound is recognised by the auditory cortex alone.

## Hearing Tests

A number of hearing tests have been described to detect hearing loss:

1. Watch test
2. Tuning fork test
3. Audiometry
4. Recording of brainstem auditory evoked potentials (BAEP)

The commonly used hearing tests in clinical practice are tuning fork tests.

# METHODS

## Watch Test

### Principle

Sound is sensed by the hair cells in the ear and conducted via auditory pathways to the auditory cortex. A defect in either perception or conduction of sound can lead to hearing loss.

### Requirement

Wrist watch

### Procedure

1. Ask the subject to close his eyes.
2. Ask him to plug one ear with a finger.
3. Slowly bring a watch from a distance to his opened ear and ask him when he hears the sound.
4. Note the distance at which the subject hears the sound of the wrist watch.
5. Repeat the same in the other ear.
6. Compare the result with a normal subject.

### Disadvantages

1. It detects only gross hearing impairment.
2. It cannot detect the nature and degree of hearing loss.

## Tuning Fork Tests

Tuning fork tests are based on the principle that sound is conducted to the ear by the air (air conduction). Therefore, deafness can be detected by testing air conduction or by directly stimulating the bone that conducts sound.

There are three types of tuning fork tests: Rinne's test, Weber's test and Schwabach test. For all these tests, tuning fork (512 Hz) is required. Tuning forks of higher frequency like 512 Hz or 256 Hz produce more sound than vibration, whereas tuning forks with lower frequency produce more vibration than sound. Therefore, 512 Hz or 256 Hz tuning forks are preferred for hearing tests.

## Rinne's test

### Principle

Rinne's test compares hearing ability through the mediums of bone and air; that means there is comparison of bone conduction with air conduction of the same ear.

### Procedure

1. Give proper instructions to the subject.

> Note: Instruct him to raise the finger when he stops hearing the sound of the vibrating tuning fork.

2. Hold the stem of the tuning fork between the thumb and the index finger in such a way that the fingers do not touch the blades of the tuning fork.
3. Make the tuning fork vibrate by suddenly stroking the blades of the fork against the hypothenar eminence or the thigh.
4. Immediately place the base of the vibrating tuning fork on the mastoid process (Fig. 35.1A) of one side and ask the subject to raise his finger when he ceases to hear the sound (Fig. 35.1B).
5. Once he stops hearing, hold the vibrating tuning fork very close to his ear (Fig. 35.1C) and ask him whether he hears the sound. When he stops hearing it, bring the tuning fork close to your ear to confirm whether the vibrating sounds have actually stopped.
6. Record your observation.

### Precautions

1. Proper instructions should be given to the subject.
2. The tuning fork should be held by the stem, taking care not to touch the blades.
3. To start the vibration in the tuning fork, the fork should be stroked against the hypothenar eminence or the thigh, not against the table or any hard surface.
4. If the subject stops hearing the sound, the vibrating tuning fork should be taken close to the examiner's ear (taking the examiner as normal) for comparison.

## Weber's Test

### Principle

Weber's test compares bone conduction of both the ears.

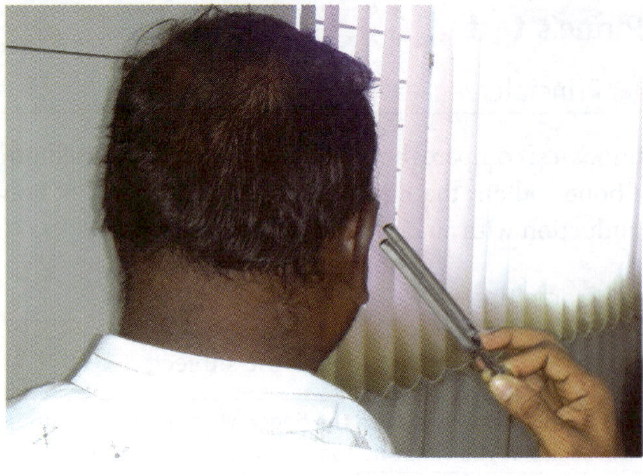

(A)

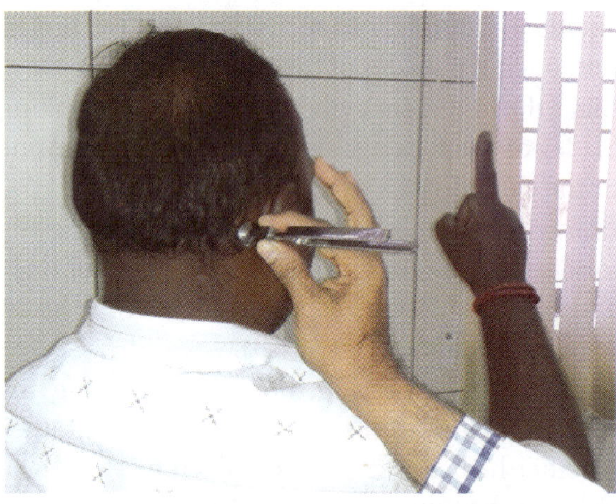

(B)

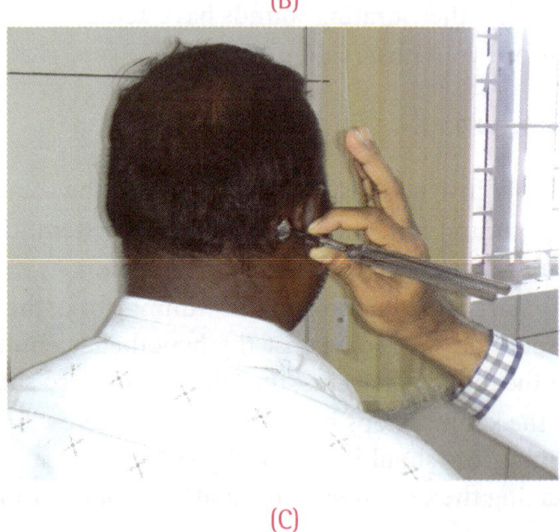

(C)

Fig. 35.1 Methodology for Rinne test. The vibrating tuning fork is placed on the mastoid process (A) and the subject is asked to raise his finger immediately after he ceases hearing (B). Then, the vibrating tuning fork is kept close to the subject's ear, and he is asked to raise his finger once he ceases hearing (C).

## Procedure

1. Give proper instructions to the subject.
2. Make the tuning fork vibrate by hitting the blades of the fork against the hypothenar eminence or the thigh.
3. Place the base of the vibrating tuning fork on the vertex of the skull (Fig. 35.2) or on the forehead of the subject (Fig. 35.3).

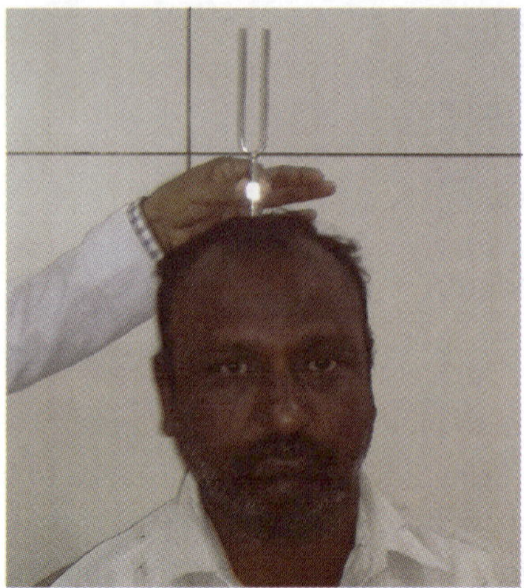

Fig. 35.2 Methodology for Weber test. The vibrating tuning fork is placed on the vertex of the skull, and the subject is instructed to indicate whether he hears equally on both sides or if the sound is better heard in one ear.

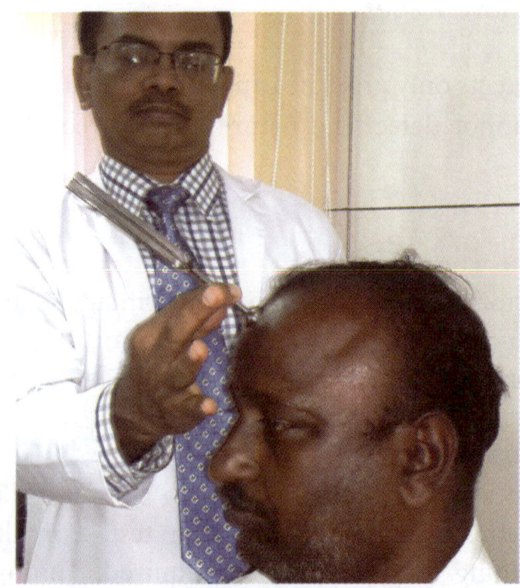

Fig. 35.3 Another methodology for Weber test. The vibrating tuning fork is placed on the forehead of the subject, and the subject is instructed to indicate whether he hears equally on both sides or if the sound is better heard in one ear.

4. Ask the subject to indicate whether he hears equally on both sides or if the sound is better heard in one ear.

### Precautions

1. Give proper instructions to the subject (subject should understand the procedure of the test).
2. To make the tuning fork vibrate, hit the blades of the fork against the hypothenar eminence or the thigh.

## Schwabach Test

### Principle

This test compares the bone conduction of the subject with that of the examiner.

### Procedure

1. Give proper instructions to the subject.
2. Make the tuning fork vibrate.
3. Place the vibrating tuning fork over the subject's mastoid process (Fig. 35.4A).
4. Ask the subject to raise his finger when he stops hearing the sound.
5. Immediately bring the tuning fork close to your own ear and check if you still hear the sound (Fig. 35.4B).

### Precautions

1. Proper instructions should be given to the subject.
2. Once the subject stops hearing the sound, a comparison should be made with the examiner by placing the tuning fork on his mastoid process.

## Audiometry

### Principle and Brief Procedure

Audiometry is an objective and accurate method to assess the degree of deafness and frequency range at which it manifests. This is done by using an audiometer which is an electroacoustic device. The test is conducted in a soundproof room. One ear is tested at a time with the help of an earphone. The subject flashes a light when a sound is heard. At each frequency the threshold intensity is determined and plotted against a graph as a percentage of normal hearing. The audiometer provides pure tones of different frequencies at various levels of loudness or intensity from an oscillator connected via an amplifier to the earphones. Routinely, the audiometer provides a minimum of 7 tones (250, 500, 1000, 2000, 3000, 4000 and 8000 Hz). The intensity of each tonal frequency can be increased. The lowest decibel at which the patient hears the tone is called the threshold. A graph is plotted showing the audiometric threshold as a function of frequency discrimination. This graph is called an audiogram.

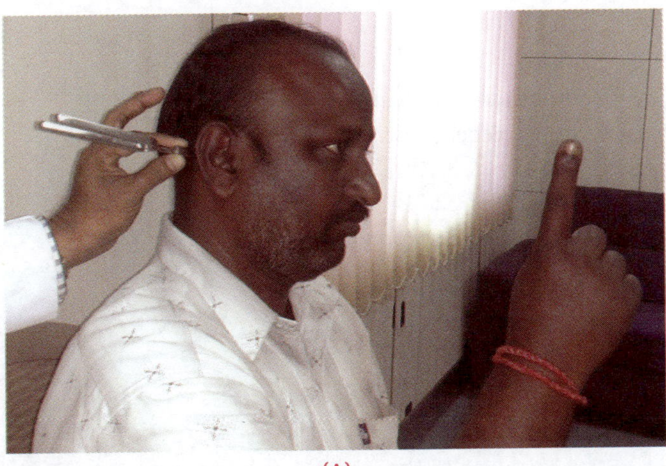

(A)

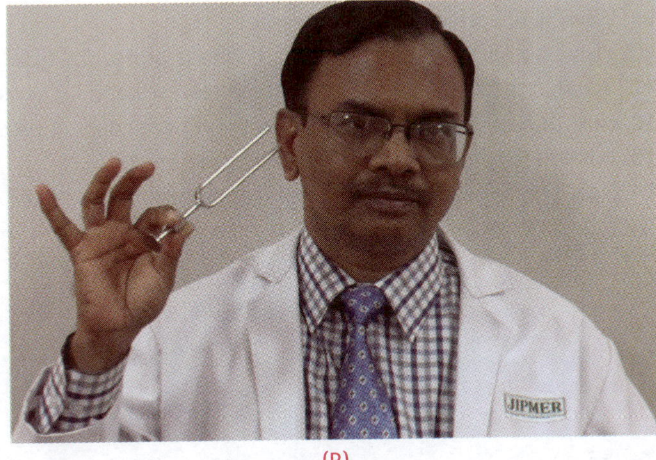


(B)

Fig. 35.4 Methodology for Swabach test. The vibrating tuning fork is placed on the mastoid process and the subject is asked to raise his finger immediately after he ceases hearing (A). Then, the examiner brings the same tuning fork close to his ear and checks comparatively if the sounds are still audible (B).

## Brainstem Auditory Evoked Potential (BAEP)

This is the most accurate method to differentiate organic deafness from functional deafness, and determine the exact site of hearing loss.

# DISCUSSION

## Rinne's Test

This test compares bone conduction with air conduction of the same ear. If the hearing is normal, the subject will hear the sound of the vibrating fork by air conduction even after he has ceased hearing by bone conduction, because air conduction is better than bone conduction. This is called Rinne-positive. In conduction deafness, vibrations in the air are not heard after bone conduction is over, that is, bone conduction is better than air conduction. This is Rinne-negative. In total nerve deafness, no sound is heard in either case. In partial nerve deafness, the Rinne test becomes false-positive (For details, refer Table of question No. 14).

## Weber's Test

Normally, sound is heard equally in both ears. If sound is heard better in the defective ear, the hearing loss is due to conduction deafness. If the sound is louder in the normal ear, the hearing loss in the defective ear is due to nerve deafness.

## Schwabach Test

If the subject is normal, bone conduction of the subject is equal to bone conduction of the examiner. In conduction deafness, bone conduction is better than normal. In nerve deafness, bone conduction is worse than normal.

# VIVA

1. What are the uses of hearing tests in clinical medicine?
2. What are the attributes of sound?
3. What are the different hearing tests?
4. What are the principles of hearing tests?
5. What are the tuning fork tests?
6. How do you perform Rinne's test? What are the precautions for this test?
7. How do you perform Weber's test? What are the precautions of this test?
8. How do you perform the Schwabach test? What are the precautions of this test?
9. What is the principle of audiometry?
10. What is BAEP? What is its use in diagnosis of hearing loss?
11. What is the significance of the Rinne test? What do you mean by Rinne-positive and Rinne-negative?
12. How do you differentiate nerve deafness from conduction deafness by using Weber's test?
13. What is the significance of the Schwabach test?
14. How are the observations of the hearing tests interpreted?

    Ans. Interpretation of tuning fork tests is performed as given in the following tabular form.

| Name of the test | Observation | Infrence |
|---|---|---|
| Rinne's test | i) Air conduction is greater than bone conduction (Rinne-positive)<br>ii) Bone conduction is greater than air conduction (Rinne-negative)<br>iii) Both air and bone conductions are absent<br>iv) Air conduction is greater than bone conduction in the defective ear (Rinne-false-positive) | i) Normal<br>ii) Conduction deafness<br>iii) Complete nerve deafness<br>iv) Partial nerve deafness |
| Weber's Test | i) Sound is heard equally in both ears<br>ii) Sound is better heard in the defective ear (lateralized to the defective ear)<br>iii) Sound is better heard in the healthy ear (lateralized to the healthy ear) | i) Normal<br>ii) Conduction deafness in the defective ear<br>iii) Partial nerve deafness in the defective ear |
| Schwabach Test | i) Bone conduction of the subject is equal to the bone conduction of the examiner<br>ii) Bone conduction of the subject is better than the bone conduction of the examiner<br>iii) Bone conduction of the subject is worse than the bone conduction of the examiner | i) Normal<br>ii) Conduction deafness in the subject<br>iii) Partial nerve deafness in the subject |

Chapter 36

# Examination of Taste and Smell

## Learning Objectives

After completing this practical, you will be able to:

- Describe the importance of examination of taste and smell in clinical physiology.
- Name the primary tastes.
- Explain the distribution of receptors for primary tastes in the tongue.
- Name the cranial nerves that carry the sensations of smell and taste.
- Examine the sensations of smell and taste.
- List the precautions taken while performing the practical.
- Name the conditions that alter the sensations of taste and smell.

You may also be able to:

- Trace the auditory pathway.
- Trace the pathway for taste and smell.
- Explain the physiological bases of the abnormalities associated with taste and smell.

## INTRODUCTION

The sensations of smell and taste are very basic to our existence as they are closely associated with ingestive behaviours. The olfactory nerve carries the sensation of smell from the nasal mucosa to the olfactory cortex of the brain. Facial, glossopharyngeal and vagus nerves carry the sensation of taste from the receptors in the tongue to the postcentral gyrus of the cortex.

### Taste

Taste receptors are present in the taste buds that are distributed in the papillae of the tongue and the mucous membrane of the oral cavity. The seventh cranial nerve carries the sensation of taste from the anterior two-thirds of the tongue, the ninth cranial nerve carries the sensation of taste from the posterior third of the tongue, and the tenth cranial nerve carries the sensation from the pharyngeal region.

#### Primary Tastes

There are four primary tastes: sweet, sour, salt and bitter. Receptors for these tastes are different and are distributed in different parts of the tongue.

*Sweet* Receptors for the sweet taste are present mainly in the tip of the tongue.

*Salt* Receptors for the salt taste are present mainly in the centre of the dorsum of the tongue.

*Sour* Receptors for the sour taste are distributed mainly in the lateral portions of the tongue.

*Bitter* Receptors for the bitter taste are distributed primarily at the back of the tongue.

#### Taste Pathway

The first order of neurons carries the sensation from the receptors in the seventh, ninth and tenth cranial nerves to the nucleus tractus solitarius (NTS) in the medulla. The second order of neurons arises from the NTS. They ascend the medial lemniscus to relay in the thalamus. The third order of neurons arises from the thalamus and projects to the lower part of the postcentral gyrus (Fig. 36.1).

### Smell

The sensation of smell is more developed in animals (macrosomatic) and less developed in humans (microsomatic). Receptors are present in the olfactory mucosa. This is the only part of the central nervous system, which is exposed to the external world.

#### Olfactory Pathway

The first-order neurons carrying the sensation pierce the cribriform plate of the ethmoid bone to reach the olfactory bulb. In the olfactory bulb, they synapse with the dendrites of the mitral and tufted cells to form the olfactory glomeruli. The glomeruli also receive inputs from the granule cells which can modulate the output from the olfactory bulb. The second-order neurons (axons of the mitral cells) form the olfactory tract that

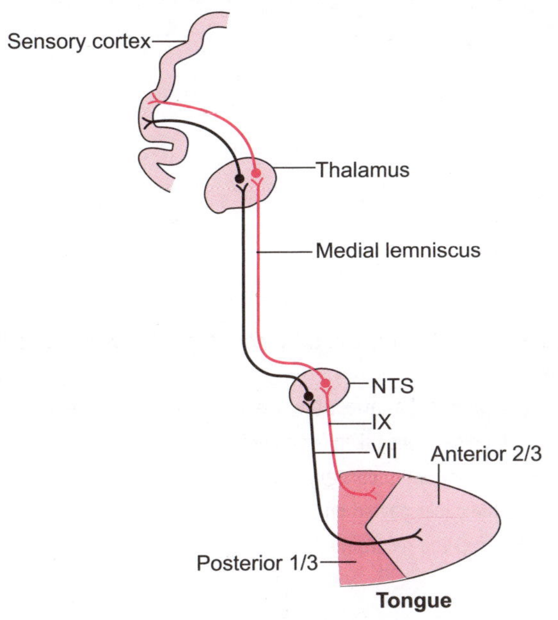


Fig. 36.1 Pathway for taste sensation. NTS: Nucleus tractus solitarius; IX: Ninth cranial nerve; VII: Seventh cranial nerve.

divides into the medial and lateral pathways. The fibres in the lateral division project to the olfactory lobe of the same side to terminate in the centres for olfaction (prepyriform cortex, amygdala and preamygdaloid areas). The fibres in the medial division project to the opposite olfactory tubercle from where they go to the dorsomedial nucleus of the thalamus and the orbitofrontal cortex.

## METHOD

This is described in Chapter 31.

## DISCUSSION

The physiological significance and clinical importance of examination of taste and smell are described in Chapter 31.

## VIVA

1. What are the primary tastes?
2. What is the distribution pattern of receptors for primary tastes in the tongue?
3. What is the pathway for the taste sensation?
4. What are the abnormalities of the taste sensation?
5. What is the pathway for the sensation of smell?
6. What are the abnormalities of the sensation of smell?

Chapter 37

# Appliances

## Learning Objectives

After completing this practical, you will be able to:

- Identify and describe the uses of appliances used in experimental physiology.
- List the advantages of using of an electrical stimulus.
- List the advantages of using frog and gastrocnemius-sciatic preparation.
- State the basic principle of the various apparatus used in amphibian practicals.
- List the factors that affect the strength of induced current.
- List the precautions taken for amphibian practicals.
- Make primary and secondary circuits.
- Smoke the paper pasted on the drum.
- Varnish (fix) the recording.

## INTRODUCTION

A student should be familiar with the apparatus that he uses in experimental physiology. The student should know the basic principle of the working of the instruments, the uses of the apparatus and the instructions for the safe use of the apparatus. As electric current is used as the stimulus to perform most of the experiments, proper earthing (grounding) and insulation of the wires must be ensured before starting the experiment.

In most experimental work, especially of the study of the response of tissues to various stimuli, four set-ups are needed: (i) the source of stimulation, (ii) a stimulating device, (iii) tissue preparation and (iv) a recording device.

**Source of stimulation** The stimulus may be mechanical, chemical, thermal or electrical. But, in most experimental procedures, electrical stimulus is usually preferred because of its many advantages:

- It is easy to deliver the stimulus. The operator can handle it conveniently.
- The apparatus for delivering the stimulus is tidy.
- The stimulus is easily controlled by the break or make of a key.
- It is possible to stimulate the tissue with the desired strength, frequency and duration, accurately and easily.
- The stimulus can be accurately localised on the tissue.
- The stimulus can be controlled from a long distance.
- This is the least injurious type of stimulus to the tissue.

**Stimulating device** Stimulating device (inductorium) is described in detail later in this chapter.

**Tissue preparation** For amphibian nerve muscle experiments, the sciatic nerve and the gastrocnemius muscle of the frog are usually used.

**Advantages of using frogs**

- It is easily available.
- It is easy to handle.
- It is harmless.
- It is less expensive.
- To maintain the tissue preparation of frogs, no extra supply of oxygen is needed as the frog muscles can directly imbibe oxygen from the environment.
- The tissue preparation of a frog can be maintained for a long duration if handled properly.
- It is easy to dissect the frog.

The advantages of using a gastrocnemius-sciatic preparation are:

- The sciatic nerve and gastrocnemius muscle are easy to locate and dissect.
- The sciatic nerve is the longest nerve and is therefore easy to place on the electrodes that are kept a short distance away from the muscle.
- The gastrocnemius muscle is a big muscle (has more cross-sectional area) and therefore on contraction, produces more force to lift the lever and records a good magnitude of contraction.

- The gastrocnemius muscle cannot be easily fatigued.

**Recording device** Recording of muscle contractions is done by using a writing lever that inscribes on the smoked surface of a moving drum fitted to a kymograph.

## DESCRIPTION AND USES OF APPLIANCES

### Source of Current

Electrical stimulation can be given either with a *direct current* (DC) source and a pair of stimulating electrodes (*galvanic current*) or by using an induction coil and the electrodes (*faradic current* or induced current). In most experiments, direct current is used. The direct current (6 volts) is available at the battery terminals of all experimental tables. To obtain an induced current, a constant current (galvanic) of low voltage is fed into the primary coil of the inductorium. To supply low-voltage direct current, a central low-voltage unit is installed in most laboratories. The output terminals feed a direct current of 3–15 volts to all the working seats in the table. This direct current is a rectified current, which comes from the central eliminator. Direct current can also be obtained from dry cells connected in series.

### Wires

Usually copper or aluminum wires are used in laboratories to carry electric current. A single thick wire is used to supply direct current. The wires are insulated by cotton, silk or enamel. For the connection or to supply current, the insulation from the tip of the wires is removed and polished with the help of fine sandpaper to give a good contact. Copper wires are usually used. The wire should not be damaged or have cracks. The wires are usually rolled on glass rods into spirals.

### Keys

The key is a device used for completing or interrupting a circuit. Two types of keys are used, the simple or tap key, and the short-circuiting key.

**The tap key** (Fig. 37.1A) This key is connected in the primary circuit in series with the DC source. The key is pressed gently and released to make and break the circuit.

**The short-circuiting key** (Fig 37.1B) This key is connected in the secondary circuit in parallel to prevent accidental leakage of current into the tissue. This also prevents unipolar induction. The key is kept closed to check unnecessary stimulation of the tissue, and when stimulation is required it is left open. Different types of short-circuiting keys are available, but the Du Bois-Reymond key (Fig. 37.1C) is usually used in the laboratory.

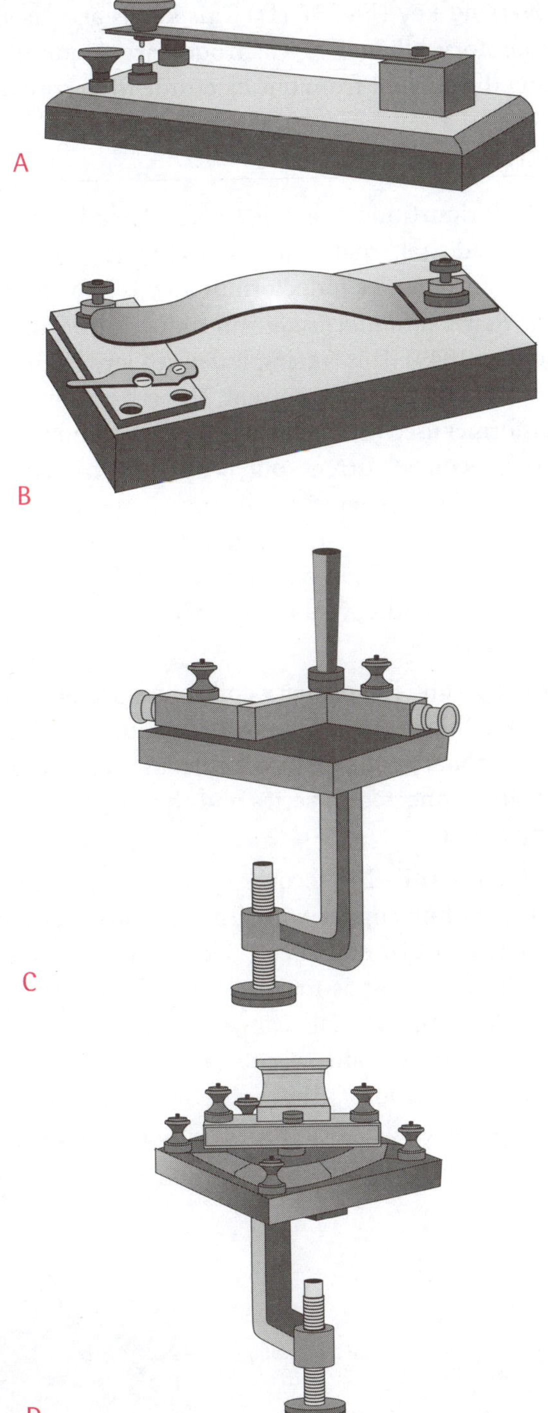

Fig. 37.1 Keys. A. Tap key; B. Short-circuiting key; C. Du Bois key; D. Reversing key.

**The reversing key** (Fig. 37.1D) This key is also used in the laboratory when two electrodes are required for shunting the current from one electrode to the other.

## Inductorium

The inductorium (induction coil) (Fig. 37.2) is a device from which a faradic (alternate) current is obtained by feeding a galvanic current. The inductorium used is known as the *Du Bois-Reymond inductorium* (introduced by Du Bois-Reymond in 1849). This is a simple device for transforming direct current into induced current. This is basically a step-up transformer used to obtain a high-voltage stimulus from a low-voltage direct current source, by using the principle of Faraday's electromagnetic induction. It consists of two separate coils: the primary coil and the secondary coil. The primary coil is fixed on a frame and the secondary coil is movable and covers the primary coil, but has no connection with it.

**The primary coil** The primary coil consists of 300 turns of insulated thick copper wire wound around a soft iron core. The primary coil, the direct current source and the tap key are connected in series and this constitutes the **primary circuit**.

**The secondary coil** The secondary coil is made of 5000 turns of very fine copper wire. The secondary coil can slide on two horizontal metal slide rods. On one of the slide rods, a scale is marked (in cm) by which the distance between the coils can be measured. The two terminals of the secondary coil are connected to the stimulating electrodes. The secondary coil and the stimulating electrodes form the **secondary circuit**.

A current is induced in the secondary coil only when there is a change in the strength of the magnetic field of the primary coil. When the strength of the current passing through the primary coil is constant, changes in the strength of the magnetic field occur only at commencement (make) and termination (break) of the current. Therefore, a current is induced in the secondary coil at make or break of the current in the primary coil. No current is induced in the secondary coil when the current passing through the primary coil is constant. The induced current is always of short duration.

The time taken by the current in the primary circuit at make to develop from zero to maximum voltage is longer than that taken by it to fall from maximum to the zero at break. This is due to the development of Faraday's extra current at make. Therefore, the *induced current in the secondary coil is stronger at break than at make.* The break stimulus is always stronger than the make stimulus. The strength of the stimulating current can be increased or decreased by changing the distance or the angle between the primary and the secondary coils. Other factors also determine the strength of the induced current.

The inductorium also has a built-in interruptor (*Neef's hammer*) which works on the same principle as that of an electric bell. When Neef's hammer is introduced in the primary circuit, the alternate make and break stimuli are rapidly repeated (40/s); this produces repeated induced current in the secondary circuit.

### *Factors that Affect the Strength of the Induced Current*

1. The distance between the two coils—when the distance between the two coils increases, the strength

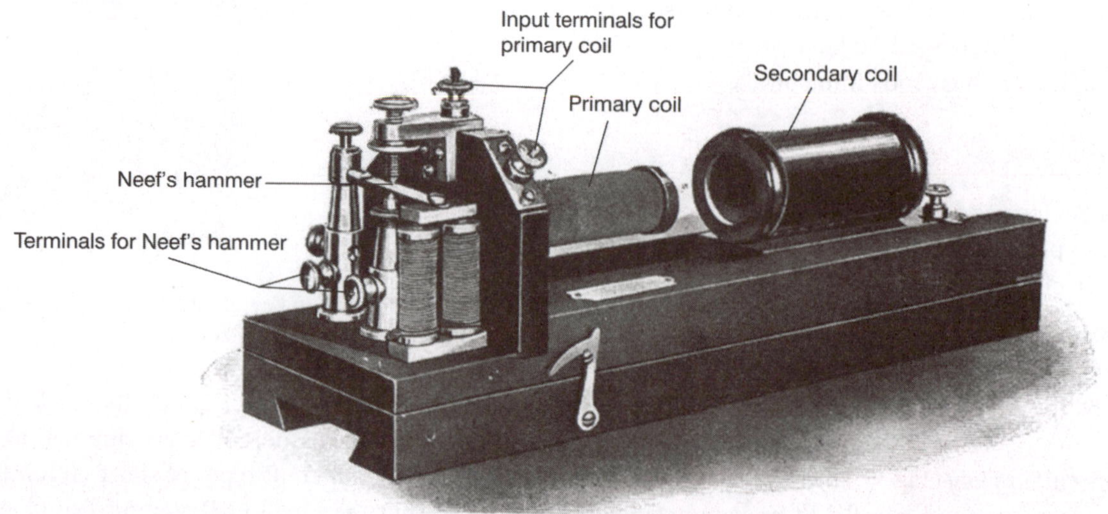


Fig. 37.2 Du Bois-Reymond inductorium.

of the stimulating current decreases and when the distance decreases, the strength of the current increases.

2. The angle between the coils—when the two coils are placed straight, the strength of the current is maximum. The strength of the current reduces by turning the secondary coil away from the primary coil. When the secondary coil is placed at right angles to the primary coil, there is no induction of current.
3. Number of turns in the coils—usually fixed.
4. The strength of direct current fed into the primary coil.

## Stimulating Electrodes

Electrodes used in biological experiments differ depending on their manufacture and use. They are designed to provide low resistance between the preparation and the amplifier input. Stimulating electrodes (Fig. 37.3) are used for delivering the electrical stimulus to the tissues. A stimulating electrode consists of two copper wires held together by a piece of perspex.

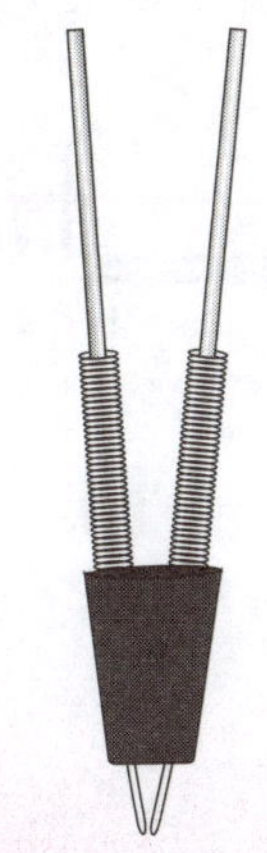

Fig. 37.3 Stimulating (simple) electrode.

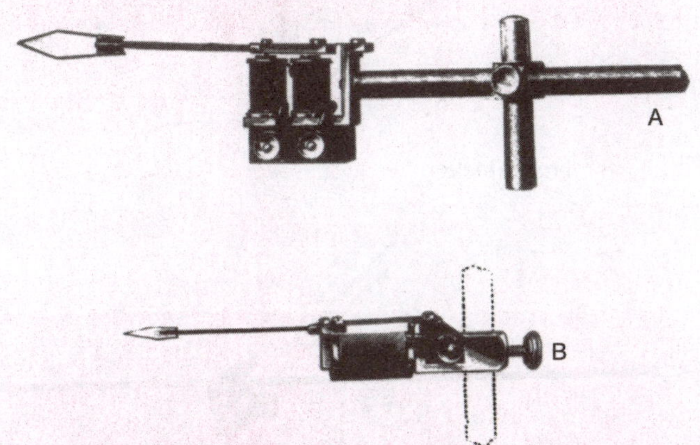


Fig. 37.4 A. Signal marker; B. Simple time-marker.

## Signal Marker

It is always better to indicate the point of application of stimulus, below the tracings. A signal marker marks (Fig. 37.4A) the moment of stimulation below the recording of the muscle contractions. It has two electromagnets and a writing lever. The lever marks the point of stimulation on the smoked paper. It is always included in the primary circuit.

This simple time-marker (Fig. 37.4B) with a single magnet can also be used for this purpose.

## Power Shaft and Pulleys

A horizontal power shaft driven by an electric motor is provided on the table. Cone pulleys with four grooves are fixed to the power shaft at each seat.

## Kymograph

Kymograph (Fig. 37.5) is the name given to any instrument that records movements on a moving surface. It consists of a metal gear box to which a vertical

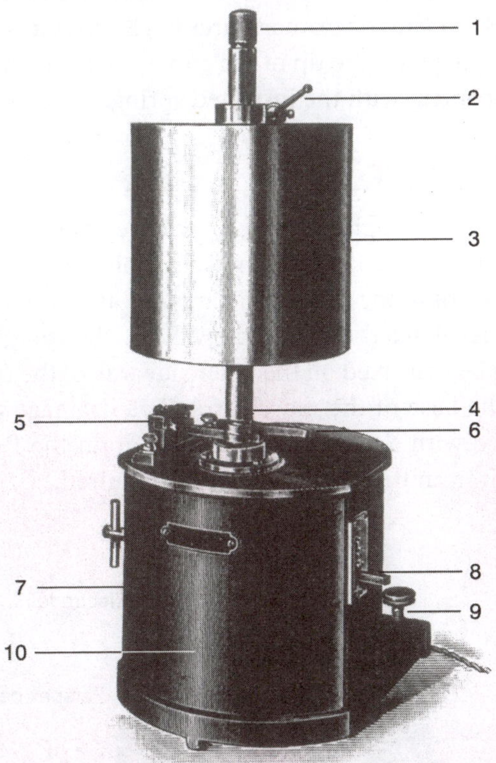


Fig. 37.5 The kymograph.1: Screw lift for cylinder; 2: Cylinder fixing lever; 3: Cylinder; 4: Spindle; 5: Contact block; 6: Contact arm; 7: Clutch lever; 8: Speed regulator; 9: Levelling screw; 10: Body of kymograph.

rotating shaft is connected. The shaft is powered by a horizontal axis running through the metal case. To this axis, on one side, a series of pulleys are attached. A belt connects one of these pulleys to one of the pulleys in the power shaft. A cylinder (6″ × 6″), also called drum, is fixed to the shaft. The drum rotates with the shaft. A gear switch on the left side of the kymograph provides high and low gears. In each gear, the drum can be made to turn at different speeds by connecting different-sized pulleys of the kymograph and the power shaft. The drum can be started or stopped by turning a clutch on the left side of the metal gear box.

There are two horizontal *contact arms* that project from the lower end of the vertical shaft. These contact arms can be separated and fixed with various angles between them. The tips of the arms, when they revolve, make contact with a spring at the left side of the top of the kymograph. The insulated carrier of the spring is adjustable and is clamped by a screw. There are two terminals for electrical connection: one is attached to the insulated spring and the other to the metal case of the gear box. By means of these connecting terminals, the insulated carrier along with the spring can be made to act as a key in the primary circuit. The circuit is 'made' or 'broken' when the tip of the contact arms makes and breaks contact with the insulated spring.

## Muscle Trough

The muscle trough (Fig. 37.6) is a perspex or plastic chamber used to keep the muscle moist and viable in Ringer's solution. A block carrying the stimulating electrodes is fixed on the side walls of the trough. The writing lever is fixed on the other side wall of the trough. From the base of the muscle trough, a drainage pipe is provided with a clamp that helps to drain the Ringer's solution from the trough whenever required.

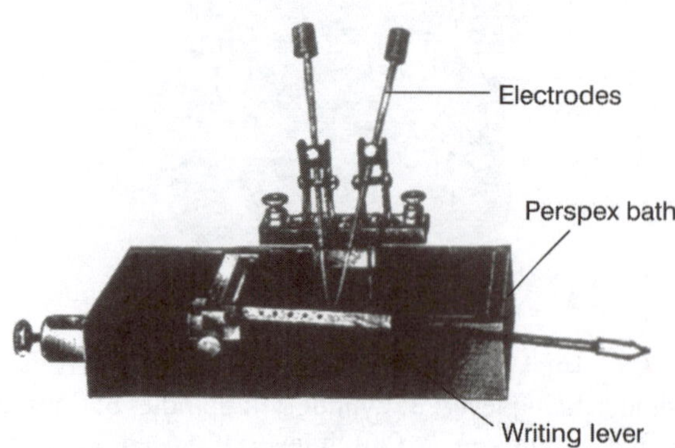


Fig. 37.6 Muscle trough.

## Levers

Different types of levers are used in experimental physiology for various purposes. Commonly used levers are the writing simple lever, the starling heart lever, the isometric lever, the afterload lever (Fig. 37.7) and the frontal lever (Fig. 37.8).

**The writing lever** This is used to magnify and record the muscle contraction on the drum. The lever consists of a horizontal arm, which bears holes and notches for hanging the weights (Fig. 37.9). The lever is fixed to the side wall of the muscle trough. The writing point of the lever is made up of a triangular piece of photographic film.

An ink writing stylus can be fitted into the writing lever, which can write on a white glazed paper instead of on a smoked drum. There is a screw (afterload screw) near the fulcrum of the lever, which limits the downward movement of the lever.

**The Starling heart lever** This is used for recording the cardiogram of a frog's heart. This lever is more sensitive than the writing lever, as it records the contractions of the heart, which are weaker than the contractions of the gastrocnemius muscle. It consists of a frame with a light

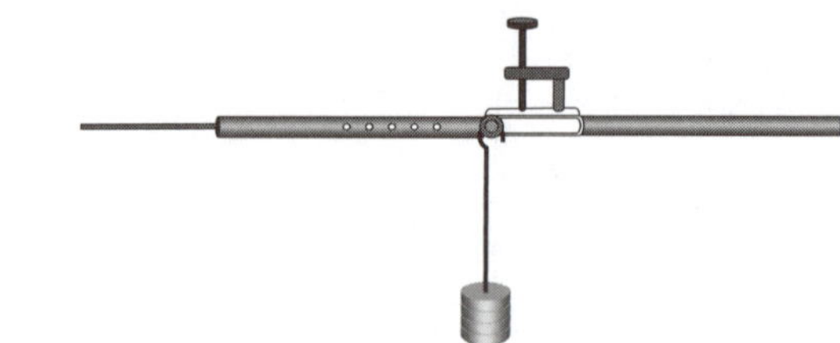

Fig. 37.7 Afterload lever.

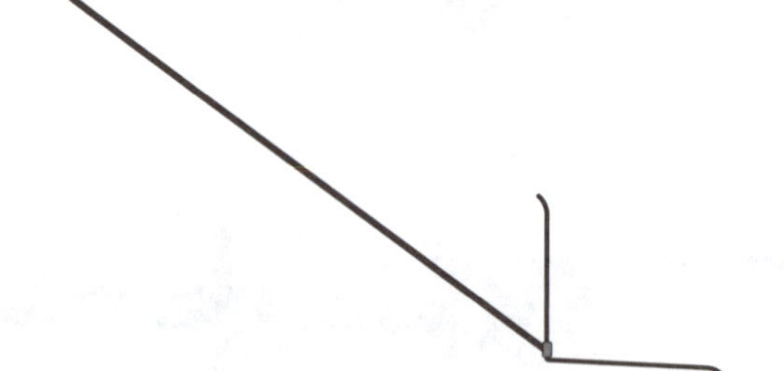

Fig. 37.8 Frontal lever.

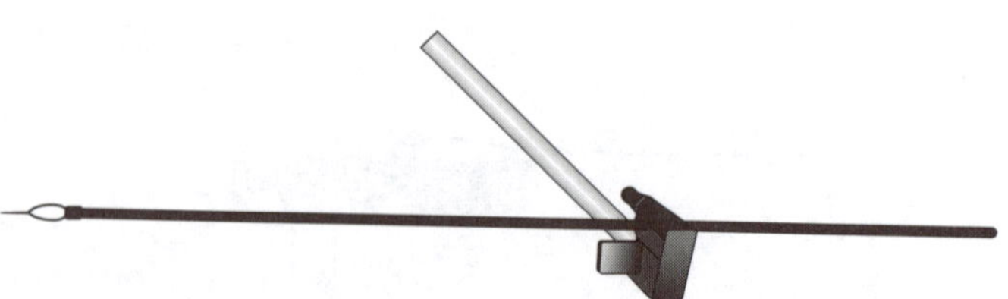

Fig. 37.9 Simple lever.

steel lever, with holes and notches, supported by a fine adjustable nickel silver spring (Fig. 37.10).

**Isometric lever** This consists of a holder that carries a steel tension spring and a flat writing lever (Fig. 37.11). It is used for recording isometric contractions.

## Myograph Stand

This is a vertical rod fixed to a heavy and triangular base (Fig. 37.12). The muscle trough can be fitted to the rod and can be moved up and down with the help of a fitted screw. The rod can be turned on its axis so that the writing point of the muscle lever can be made to touch or be removed from the drum without disturbing other adjustments.

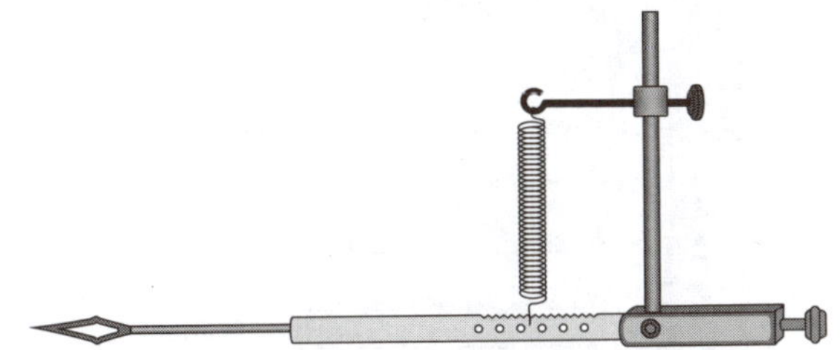

Fig. 37.10 Starling heart lever.

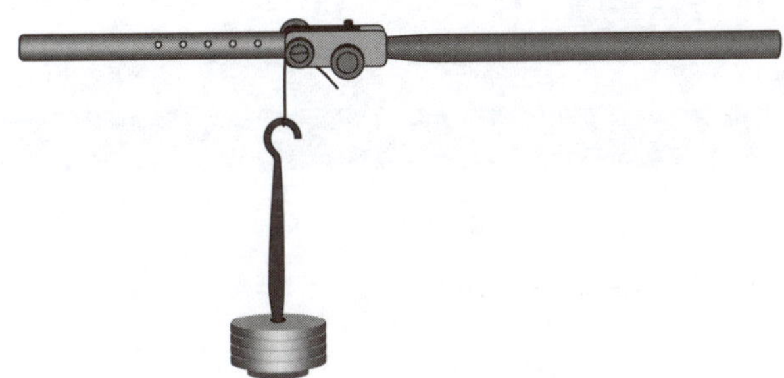

Fig. 37.11 Isometric lever.

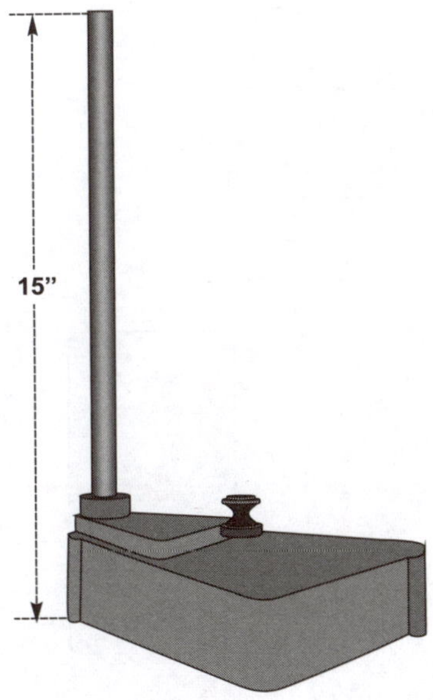


Fig. 37.12 Myograph stand.

## Tuning Fork

A tuning fork (Fig. 37.13) with a frequency of 100 vibrations per second (100 Hz) is used for measuring different time intervals. To the end of one arm of the tuning fork, a writing point is attached. The tuning fork is set to vibrate and is then made to write on the fast rotating drum to obtain a tracing. This tracing consists of different waves. Each wave of the tracing (from crest to the crest) measures 0.01 seconds (10 ms).

## Pohl's Commutator

This is used to change the direction of current. It consists of a vulcanite base on which a rocking metallic cradle is mounted (Fig. 37.14). There are six cup-like depressions filled with mercury, and six terminals are attached to these cups. Two narrow copper strips connect the diagonally opposite corner cups.

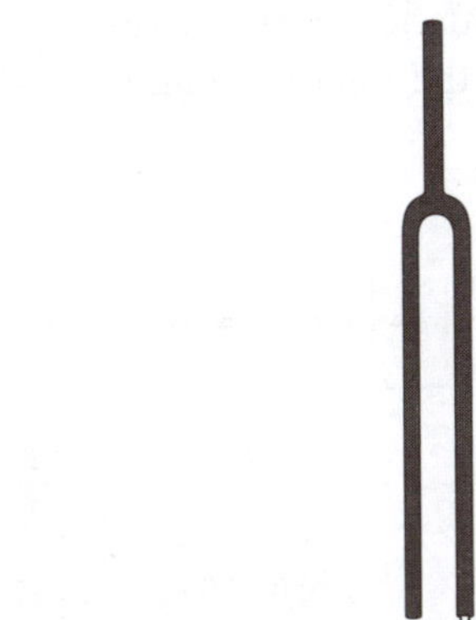

Fig. 37.13 Tuning fork.

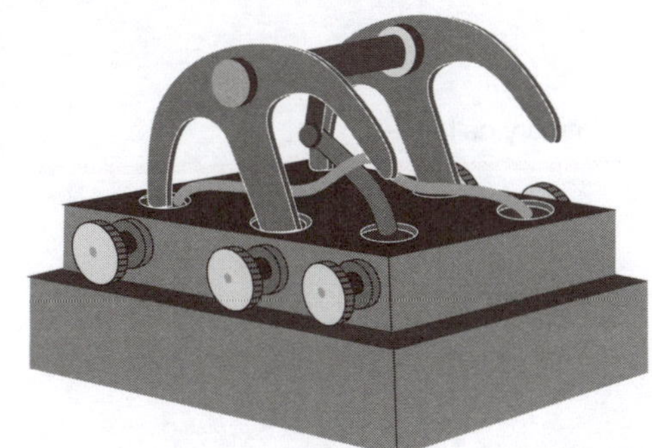

Fig. 37.14 Pohl's commutator.

### *Student's Stimulator*

This is an electronic stimulator with a DC output of 0–15 volts. The strength (volts), frequency and duration of the stimulus are indicated on the apparatus. More advanced stimulators, which are required for special experiments and research, are also available.

## EXERCISES

### Making Electrical Connections

Make the primary and secondary circuits as depicted in Figs. 37.15A and B. Check whether the primary and secondary circuits are made correctly.

1. To check the primary circuit, connect a short piece of wire to one of the low volts terminals and strike the other terminal with its free end. A spark indicates the presence of current. Check the simple key and the contact block on the kymograph. Each time the striker makes contact a spark is produced.
2. To check the secondary circuit, place the tissue on the wires connected to the secondary coil terminals. If twitchings occur in the tissue with each revolution of the spindle, the connection is correct. If the muscle does not contract, place the electrodes directly on the muscle. If the muscle contracts due to direct stimulation, check if the nerve is damaged during the dissection.

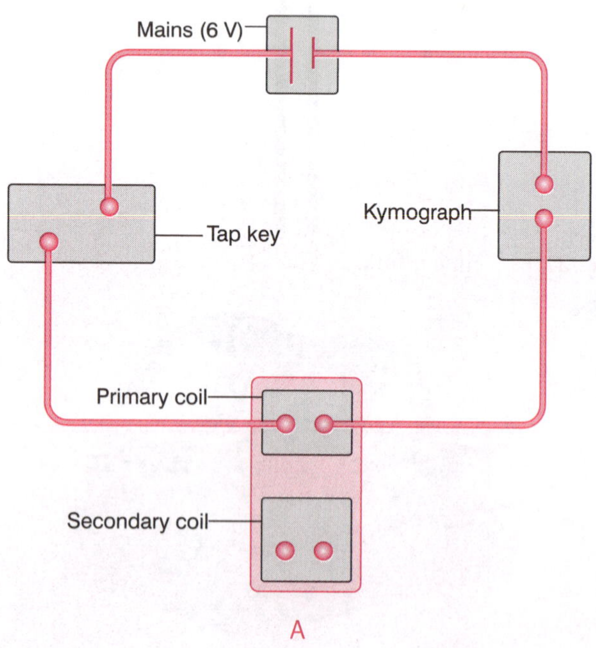


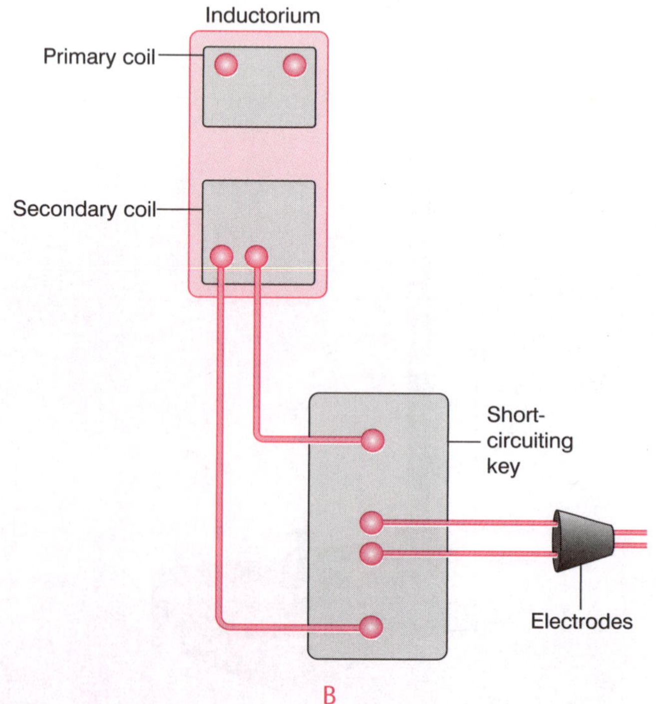


Fig. 37.15 A. Primary circuit; B. Secondary circuit.

### Smoking

Before smoking the drum, a piece of a glazed paper is properly pasted on the drum. Then the drum is placed on the horizontal arm of the smoking stand (Fig. 37.16). The burner is put on and the drum is smoked uniformly by rotating manually on the flame. A thin and uniformly black smoking is aimed at.

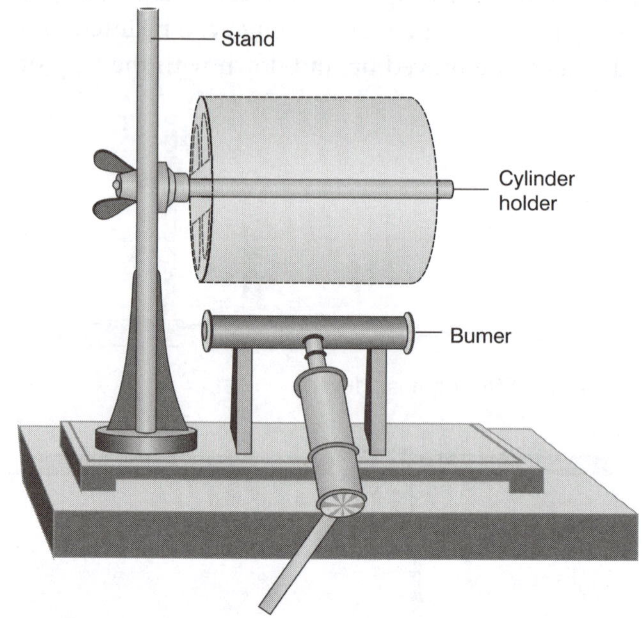


Fig. 37.16 Smoking stand.

## Varnishing

Varnishing is done to fix the recording on the smoked paper. Labelling of the recording is done before varnishing. The paper is cut at the jointed portion and taken out of the drum and dipped in the 2 per cent solution of resin or methylated spirit. Then the paper is clipped and hung till it is completely dry.

## Precautions

1. The primary and secondary circuits should be made perfectly.
2. Loose connections in the circuits should be detected and dealt with.
3. The wires used for making the circuit should be as short as possible. Long wires can be shortened by winding them around a glass rod or a pencil.
4. The kymograph should be properly levelled by using the levelling screws at its base.
5. The drum should be tightly fixed to the vertical shaft.
6. The drum should always be rotated clockwise.
7. The writing lever should always be arranged on the right side of the drum.
8. The writing lever should be tangential with the recording surface.
9. The tip of the writing lever should touch the smoked surface evenly and lightly.
10. The initial and resting positions of the writing lever should always be horizontal.
11. The tracing should be taken at least one inch above the lower edge of the drum.
12. The contact arm should be tightly fixed.

## VIVA

1. What are the different types of stimuli and why is the electrical stimulus usually preferred?
2. Why is the frog selected for amphibian practicals?
3. What are the advantages of using the gastrocnemius-sciatic preparation for frog experiments?
4. What are the types of keys used in amphibian experiments and what are their uses?
5. What is the principle of working of the inductorium?
6. What are the factors that determine the strength of induced current?
7. Why is the break stimulus stronger than the make stimulus?
8. What is the use of the short-circuiting key?
9. What is the use of a signal marker?
10. What is the principle used in the working of a kymograph?
11. How is the speed of the kymograph regulated?
12. What is the use of the contact arm of the kymograph?
13. How is the time tracing obtained in the recording?
14. What are the precautions taken for making electrical circuits?
15. How are the recordings fixed?

Chapter 38

# Nerve-Muscle Preparation

## Learning Objectives

After completing this practical, you will be able to:

- Hold a living frog.
- Pith the frog.
- Dissect the frog to isolate the sciatic nerve and gastrocnemius muscle.
- List the precautions taken during pithing and making the nerve-muscle preparation.
- List the reasons why the gastrocnemius muscle and sciatic nerve of frogs are preferred for amphibian nerve muscle experiments.
- State the composition of Ringer's solution.

## INTRODUCTION

For any amphibian nerve-muscle experiment, the sciatic nerve and the gastrocnemius muscle of the frog are used for of the following reasons:

1. The sciatic nerve is a long nerve, and is therefore easy to mount in the muscle trough.
2. The gastrocnemius muscle is a bulky muscle and therefore it gives good amplitude of contraction on stimulation. It cannot be fatigued easily.

Before making the nerve-muscle preparation, the frog should be pithed by destroying the brain and spinal cord.

## METHODS

### Nerve-Muscle Preparation

#### Principle

A pithed frog is dissected to isolate the intact sciatic nerve and gastrocnemius muscle. This nerve-muscle preparation is mounted on the muscle trough to perform various experiments.

#### Requirements

1. Frog (living)
2. Pithing needle
3. Dissecting set
   Dissection board
   A pair of scissors with blunt ends (8″)
   A pair of scissors with sharp ends (6″)
   A pair of pointed forceps
   A glass rod
4. Ringer's solution

#### Procedure

There are two broad steps in nerve-muscle preparation: pithing of the frog and dissection to make the nerve-muscle preparation.

*Pithing*

1. Hold the frog gently but firmly with the help of cloth or cotton.

> Note: The skin of the frog is slippery. Therefore, the animal should be held with a dry cloth or cotton.

2. Hit a blow on its head to make the animal unconscious.

> Note: This procedure is called *stunning*.

3. Hold the unconscious frog in your hand and ventroflex its head.
4. Feel the depression at the junction of the skull and vertebral column.

> Note: This corresponds to a point in the middle of the line joining the posterior borders of the tympanic membranes.

5. Insert a pithing needle firmly through the skin, muscle and bone tissue into the spinal cord.
6. Manipulate the needle anteriorly into the skull and rotate it to destroy the brain.

7. Withdraw the needle and direct it backwards into the spinal cord and rotate the needle to destroy the cord.

> **Note:** Immediately after the needle is directed into the spinal cord, the muscles of the lower limb and trunk become spastic. they become flaccid after destruction of the spinal cord. This procedure is called pithing. After pithing, the animal loses its voluntary and reflex movements, but is still alive and can be used for experiments.

*Dissection*

1. Cut the skin of the frog around the middle of the trunk and strip off the skin from the trunk and hind limbs.
2. Place the frog on the frog board on its abdomen.
3. Pick up the tip of the urostyle with the forceps and lift it carefully. Cut the pelvic girdle on its sides taking care not to injure the underlying sciatic nerve.
4. Identify the sciatic plexus.
5. Isolate a 2 cm long piece of vertebral column from where the sciatic plexus originates by cutting the vertebral column above and below the exit of the sciatic nerve with scissors.
6. Bisect the vertebral column vertically into two halves with the help of the bone cutting scissors.
7. Expose the sciatic nerve in the thigh between the muscle mass posteriorly by separating the muscle with the help of the blunt glass probe (Fig. 38.1).
8. Clean the nerve from its surrounding fascial attachments.

> Note: Do not pull the nerve; do not touch it with any metal object. Use only a glass rod for handling the nerve.

9. Identify, separate and cut the gastrocnemius tendon from its attachment and tie a long thread around the tendon.
10. Free the muscle from the tibia and cut the tibia close to the knee joint, then cut the femur close to the knee joint. The knee joint should be kept intact.
11. Remove all redundant muscles (other than the gastrocnemius).
12. Lift the nerve-muscle preparation (Fig. 38.2) carefully and transfer it to a container filled with Ringer's solution.
13. Keep the nerve-muscle preparation immersed in Ringer's solution until it is used for the experiment.

> Note: If required, a nerve-muscle preparation from the other side can be obtained.

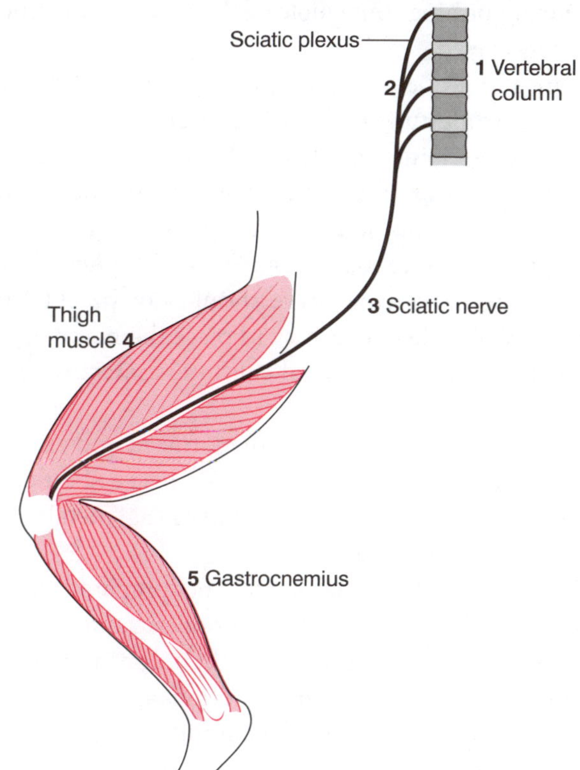


Fig. 38.1 Anatomical position of the sciatic nerve and gastrocnemius muscle of frog.

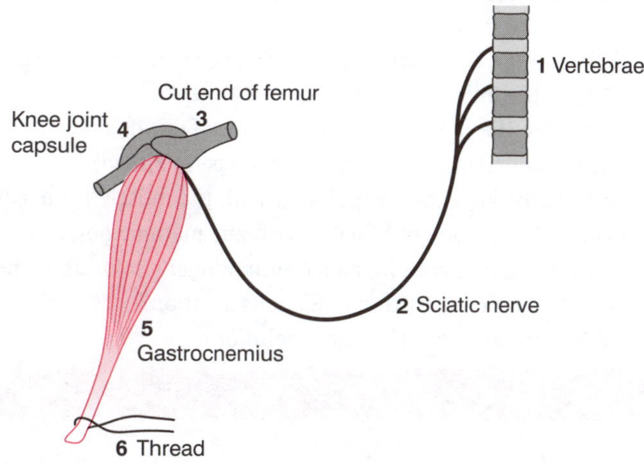


Fig. 38.2 The sciatic-gastrocnemius preparation. Note that a thread is tied to the tip of the tendon and that a portion of the vertebral column is kept intact with the nerve.

## Precautions

1. The frog should be stunned before pithing (pithing of a conscious frog is painful for the frog).
2. The frog should be held by wrapping it with a cloth piece or cotton as the skin is slippery.

3. During pithing, the whole of the spinal cord should be destroyed.
4. Care should be taken not to injure the sciatic nerve plexus while cutting the pelvic girdle.
5. The knee joint should be kept intact with the preparation as it becomes easy to fix the muscle through the knee joint in the muscle trough.
6. A piece of vertebral column should be kept intact with the nerve (the nerve should not be cut from its origin). It becomes easy to place the nerve on the electrodes if the vertebral column is intact with the nerve.
7. The nerves should be identified, traced and exposed with the help of a glass rod. The nerve should not be handled with metallic objects, as metals may stimulate the nerve.
8. While dissecting, to obtain the preparation, the nerve and the muscle should not be strained.
9. The nerve-muscle preparation should be immediately transferred into Ringer's solution as soon as the dissection is over. The preparation should not be allowed to dry.
10. Once the preparation is ready, mount in the muscle trough to start the experiment. Otherwise, the muscle may be fatigued.

## DISCUSSION

Once the nerve-muscle preparation is made, it should be immediately immersed in Ringer's solution. The preparation should be mounted in the muscle trough as early as possible and the experiment should be started.

### Composition of Ringer's solution

NaCl : 0.6% (isotonic with frog plasma)

KCl : 0.014% (maintains membrane potential)

$CaCl_2$ : 0.012% (maintains muscle excitability)

$NaHCO_3$ : 0.02% (maintains pH)

$NaH_2PO_4$ : 0.001% (maintains pH)

Dextrose : 0.1% (provides nutrition)

## VIVA

1. Why is the frog chosen for amphibian experiments?
2. Why are the gastrocnemius muscle and sciatic nerve selected for nerve-muscle experiments?
3. Why is the animal stunned before pithing?
4. What are the precautions to be followed during dissection for the nerve-muscle preparation?
5. How can you assess that a frog is properly pithed?
6. Why is the knee joint kept intact with the muscle for making the preparation?
7. Why is the nerve not handled with any metallic objects?
8. Why is the preparation immersed in Ringer's solution immediately after dissection?
9. What is the composition of Ringer's solution?
10. What are the uses of Ringer's solution?

Chapter 39

# Simple Muscle Twitch

## Learning Objectives

After completing this practical, you will be able to:

- Dissect and make a sciatic nerve and gastrocnemius muscle preparation.
- Make primary and secondary circuits.
- Record the response of the muscle in response to a single electrical stimulus to the nerve.
- Record the time-tracing below the recording of the simple muscle curve.
- Calculate the latent period, contraction period and relaxation period from the recording.

## INTRODUCTION

When a muscle is stimulated with a single induction shock, it exhibits a momentary twitch like a contraction. This momentary contraction of the muscle in response to electrical stimulation is called **simple muscle twitch**. The contraction recorded on a moving kymograph is known as a **simple muscle curve**. The simple muscle curve is recorded to study the latent period, contraction period and relaxation period of the skeletal muscles (Fig. 39.1).

The **latent period** is the period from the point of stimulus to the point of onset of contraction. The **contraction period** is the period between the point of onset of contraction to the point that corresponds to the peak of contraction. The **relaxation period** is the period from the peak of contraction to the end of relaxation.

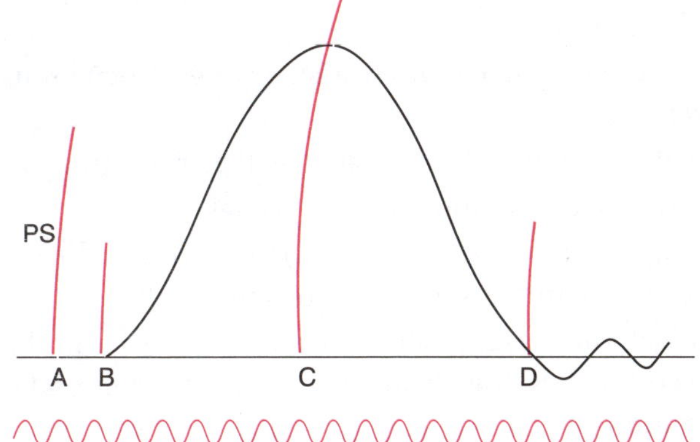


Fig. 39.1 Simple muscle twitch with time-trace below the curve. PS: Point of stimulation; AB: Latent period; BC: Contraction period; CD: Relaxation period.

## METHODS

### Method to Study Simple Muscle Twitch

#### Principle

When a muscle is stimulated with a single induction shock, the muscle contracts. This lifts the lever to record a curve on a revolving smoked drum.

#### Requirements

1. Dissection instruments
2. Kymograph
3. Muscle trough
4. Inductorium
5. Short-circuiting key
6. Tap key
7. Ringer's solution
8. Smoked drum
9. Low-resistance wires
10. Electrodes
11. Tuning fork (100 Hz)
12. Thread
13. Hook and weights (Fig. 39.2)

#### Procedure

1. Arrange the primary and secondary circuits for recording a muscle twitch (*Refer* Fig. 37.15).
2. Include the kymograph in the primary circuit.

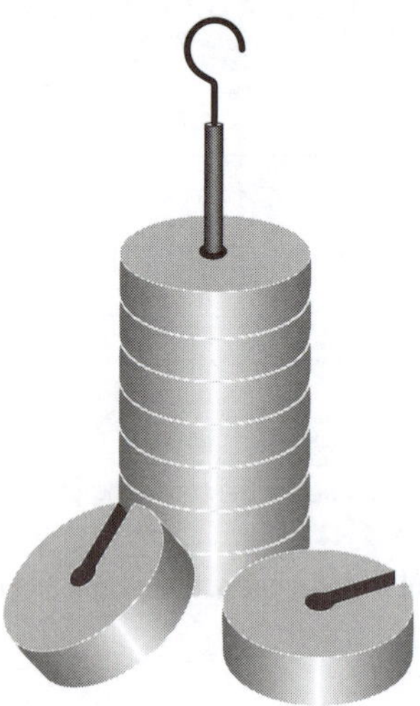

Fig. 39.2 Hook with weights.

3. Select the fastest speed of the kymograph (first gear; pulleys 4 : 1).
4. Dissect a frog to obtain a sciatic nerve-gastrocnemius preparation.
5. Fix the nerve-muscle preparation in the muscle trough.
6. Pour Ringer's solution into the trough.
7. Hang a 10 g weight from the writing lever and keep the muscle in the afterloaded position.
8. Adjust the writing lever in such a way that the lever touches the drum lightly in the horizontal position.
9. Adjust the secondary coil to obtain a contraction at break stimulus only.
10. Set the drum in motion and record a baseline.
11. Press the tap key and release it as soon as you record the first contraction.
12. Vibrate the tuning fork by hitting against the thigh or against the hypothenar eminence of the hand and record a time-tracing below the simple muscle curve.
13. Stop the drum and close the short-circuiting key.
14. Rotate the drum manually so that the contact arms touch the kymograph key.

> NoteThis marks the instant when the primary circuit will be complete if the tap key is closed, which results in a stimulus from the secondary coil.

15. Mark the point of stimulation by moving the writing lever over the smoked drum.
16. Mark the beginning of contraction, peak of contraction and end of relaxation by moving the lever vertically on the drum manually on the corresponding points in the curve.
17. Calculate and record the duration of latent period (LP), contraction period (CP) and relaxation period (RP).

## Precautions

In addition to the precautions described for 'nerve-muscle preparation' in Chapter 38, the following precautions should be observed:

1. The stimulus should be given briefly for a single induction shock.
2. The point of stimulus should be accurately marked.
3. While marking for latent period, contraction period and relaxation period, the lever should be placed exactly on the points.
4. Time-tracing should be taken just below the recording.

## Observations and Results

Observe and study the simple muscle curve ( Fig. 39)1 Express the duration of LP, CP and RP in ms; and also calculate the CP and RP as a percentage of the total muscle curve (CP + RP) duration.

# DISCUSSION

The latent period, contraction period and relaxation period vary according to the type of muscle.

The latent period is due to:

- Time taken for the stimulus to travel along the nerve to the neuromuscular junction.
- Time taken for the impulse to cross the neuromuscular junction, to stimulate the muscle.
- Time taken for the excitation–contraction coupling to occur.
- Time taken by the lever to overcome the inertia of rest.
- Time taken to overcome the viscous resistance of the muscle.

The latent period is normally about 10 ms. The contraction period represents the duration of mechanical contraction. It normally ranges between 20 and 40 ms.

The relaxation period represents the time taken by the muscles to relax. It is normally more than the contraction period and ranges between 30 and 50 ms.

## VIVA

1. What are the causes of the latent period?
2. What is isometric contraction and how does it differ from isotonic contraction?
   Ans. See Chapter 27.
3. Give examples of isometric and isotonic contractions.
   Ans. See Chapter 27.
4. What is the normal duration of the contraction and relaxation periods of the frog skeletal muscle and what do they represent?
5. Can you determine the duration of LP, CP and RP without obtaining the time-tracing below the curve?
   Ans. Yes, it can be derived from the speed of the drum.
6. Why is induced current used for recording a simple muscle twitch?
   Ans. Induced current gives a stimulus of short duration of desired intensity.
7. Why is a 10 g weight placed on the lever?
   Ans. The weight placed on the lever checks the amplitude of the contraction, overcomes the inertia of the lever, and keeps the lever horizontal.

Chapter 40

# Effect of Temperature on Simple Muscle Twitch

**Learning Objectives**

After completing this practical, you WILL be able to:

- Demonstrate the effect of temperature on muscle contraction.
- State the precautions taken for recording the effects of temperature on muscle contraction.
- Explain the effect of temperature on muscle contraction.

## INTRODUCTION

A change in temperature in Ringer's solution causes a change in muscle contraction. With a change in temperature, there is a change in amplitude and the duration of different periods of contraction (latent, contraction and relaxation periods). The changes are mainly due to change in rate of conduction velocity in the nerve, enzymatic and chemical activities in the muscle and a change in the viscosity of the muscle.

## METHODS

### Method to Study Effect of Temperature on Muscle Contraction

#### Principle

A change in the temperature of the environment affects muscle contraction. The effects of temperature on muscle contraction are studied by changing the temperature of Ringer's solution. The effects are studied on the same point of stimulus and same baseline. The change in amplitude of contraction, the duration of latent period, contraction period and relaxation period are noted.

#### Requirements

1. Same as for 'simple muscle twitch'
2. Cold Ringer's solution (10°C)
3. Warm Ringer's solution (40°C)
4. Centigrade thermometer

#### Procedure

1. Pith and dissect the frog to make the nerve-muscle preparation.
2. Set up the nerve-muscle preparation for recording the simple muscle curve.
3. Record a simple muscle curve on the revolving drum with Ringer's solution in the muscle trough at room temperature.
4. Drain the Ringer's solution from the muscle trough and replace with warm Ringer's solution and wait for 1–3 minutes to allow the muscle to warm up.
5. Using the same baseline, same point of stimulation and same strength of stimulus, record the effect of warm Ringer's solution on the simple muscle curve.
6. Note the temperature of the Ringer's solution and drain the solution from the muscle trough.
7. Pour the normal Ringer's solution and wait for some time for the preparation to come back to normal temperature. Pour cold Ringer's solution into the muscle trough and wait for 2–5 minutes to allow the muscle to cool.
8. Using the same baseline, point of stimulation and strength of stimulus, record the effect of cold Ringer's on muscle contraction.
9. Record a time-tracing below the recordings with the help of a tuning fork.
10. Calculate the latent period, contraction period and relaxation period of the muscle contraction with different temperatures.
11. Record your observations in a tabular form (Table 40.1).

Table 40.1 Tabulation of experimental recordings.

| Temperature of Ringer's soln. | L P (ms) | C P (ms) | R P (ms) | Height of Contraction (cm) |
|---|---|---|---|---|
| 1. Normal (25°C) | | | | |
| 2. Warm (40°C) | | | | |
| 3. Cold (10°C) | | | | |

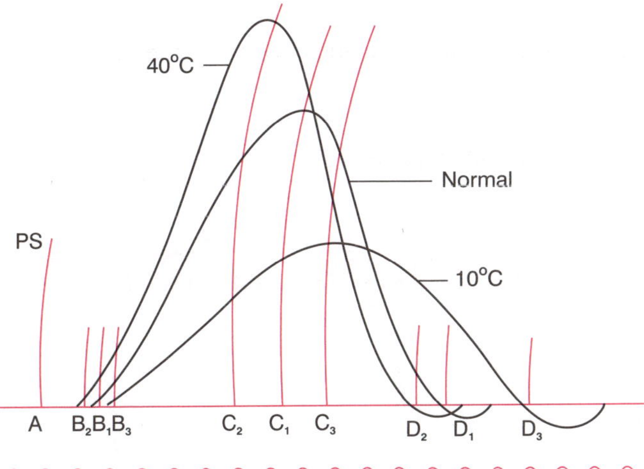


Fig. 40.1 Effect of temperature on simple muscle twitch. $AB_1$, $AB_2$ and $AB_3$ are the latent periods; $B_1C_1$, $B_2C_2$ and $B_3C_3$ are the contraction periods; $C_1D_1$, $C_2D_2$ and $C_3D_3$ are the relaxation periods of normal, high (40°C) and low (10°C) temperatures respectively.

## Observation

Compare the recordings of the three muscle curves recorded at three different temperatures of Ringer's solution. Study the height and slope of contraction, and the duration of latent period, contraction period and relaxation period of each curve ( Fig. 40.1).

## Precautions

The precautions are the same as those for 'simple muscle twitch'. In addition to these, the following precautions are also to be kept in mind:

1. The point of stimulation, the baseline and the strength of stimulation for all the recordings should be kept constant.
2. The temperature of Ringer's solution should not exceed 42°C.

> Note: When the temperature of the solution is 43°C or more, the muscle proteins are denatured. Muscles remain in a state of sustained contraction. This phenomenon is known as heat rigor.

3. The temperature of the cold solution should not be less than 4°C.

> Note: When the temperature of the solution is very low, the muscle proteins are coagulated. This prevents muscle contraction.

4. The temperature of the solution should be recorded just prior to or immediately after muscle contraction.
5. The effects of the warm solution should be recorded before recording the effects of cold Ringer's, because cold Ringer's inhibits all enzymatic and metabolic activities of the muscle. It may be difficult to revive muscle activities from the effects of cold Ringer's.

## DISCUSSION

When muscle contraction is recorded with higher temperature of Ringer's solution, the latent period, contraction period and relaxation period decrease, and the height of contraction increases. The decrease in latent period is due to:

- Increase in conduction velocity in the nerve
- Increased rate of neuromuscular transmission
- Inertia of the lever is overcome faster

The shortening of the contraction and relaxation periods is due to faster contraction and relaxation. This occurs due to activation of myosin ATPase activity and decreased resistance of the muscle to contractions as the viscosity of the muscle decreases with increased temperature. The amplitude of contraction increases due to increased enzymatic and chemical activities in the muscle.

When muscle contraction is recorded with low temperature of Ringer's solution, the opposite effects are observed. They are due to decreased rate of conduction of impulse in the nerve and through the neuromuscular junction, increased viscosity of the muscle, decreased enzymatic and chemical activities in the muscle.

The change in the muscular activities of human beings due to change in environmental temperature, though similar, may be different from these experimental observations. This is because physical efficiency depends on various factors like training, motivation, state of nutrition, environmental temperature, humidity and so on. However, the body temperature never rises to the extent of causing heat rigor. But, if a person is exposed to a high temperature for a long duration, a phenomenon akin to heat rigor occurs; if a person is exposed to very low temperatures, muscle contraction is inhibited.

## VIVA

1. What are the precautions taken when recording the effects of temperature on muscle contraction?
2. What are the changes in muscle contraction, which occur in response to warm Ringer's solution? What are the causes of these changes?
3. What are the changes in muscle contraction, which occur in response to cold Ringer's solution? What are the causes of these changes?
4. What is heat rigor?
5. Why is the effect of warm Ringer's recorded before recording the effect of cold Ringer's?
6. What is the effect of temperature on performance in human beings?

Chapter 41

# Genesis of Tetanus

## Learning Objectives

After completing this practical, you will be able to:

- Define treppe, clonus and tetanus.
- Demonstrate the effects of increasing frequency of stimulation on muscle contraction.
- List the precautions taken during genesis of tetanus in this experiment.
- Calculate the minimal tetanisable frequency (MTF).
- List the factors that affect MTF.
- Explain the physiological basis of treppe, clonus and tetanus.
- Differentiate between experimental and clinical tetanus.
- List the causes, features and prevention of tetanus (the disease).

## INTRODUCTION

Tetanus refers to a state of sustained tonic contraction of the muscle (without relaxation) due to rapidly repeated stimulation. It does not occur if the muscle is stimulated at a lower rate (lower frequency). If the rate of stimulation increases (higher frequency), tetanus ensues. When the muscle is stimulated below the tetanising frequency, incomplete tetanus (clonus) occurs.

## METHODS

### Method to Study Genesis of Tetanus

#### Principle

If a muscle is stimulated at higher frequencies there is sustained tonic contraction of the muscle (tetanus). The nerve-muscle preparation is stimulated at different frequencies using a vibrating interrupter till tetanus ensues.

#### Requirements

1. Same as for 'simple muscle twitch'.
2. Vibrating variable interrupter (Fig. 41.1). The reed is calibrated to vibrate at a frequency of 5, 7, 10, 20, 30 and 40 vibrations per sec. This is achieved by sliding the clamping plate along the metal guides fixed to the base board.
3. Signal marker.

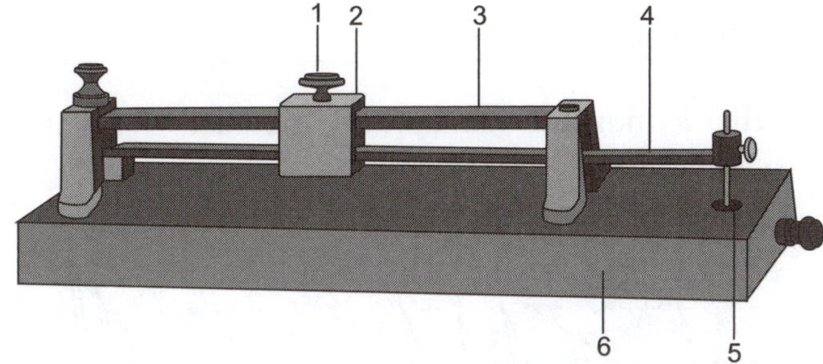


Fig. 41.1 Vibrating reed. 1: Clamping plate; 2: Thumb screw; 3: Vibration scale; 4: Metal guide; 5: Mercury cup; 6: Base board.

#### Procedure

1. Arrange an electrical circuit for single induced shocks, including vibrating interrupter and signal marker in the primary circuit. Exclude kymograph from the circuit.
2. Set up the kymograph and nerve-muscle preparation as for the recording of the simple muscle curve.
3. Adjust the inductorium for weak break shocks.
4. Adjust the length of vibrating reed of the interrupter to provide five interruptions (stimuli) per second.
5. Start the kymograph using slow speed (fast gear; pulley 1:4) and set the reed vibrating. Open the short-circuiting key to stimulate the muscle and close it after recording 5–7 contractions on the drum.
6. Now increase the rate of interruptions (stimulation) to 10, 15, 20, 30 and 40 per second and take a record of each stimulation, using fresh space on the smoked paper. Avoid unnecessary stimulation.

> **Note:** If high frequency for obtaining tetanus is not available, use Neef's hammer by including it in the primary circuit.

7. Note the frequency of stimulation, which produced complete tetanus in your experiment.
8. Above each set of recordings indicate the rate of stimulation as given in the figure.
9. Fix the recording by varnishing the paper.

### Observation

Observe and study the graph (Fig. 41.2). Observe the staircase phenomenon (treppe) of the first initial stimuli. At the low frequency of stimulation single contractions occur, with increasing frequency, first clonus (partial tetanus) and then tetanus occur.

### Precautions

1. The kymograph should be excluded from the circuit.

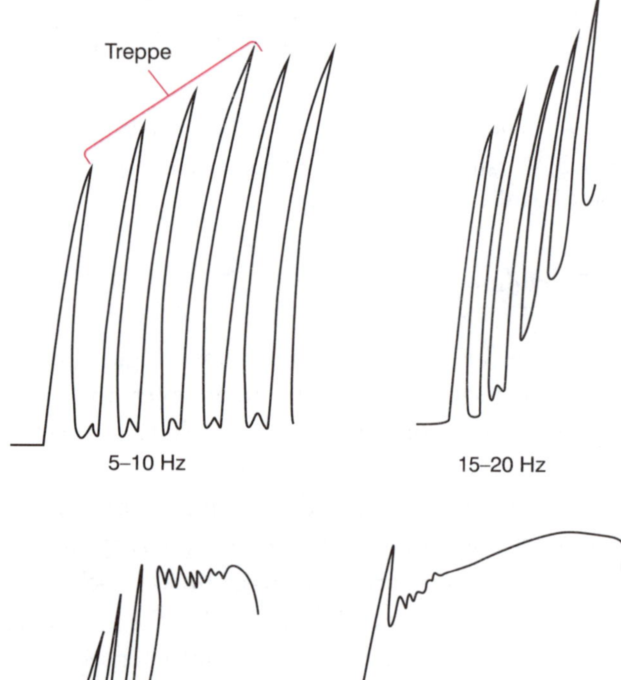


Fig. 41.2 Genesis of tetanus.

2. The inductorium should be adjusted for weak break shocks.
3. The preparation should be stimulated from lower frequency to the higher frequency.
4. Unnecessary stimulation should be avoided.
5. If tetanising frequency in not obtained, Neef's hammer should be included in the primary circuit.

## DISCUSSION

### Minimal Tetanisable Frequency

The minimal tetanisable frequency (MTF) of a muscle can be calculated from the simple muscle curve (measuring the contraction period) by using the following formula:

$$\text{MTF} = \frac{1}{\text{Contraction period}}$$

For example, if the contraction period is 0.04 seconds, the MTF = 1/0.04 = 25 Hz.

#### Factors that Affect MTF

1. **Type of muscle** In slow muscles, the MTF is low because they produce slow, sustained contractions (longer contraction period). In fast muscles, the MTF is greater because the contraction period is less. An example of a slow muscle is soleus, and examples of fast muscles are the muscles of the eye.
2. **Temperature of the environment** Tetanisable frequency is lower in a hot environment and higher in a cold environment.
3. **Load acting on the muscle** If the load acting on the muscle is greater, the tetanisable frequency decreases.

### Treppe

Treppe is also known as the **staircase phenomenon**; it is the progressive increase in the force of contraction for the first two to three contractions when a muscle is stimulated repeatedly. This occurs due to the accumulation of calcium in the sarcoplasm due to application of repeated stimuli. Treppe is also seen in cardiac muscles. However, the cardiac muscle cannot be tetanised because of a longer refractory period.

## Clonus

Clonus is a state of partial tetanus observed in experimental conditions (experimental clonus). This should not be confused with the clinical clonus, for example, ankle clonus, seen in upper motor neuron type of paralysis. In experimental clonus, relaxation is incomplete.

## Tetanus

Tetanus is a state of sustained contraction. The muscle remains in a state of tonic contraction without relaxation. This occurs when a nerve-muscle preparation is stimulated at a higher frequency. Rapid and repeated stimulation leads the stimuli to fall during the contraction phase so that the contractile processes are repeatedly activated. The muscle does not get time to relax. Therefore, with each stimulation, the muscle contracts without relaxation. Individual responses fuse to give a state of sustained contraction (tetanus). The muscles of our body, which are involved in the maintenance of posture exhibit tetanic contraction (sustained contraction). An erect posture is maintained due to sustained contraction of the antigravity muscles. Tetanic contraction of the skeletal muscles is also observed during an isometric exercise.

Tetanus is also seen clinically when a person is infected by a group of bacteria called *Clostridium tetani*. Tetanus usually occurs following an injury (cut, wound) through which the bacteria enter the body. The tetanus toxin released by the bacteria stimulates the motor neurons repeatedly at a higher frequency and results in tetanus. The facial muscles are commonly affected. In severe cases, all the skeletal muscles of the body may be affected. The disease can be prevented by prior immunisation with the tetanus vaccine or receiving the vaccine within twelve hours of injury.

## VIVA

1. Define treppe, clonus and tetanus.
2. What is the mechanism of the staircase phenomenon?
3. How is tetanus produced experimentally?
4. What is minimal tetanisable frequency (MTF)? How is the MTF calculated and what are the factors that affect MTF?
5. Explain why the cardiac muscle cannot be tetanised.
6. Give an example of tetanic contractions in our body.
7. Why is the tension developed by a tetanically contracting muscle more than the tension developed by the muscle during a single twitch?

   Ans. During a single contraction of the muscle, any calcium released into the sarcoplasm is quickly taken back into the cisterns during relaxation. But if the muscle is stimulated repeatedly, there is accumulation of calcium in the sarcoplasm as calcium cannot be pumped back fully into the cisterns. This increases the tension in the muscle.
8. What is the cause of tetanus (disease) and how is the disease prevented?
9. What is tetany?

   Ans. Tetany occurs due to hypocalcemia, for example, hypoparathyroidism. It is not connected with tetanus.

CHAPTER 42

# Genesis of Fatigue

**LEARNING OBJECTIVES**

After completing this practical, you will be able to:
- Define fatigue.
- Demonstrate the site of fatigue in the nerve-muscle preparation.
- List the precautions taken during the recording of the genesis of fatigue.
- Name the site of fatigue in isolated and intact preparations.
- Explain the causes of fatigue in isolated preparations.
- Explain how recovery can be expedited.

## INTRODUCTION

Fatigue is defined as decrease in performance due to continuous and prolonged activity. It can occur in the whole organism or in isolated preparations. The mechanism of fatigue is different in an intact organism and in an isolated preparation. Fatigue is a reversible phenomenon and there is no permanent functional or structural damage to the tissues. In humans, fatigue first occurs in the central nervous system whereas in isolated preparations, the neuromuscular junction is the first site of fatigue.

## METHODS

### Method to Study Genesis of Fatigue

#### Principle

A muscle is fatigued when it is stimulated repeatedly and continuously. The phenomenon of fatigue is recorded by stimulating the preparation without changing the baseline, the point of stimulation and the strength of the stimulus.

#### Requirements

The requirements are the same as for 'simple muscle twitch'.

#### Procedure

1. Dissect the frog to make the nerve-muscle preparation.
2. Mount the preparation in the muscle trough and set it up for recording a simple muscle curve. Mark the point of stimulation.
3. Repeatedly stimulate the nerve and record the first, second and third contractions on a fast-moving drum without changing the point of stimulation. Note the beneficial effect.
4. Move the writing lever away from the drum.
5. Without changing the point of stimulation, stimulate the nerve repeatedly by keeping the tap key pressed and record every tenth contraction by applying the writing lever to the drum.

> Note: The drum rotates without recording the muscle contraction. Only the tenth contraction is recorded on the drum. This is done to avoid overlapping recordings. Recording can be made with each stimulation, but overlapping of the recordings will make it difficult to study the graph.

6. Continue to record every tenth contraction till the contractions are too feeble to be recorded.
7. Change the point of stimulus to record a muscle contraction at a different place adjacent to the fatigue curve and on the same baseline.
8. Stimulate the muscle directly and record the contraction on the changed point of stimulus.
9. Drain the Ringer's solution and replace with fresh solution.
10. Allow the nerve-muscle preparation to rest for five minutes.
11. Again change the point of stimulus on the same baseline in such a way that the next recording will be adjacent to the previous recording.

12. Stimulate the nerve to record the muscle contractions.

## Observation

Record the amplitude and duration of the phases of the first three contractions and the subsequent contractions. Note that with the onset of fatigue, the relaxation period of the muscle twitches is prolonged and the baseline goes up (Fig. 42.1A). Muscle contraction occurs by direct stimulation of the muscle (Fig. 42.1B) following fatigue. Muscle contraction also occurs in response to nerve stimulation following recovery (Fig. 42.1C).

## Precautions

1. All the precautions described for the recording of simple muscle twitch (Chapter 39).
2. All the contractions should be recorded on the same point of stimulus and on the same baseline for the fatigue curve (fatigue produced by stimulation of nerve).
3. The muscle should be directly stimulated immediately after recording the fatigue by stimulating the nerve, and the contraction should be recorded on a different point of stimulus but on the same baseline.
4. The preparation should be allowed a minimum of five minutes for recovery before stimulating the nerve, to record the effect of recovery.
5. To facilitate recovery, the old Ringer's solution should be removed and replaced by the fresh solution.

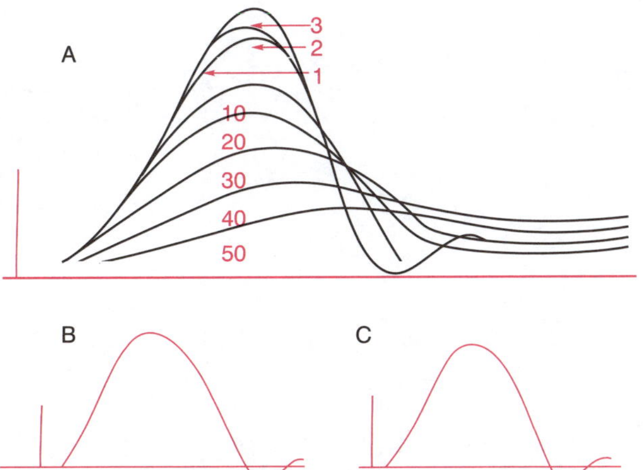


Fig. 42.1 Demonstration of the phenomenon and site of fatigue. A: Genesis of fatigue following repeated stimulation of the nerve. Numbers depicted with the curves indicate the number of stimuli. Note the beneficial effects with the first three contractions. Also, note the decrease in amplitude, prolongation of relaxation period and rise in baseline with the onset of fatigue. B: Recording of the curve by directly stimulating the muscle immediately following onset of fatigue. C: Recording of the curve by stimulating the nerve following recovery.

# DISCUSSION

In isolated preparations, fatigue can occur at three sites: the muscle, the neuromuscular junction and the nerve. The nerve is theoretically unfatiguable, therefore the possible sites may be either the muscle or the neuromuscular junction. But the muscle contraction recorded by directly stimulating the muscle following the genesis of fatigue indicates that the muscle is not fatigued. Therefore, it can be inferred that the site of fatigue is the neuromuscular junction. The cause of this fatigue is the depletion of acetylcholine, the neurotransmitter from the myoneural junction. If the preparation is allowed to rest for some time and fresh Ringer's solution is supplied to the preparation, the muscle contracts in response to the stimulation of the nerve (following the period of recovery). This again proves that the site of fatigue was the neuromuscular junction, as recovery allows re-synthesis of neurotransmitters at the nerve endings. The Ringer's solution supplies nutrition and facilitates recovery. If the muscle is directly stimulated continuously, it can also be fatigued due to exhaustion of glycogen storage. But in this condition, there will be no recovery, as the utilised glycogen cannot be replaced.

An early sign of fatigue is the prolongation of the relaxation period. When a muscle is fatigued, the relaxation becomes incomplete and then it remains in a state of partial contraction. This is called *contraction remainder*. It occurs due to a decrease in the ATP content and accumulation of the metabolites in the muscle. The baseline increases due to contraction remainder.

In human beings, the first site of fatigue is the CNS, not the neuromuscular junction.

## VIVA

1. Define fatigue.
2. What is the difference between the fatigue of an intact animal and that of an isolated preparation?
3. What is the site of fatigue in an isolated preparation and how do you demonstrate it?
4. What is the mechanism of fatigue in an isolated preparation?
5. How can the recovery be facilitated?
6. What is contraction remainder?
7. What is the early sign of fatigue in an isolated preparation?

Chapter 43

# Normal Cardiogram of Frog

## Learning Objectives

After completing this practical, you will be able to:

- Dissect and open the thorax, open the pericardium, pin the apex of the heart and fix the heart to the lever.
- Identify the different parts of the heart.
- Record a normal cardiogram.
- Explain the different waves in the cardiogram.
- List the properties of the heart demonstrated in this experiment.
- List the differences between amphibian and mammalian hearts.

## INTRODUCTION

The normal cardiogram of a frog is the recording of the mechanical activities of the heart of the frog on a smoked drum. Since the cardiogram is the recording of the mechanical activities, it records the systole and diastole of the different chambers of the heart. In a frog, the atria are called auricles, the ventricles are single-chambered, and the electrical rhythm for generating an impulse is located in the sinus venosus instead of the SA node, as seen in the mammalian heart (Table 43.1 ). Therefore, in an ideal tracing, the mechanical activities of the sinus venosus, auricles and ventricles are recorded. A **white crescentic line** is present between the auricles and the sinus venosus (Fig. 43.1 ). The normal heart rate of a frog is 40–50 beats per minute.

## METHODS

### Method of Recording Normal Cardiogram of Frog

#### Principle

The mechanical activities of the amphibian heart are directly recorded by connecting the heart to the

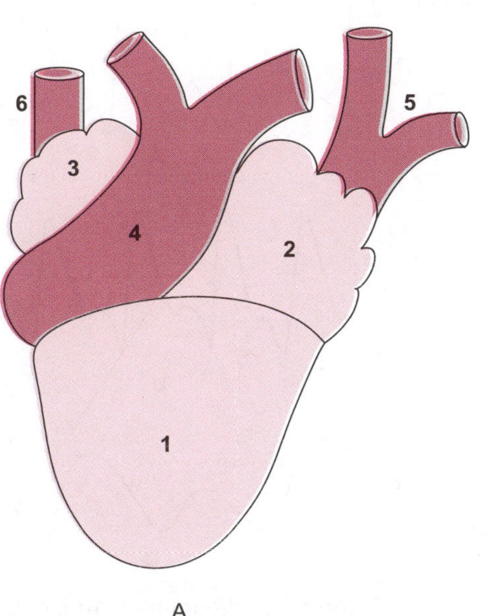


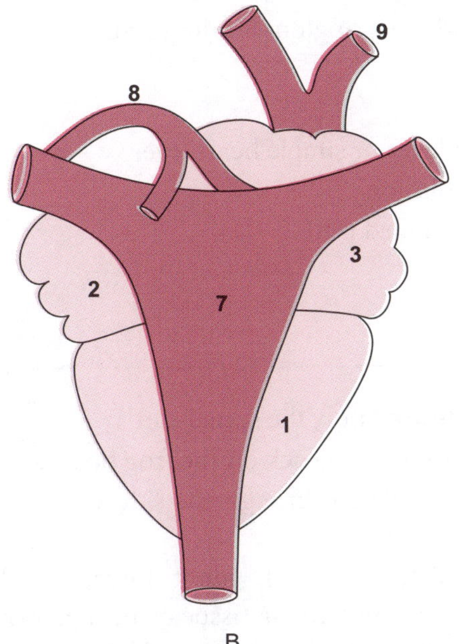


Fig. 43.1 Frog's, heart. A. Dorsal view; B. Ventral view. 1: Ventricle; 2: Left auricle; 3: Right auricle; 4: Truncus arteriosus; 5: Left anterior caval vein; 6: Right anterior caval vein; 7: Sinus venosus; 8: Pulmonary vein; 9: Right systemic arch; 10: Posterior caval vein.

Table 43.1 Differences between amphibian and mammalian heart.

| | Amphibian heart | Mammalian heart |
|---|---|---|
| 1. Heart chambers | Three-chambered heart; two auricles and a ventricle | Four-chambered heart; two atria and two ventricles |
| 2. Sinus venosus | Present; receives venous blood atrium | Absent; venous blood directly drains to right |
| 3. Coronary arteries | Not well developed | Well developed |
| 4. Blood in ventricle | Mixed (arterial and venous) | Not mixed |
| 5. Myocardial perfusion | Directly from the blood present in the ventricle | Through coronaries |
| 6. Pacemaker | Pacemaker is present in sinus venosus | SA node is the pacemaker, which is present in the right atrium |
| 7. White crescentic line | Present; works as parasympathetic ganglion | Absent |

writing lever with a thread which transmits the waves of contraction and relaxation from the heart to the lever. The cardiac activities are recorded on a moving drum.

## Requirements

1. Kymograph with Sherrington–Starling drum
2. Frog board
3. Myograph stand
4. Starling's heart lever or simple heart lever
5. Frog Ringer's solution
6. Pins (also one hooked pin)
7. Thread

## Procedure

1. Pith the frog (destroy only the spinal cord).
2. Lay the pithed frog on its back on the frog board.
3. Make a median incision through the skin over the sternum.
4. Raise the xiphisternum with blunt forceps and separate it from the underlying tissue using a pair of blunt scissors, taking care not to injure the heart.
5. Insert one of the blades of the scissors under the pectoral girdle and cut on both sides so that the anterior wall of the thorax can be removed.
6. Pull the forelimbs laterally and fix them on to the board with pins so as to keep the chest wide open.
7. Identify the heart, beating inside the thin membrane (pericardium).
8. Observe that at the apex of the heart, there is a small clear space between the heart and pericardial membrane. With the help of forceps, pinch and lift the pericardium at the apex at this clear space, taking care not to touch the heart.
9. Make a slit in the pericardium with the help of a pair of fine scissors and then cut the pericardium up to the base of the heart, taking care not to injure the heart.
10. Study the different parts of the heart (Fig. 43.1).

> Note: On the ventral aspect of the heart, the initial dilated portion of the aorta, which is known as bulbus arteriosus, divides into two aortae. On the dorsal aspect (lift the ventricle), identify the sinus venosus separated from the auricles by a white crescentic line. Note that two superior vena cavae and the inferior vena cava enter the sinus venosus. Observe the change in colour of the chambers during systole (contraction) and diastole (relaxation).

11. Fix the pericardium through the base of the heart to the frog board with a pin.

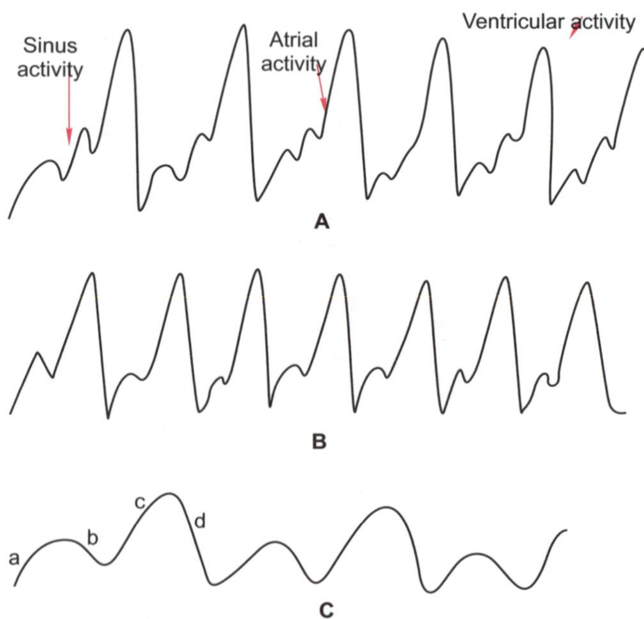


Fig. 43.2 Normal cardiogram of frog. A. Ideal recording (at slow speed; 1.2 mm/s); B. Usual recording (at slow speed; 1.2 mm/s); C. Usual recording at fast speed (a: atrial systole; b: atrial relaxation; c: ventricular contraction; d: ventricular relaxation).

12. Hook a bent pin through the apex of the heart taking care not to puncture the chambers of the ventricle.
13. Tie one end of the thread to the pin and lift the ventricle by the thread. Tie the other end of the thread to the heart lever.

> Note Keep the thread vertical and taut enough to transmit the contraction of the heart to the writing point of the lever.

14. Keep the writing arm of the lever horizontal.
15. Touch the writing point of the heart lever lightly to the smoked paper on the drum in the lower third (about 5 cm from the lower margin) of the drum.
16. Set the drum to rotate at a slow speed (1.2 mm/s) and record the cardiogram starting from just after the joint of the paper on the drum.
17. Take a time-tracing below the recording.
18. Repeat the recording of the cardiogram at a higher speed (2.5 mm/s).

> Note Recording at a faster speed will clearly show the different components of the cardiogram.

## Observation

Identify the different components of the cardiogram recorded at slow and fast speeds as given in Fig. 43.2. Observe the rhythmicity (whether regular or irregular) and calculate the heart rate.

## Precautions

1. While cutting the sternum of the frog with a median incision, care should be taken not to damage the heart.
2. The heart should be exposed by cutting the pericardium.
3. While cutting the pericardium, take care not to damage the heart.
4. The hooked pin should be introduced at the apex of the heart through the wall of the ventricle. While introducing the hooked pin, take care not to puncture the ventricle (the pin should not enter the ventricular cavity).
5. The thread connecting the heart and the lever should be placed vertically.
6. The lever should be placed horizontally.
7. The base of the heart should be fixed. It increases the amplitude of recording as the force of contraction is directly transmitted to the lever due to pulling of apex towards the fixed base during each systole.
8. Frog Ringer's solution should be poured on the heart at regular intervals to prevent it from drying.

# DISCUSSION

The properties of the heart, which are studied in this experiment, are automaticity, rhythmicity, conductivity and contractility. Automaticity is studied by observing the automatic beating of the heart, which occurs due to the impulse generated automatically in the heart; rhythmicity is studied by rhythmical beating of the heart; conductivity is studied by conduction of impulse from the sinus venosus to the ventricles (better demonstrated by Stannius ligatures); and contractility is recorded by observing the contraction of the heart and recording the systole and diastole in the tracings.

In the heart of a frog, the cardiac impulse is generated in the sinus venosus. Impulse is transmitted from the sinus venosus to the auricles and then to the ventricles. A slight pause is seen between auricular and ventricular contraction and this is due to the delay (partial conduction block) in conduction of the impulse from the auricles to the ventricles. In a frog, the rate of impulse generation is maximum in the sinus venosus. Therefore, the sinus venosus is the natural pacemaker of the heart.

## The Cardiogram

Different waves in the cardiogram represent the activities of different chambers of the heart. Usually only two types of waves are seen. The 'a' wave represents auricular systole (upgoing) and diastole (downgoing), and the 'v' wave represents ventricular systole and diastole. In an ideal recording, the 's' wave is what appears before the 'a' wave also seen. The 's' wave represents the systole and diastole of the sinus venosus.

## VIVA

1. What is the difference between the cardiogram (recorded in this experiment) and the electrocardiogram?
2. What is the normal heart rate in a frog?
3. What are the properties of the cardiac muscle? What properties of the cardiac muscle are demonstrated in this experiment?
4. What are the differences between the amphibian and mammalian hearts?
5. Where is the pacemaker of a frog's heart situated?
6. What does the crescentic line represent?
7. What are the different waves recorded in a normal cardiogram of a frog's heart? How are these waves produced?
8. What are the precautions taken during dissection to expose the heart?
9. Why is the base of the heart fixed?
10. Why should only the spinal cord be destroyed during pithing?

    Ans. Cardiovascular centres are present in the brain. Therefore, if the brain is destroyed with pithing, there may be an alteration in heart function.

Chapter 44

# Effect of Temperature on Frog's Heart

## Learning Objectives

After completing this practical, you will be able to:

- State the physiological importance of performing this practical.
- Demonstrate the effect of cold and warm Ringer's solution on the sinus venosus and the ventricle.
- List the precautions taken for studying the effect of cold and warm Ringer's solution on the sinus venosus and the ventricle.
- Explain the changes in cardiac activities following the application of cold and warm Ringer's solution on the sinus venosus and the ventricle.

## INTRODUCTION

The application of cold and warm Ringer's solution on the sinus venosus changes the heart rate by changing the pacemaker activity, which is present in the sinus venosus in frogs. The application of cold and warm Ringer's solution on the ventricle changes the force of contraction by directly affecting the contractile machinery of the myocardium.

This experiment is carried out to study the effect of temperature on the sinus venosus and the ventricle, and to know the site of impulse generation in the frog's heart.

## METHODS

### Method to Study Effect of Temperature on Frog's Heart

#### Principle

The application of cold and warm Ringer's solution on the sinus venosus changes the heart rate and that on the ventricle changes the force of contraction. These changes are observed by applying cold and warm Ringer's solution separately on the sinus venosus and on the ventricle, and recording the effect on a moving drum.

#### Requirements

1. Same as for Chapter 43.
2. Cold Ringer's solution (15°C)
3. Warm Ringer's solution (35°C)
4. Dropper
5. Blotting paper

#### Procedure

Expose the heart of a pithed frog and record a normal cardiogram as described in Chapter 43. Then carry out the experiment separately on the sinus venosus and on the ventricle as described below.

*On the Sinus Venosus*

1. Record a normal cardiogram (about 10 beats).
2. Apply cold (15°C) Ringer's solution to the sinus venosus with the help of a dropper and record its effect on the cardiogram (about 10 beats).
3. Apply Ringer's solution at normal room temperature and record a normal cardiogram (about 10 beats).
4. Apply warm Ringer's (35°C) to the sinus venosus with the help of a dropper and record its effect on the cardiogram (about 10 beats).
5. Apply Ringer's solution at normal room temperature and record a normal cardiogram (about 10 beats).

*On the Ventricle*

1. Record a normal cardiogram (about 10 beats) at room temperature.
2. Apply cold (15°C) Ringer's solution to the ventricle with a piece of blotting paper and record its effect on the ventricle.

> Note: The small piece of blotting paper is soaked in cold Ringer's solution and the paper then is placed on the ventricle with the help of forceps, taking care not to allow the solution to trickle down to the sinus venosus.

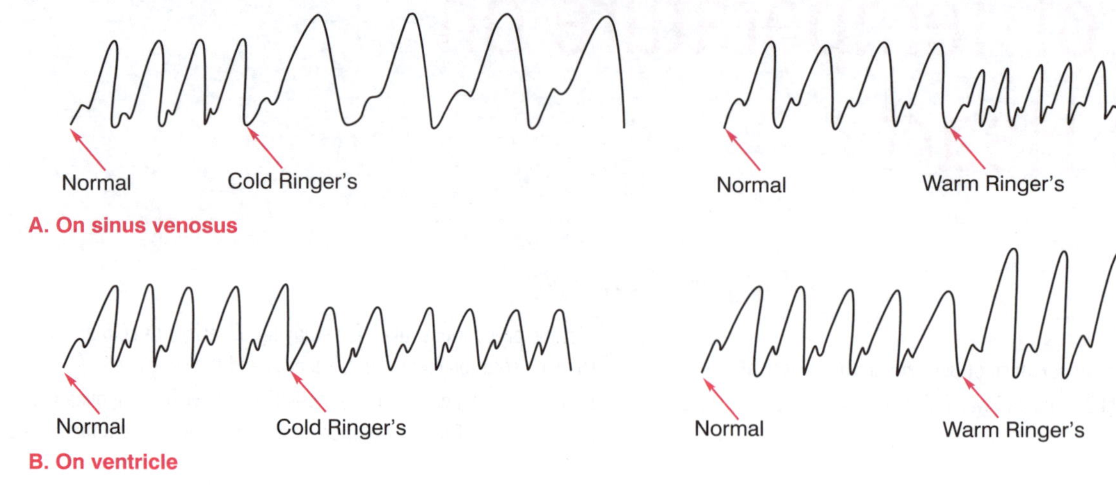


Fig. 44.1 Effect of temperature on frog's heart.

3. Apply Ringer's solution at normal room temperature and record a normal cardiogram (about 10 beats).
4. Apply warm Ringer's (35°C) to the ventricle with blotting paper and record its effect on the ventricle.

> Note: The blotting paper is soaked in warm Ringer's solution and then placed on the ventricle with forceps, taking care not to allow the solution to trickle down to the sinus venosus.

5. Apply Ringer's solution at normal room temperature and record a normal cardiogram (about 10 beats).

Tabulate the effects of temperature on the sinus venosus and on the ventricle with reference to heart rate and force of contraction.

## Observation

Study the effect of temperature on the sinus venosus and the ventricle. Note that cold Ringer's decreases the heart rate but increases the force of contraction, and warm Ringer's increases the heart rate but decreases the amplitude of contraction when applied to the sinus venosus. Cold Ringer's decreases the amplitude of contraction without changing the heart rate and warm Ringer's increases amplitude of contraction without changing the heart rate when applied to the ventricle (Fig. 44.1).

## Precautions

1. The normal cardiogram should be recorded prior to the recording of the effects of cold and warm Ringer's solution on the sinus venosus and the ventricle.
2. The temperature of cold Ringer's should be 15°C and temperature of warm Ringer's should be 35°C. If the solution is very cold or very hot, the heart may be damaged.
3. The temperature of the solutions should be recorded just before their application.
4. Care should be taken to apply the solution only on the sinus venosus when the effect of cold and warm Ringer's solution is carried out.
5. Care must be taken to prevent the trickling down of the solution to the sinus venosus from the ventricle, when the effect of cold and warm Ringer's is carried out. For recording the cardiogram, the ventricle is placed above the sinus venosus, blotting paper (not the dropper) is used to pour cold and warm Ringer's solution on the ventricle so that the solution does not trickle down to the sinus venosus.
6. The heart should be moistened with normal Ringer's solution frequently to prevent drying.
7. When not recording, the lever of the heart should be lowered to prevent deterioration of the function of the heart.

# DISCUSSION

## Cold Ringer's on the Sinus Venosus

The application of cold Ringer's solution on the sinus venosus decreases the heart rate and increases the amplitude of contraction. The heart rate decreases because the cold Ringer's directly inhibits the pacemaker activity of the heart. This is the **primary effect**. The increase in amplitude of contraction is due to the Frank–Starling law. When the heart rate decreases, the ventricular end diastolic volume increases as the ventricle gets more time to fill. The increased ventricular filling increases the length of the ventricular muscle fibre prior to onset of systole. Therefore, the force of the contraction increases. This is the **secondary effect**.

## Warm Ringer's on the Sinus Venosus

The application of warm Ringer's solution on the sinus venosus increases the heart rate and decreases the force of contraction. The increase in heart rate is the primary effect and the decrease in the force of contraction is the secondary effect. The heart rate increases due to stimulation of the pacemaker activity in the sinus venosus by the warm solution. The force of contraction decreases due to less filling of heart (decreased end diastolic volume) as the heart gets less time to fill.

## Cold Ringer's on the Ventricle

The application of the cold Ringer's solution to the ventricle decreases the force of contraction due to the inhibition of myocardial contractility by the cold solution. The heart rate does not change as the pacemaker of the heart is present in the sinus venosus, which remains unaffected in this experiment. The myocardial activity is depressed by the cold Ringer's solution because at the low temperature, the enzymatic activity of the myocardium decreases and the viscosity of the myocardial tissue increases.

## Warm Ringer's on the Ventricle

The application of warm Ringer's solution to the ventricle increases the force of contraction due to the accentuation of myocardial activity by the direct action of warm solution on it. The heart rate remains unchanged as the pacemaker is present in the sinus venosus. Warm Ringer's stimulates myocardial contractility by increasing the enzymatic activity and decreasing the viscosity of the myocardial tissue.

These experiments prove that the sinus venosus is the pacemaker of the frog heart.

## VIVA

1. What is the effect of cold Ringer's on the sinus venosus and the ventricle? What is the physiological basis?
2. What is the Frank–Starling law of the heart?
3. What is the effect of warm Ringer's solution on the sinus venosus and the ventricle? What is the physiological basis?
4. What are the precautions taken for demonstrating the effect of cold and warm Ringer's on the sinus venosus and the ventricle?
5. What is the physiological basis of the difference between the cold and warm Ringer's on the sinus venosus and the ventricle?

# Chapter 45

# Effect of Stannius Ligatures on Frog's Heart

### Learning Objectives

After completing this practical, you will be able to:
- Explain the clinical implication of this practical.
- Demonstrate the effect of Stannius ligature on the frog heart.
- Explain the effect of Stannius ligatures.
- State the rate of discharge of different potential pacemakers of the heart.
- Classify heart blocks.

## INTRODUCTION

In humans, the cardiac impulse is generated in the SA node and conducted to all parts of the heart. Therefore, the SA node is the pacemaker of the heart. In a frog's heart, the pacemaker is present in the sinus venosus. The cardiac muscle has the property of automaticity, that is, it has the power to generate its own impulse. Though normally an impulse is generated in the SA node (primary pacemaker), automaticity is not limited to the SA node alone. When the SA node is diseased, the other potential pacemakers of the heart take over the responsibility to generate the impulse. The first to take over the work of the SA node is the AV node. The next in the hierarchy are bundle of His, the Purkinje system and the ventricular muscle. The rate of discharge is maximum in the SA node as it is the natural pacemaker of the heart. The rate of discharge gradually decreases in the hierarchy of the pacemakers.

In humans, the rate of discharge of the different pacemakers is as follows:

| | | |
|---|---|---|
| SA node | : | 60–100/min |
| AV node | : | 50–70/min |
| His bundle | : | 40–60/min |
| Purkinje system | : | 30–50/min |
| Ventricular muscle | : | 15–40/min |

This practical demonstrates the hierarchy of pacemaking activity of the different tissues of the heart.

## METHODS

### Method to Study Effect of Stannius Ligatures on Frog's Heart

#### Principle

The rate of discharge of impulses is different in different potential pacemakers of the heart. Their rhythms are demonstrated by separating (appropriately placing ligatures) them from each other.

#### Requirements

1. Same as for Chapter 43
2. Aneurysm needle
3. Thread

#### Procedure

1. Set up the experiment as for recording a normal cardiogram.
2. Pass a threaded aneurysm needle between the truncus arteriosus and the atria.
3. Hook up the heart and record the normal cardiogram on a slow-moving drum.
4. Bring forward the thread under the truncus arteriosus and tie it at the junction of the sinus venosus and the atria (on the white crescentic line).

Note: This is the first Stannius ligature (Fig. 45.1). It records the atrial rhythm.

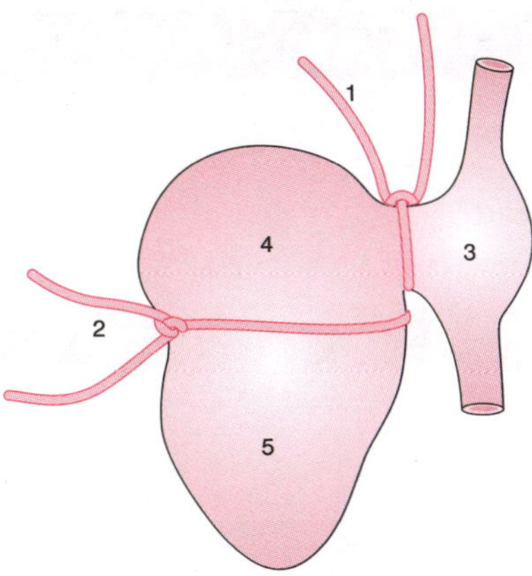


Fig. 45.1 Position of Stannius ligatures as seen in the side view of the heart. 1: First Stannius ligature; 2: Second Stannius ligature; 3: Sinus venosus; 4: Auricles; 5: Ventricle.

5. Record the effect of ligation on the cardiogram.
6. Apply the ligature at the atrioventricular junction and record the effect of ligation on the cardiogram.

> Note: This is the second Stannius ligature. It records the ventricular rhythm. Note that the ventricle starts beating after a pause, and at a much slower rate (idioventricular rhythm).

## Observation

Note that the frequency of heart beat after placing the first Stannius ligature is significantly less than the normal rhythm. The frequency of heart beat is much lower after placing the second Stannius ligature (Fig. 45.2).

## Precautions

1. The first Stannius ligature should be tied between the truncus arteriosus and the atria.
2. The second Stannius ligature should be tied between the atria and ventricle.
3. Recording should be done immediately after placing the ligatures.

# DISCUSSION

The sinus venosus (SA node in humans) is the primary pacemaker of the heart. Therefore, the first Stannius ligature, which prevents transmission of impulses from the sinus venosus to atria, decreases the heart rate as the impulse is now generated by the atria (atrial rhythm). After placing the second Stannius ligature, which prevents transmission of impulse from the atria to the ventricle, the heart rate decreases further as the impulse is now generated by the ventricle (ventricular rhythm). This indicates that the primary pacemaker in frog heart is present in the sinus venosus.

## Clinical Significance

### Heart Blocks

As already noted, the SA node normally controls the heart rate. Interruption of impulse transmission from the atria to the ventricle is called heart block. There are three degrees of heart blocks: first, second and third. In first degree and second degree heart blocks, impulse transmission is not completely interrupted between the atria and the ventricle, therefore these are called **incomplete heart blocks**. However, impulse transmission is completely blocked between the atria and the ventricle in the third degree heart block, and therefore it is called **complete heart block.**

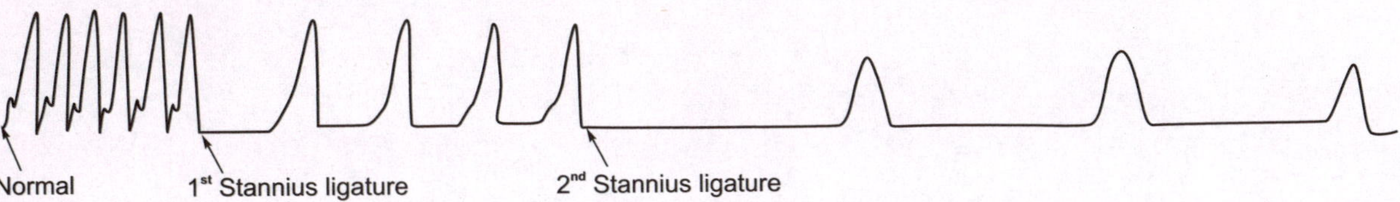


Fig. 45.2 Recording of the effects of Stannius ligature on frog's heart.

## VIVA

1. What is the effect of the first Stannius ligature on the heart?
2. What is the effect of the second Stannius ligature on the heart?
3. What is the rate of discharge of the different potential pacemakers of the heart?
4. What is heart block? What are the different types of heart blocks?

Chapter 46

# Postural Reflexes in the Frog

### Learning Objectives

After completing this practical, you will be able to:

- Explain the importance of studying the postural reflexes of the frog in practical physiology.
- List the postural reflexes integrated at different levels of the CNS.
- Explain the role of different parts of the neuraxis in the regulation of motor activities.

## INTRODUCTION

Motor activities are controlled at different levels in the CNS. These activities include voluntary activities and reflex activity. There are many reflexes that help maintain erect posture and balance, and coordinate activities at different joints to perform a particular movement. These are called **postural reflexes**. According to their site of integration, the reflexes are classified into spinal, medullary, midbrain and cortical reflexes. By making a section at the relevant part, we can isolate a portion of the CNS from its higher regions and study the motor activities of the animal, which are controlled by that isolated portion of the CNS.

## METHODS

### Method to Study Postural Reflexes in the Frog

#### Principle

The reflexes integrated at different parts of the CNS can be studied separately by making a section at the upper level of that part which isolates the part from its higher regions of the CNS. This enables us to study the motor activities integrated in that part of the CNS.

#### Requirements

1. A pair of scissors
2. A living frog

#### Procedure

1. Study the normal behaviour of an intact frog, for example, how a frog jumps, respires, swims and so on, and observe the attitude of jumping, righting, and other behaviour. Study the withdrawal reflex by applying a noxious stimulus like pinching or pricking a part of the limb.

> Note: Swimming can be studied by placing the frog in a bowl of water. Righting can be studied by placing it on its back and observing whether it is capable of righting itself.

2. Pith the frog to destroy only the cerebral hemisphere (do not destroy the spinal cord) or remove the cerebral hemisphere by cutting with a pair of sharp scissors along a line (Fig. 46.1) passing through the caudal border of the eyeball (the upper blade of the scissors is placed on this line, whereas the lower blade remains inside the mouth).

> Note: This type of preparation is called a *decerebrate preparation* and the animal is known as a *decerebrate frog*. In higher animals, a decerebrate preparation is made by making a midcollicular lesion.

3. Observe the frog's behaviour after removing the cerebral hemisphere and note whether it maintains normal posture, whether respiration continues, whether it is able to swim and right itself. Apply noxious stimuli by pinching and observe the response of the frog to the stimulus.
4. Cut and remove the head in front of a line passing behind the tympanic membranes.

> Note: This preparation is called a *spinal preparation* and the animal is known a *spinal animal*. In humans or higher animals, the spinal preparation is done by making a section at the upper segments of the spinal cord.

5. Study all the parameters as observed after making the first section.

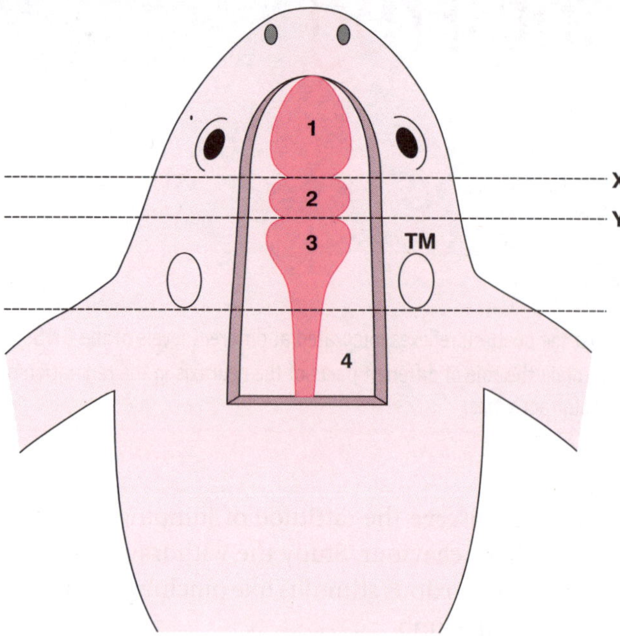


Fig. 46.1 Position of incision for decerebrate (X) and spinal (Y) preparation. TM: Tympanic membrane; 1: Cerebral hemisphere; 2: Midbrain; 3: Hindbrain; 4: Spinal cord. (Brain is exposed dorsally to identify the position of different parts).

> Note: Immediately after the section is made, the frog becomes completely flaccid (loss of muscle tone) but within minutes this stage of flaccidity disappears and postural reflexes reappear.

6. Destroy the spinal cord by pithing (pushing the pithing needle down the vertebral column and rotating the needle) and study the effect on various parameters.

> Note: The animal becomes permanently flaccid and loses all postural reflexes.

## Observation

Record your observation in a tabular form as given below:

| | Spontaneous behaviour (normal attitude, respiration, etc.) | Withdrawal reflex | Righting reflex |
|---|---|---|---|
| 1. Intact | ++ | ++ | ++ |
| 2. Decerebrate frog | ++ | ++ | Present |
| 3. Spinal frog | Absent | ++ | Absent |
| 4. Frog with no spinal cord | Absent | Absent | Absent |

## Precautions

1. While making the frog decerebrate, the section should be made at the caudal border of the eyeball.
2. For making a spinal frog, the section should be made on the line passing behind the tympanic membranes.
3. All the reflexes should be studied carefully.

# DISCUSSION

The different motor and reflex activities are integrated at different levels of the CNS. These activities are studied by making sections at different levels of the neuraxis. The reflex activities below the levels of lesion become hyperactive due to different mechanisms. These mechanisms involve loss of inhibitory control from the higher centres and the development of denervation hypersensitivity to the mediators released by the remaining spinal excitatory endings and also due to the development of collaterals from the existing neurons.

## Decerebrate Preparation

The decerebrate preparation is made in higher animals (dogs, cats and monkeys) by making a midcollicular lesion. It is difficult to produce decerebrate preparation in frogs as the brain structures are not well developed (colliculi may not be present). Therefore, such preparation is actually a *decorticate preparation*. In such preparations, all the reflexes may be present. But, in humans, in decorticate preparation, the initiative memory and placing and hopping reactions will be lost. As the memory, hopping and placing reactions are not encountered in a normal frog, these parameters cannot be studied in the decorticate frog. In decerebrate preparations in higher animals like dogs and cats, the righting reflexes are lost as these reflexes are integrated at the level of the midbrain. As decerebrate preparation is difficult to obtain in frogs, the righting reflexes will be present in this preparation.

## Spinal Preparation

A spinal preparation is made by making a section at the upper border of the spinal cord (upper cervical segment). As soon as the section is made, the animal becomes totally flaccid and all the reflex activities are lost. This phase is known as the **phase of spinal shock.** The spinal shock is due to loss of tonic bombardment of spinal neurons by excitatory impulses in the descending pathways from the supraspinal segments of the CNS. The phase of spinal shock passes off very quickly in the frog (within minutes) following which the reflex activities reappear. In spinal animals, all the reflexes will be lost except the reflexes that are integrated at the level of the spinal cord (spinal reflexes). Spinal reflexes include stretch reflex, supporting reactions (positive and negative) and withdrawal reflex. In frogs, the supporting reactions and stretch reflexes (tendon reflexes) cannot be elicited. The withdrawal reflex is present in a spinal frog.

### Destruction of the Spinal Cord

After the spinal cord is destroyed, all the above reflexes and motor activities are lost. Because the cell bodies of the lower motor neurons (which are the final common pathway for transmission of impulses from the spinal and supraspinal segments) are destroyed, no reflex activities take place.

## VIVA

1. Name the reflexes integrated at the level of the spinal cord (spinal reflexes), medulla, midbrain and cortex.
2. What is a decerebrate preparation? What are the reflexes present in a decerebrate animal?
3. How is a decerebrate preparation made in higher animals?
4. What is a spinal preparation? What are the reflexes seen in a spinal preparation?
5. What are antigravity reflexes? What is the role of these reflexes in the integration of motor activities?
6. What are righting reflexes? In which part of the CNS are these reflexes integrated?
7. What is spinal shock and what is its mechanism?
8. What are the differences between the postural reflexes of humans and frogs?

# Index of Normal Values

## A. Blood

### 1. Hemogram

| Test | Normal value |
|---|---|
| Total RBC count | |
| Men | 4.5–6 million/$mm^3$ |
| Women | 4–5.5 million/$mm^3$ |
| Hemoglobin | |
| Men | 14–18 g/dl |
| Women | 12–16 g/dl |
| Packed cell volume | |
| Men | 40–50% |
| Women | 37–47% |
| Mean corpuscular volume | 78–96 fl |
| Mean corpuscular hemoglobin | 27–33 pg |
| Mean corpuscular Hb conc | 30–37% |
| Total leucocyte count | 4000–11,000/$mm^3$ |
| Differential count | |
| Neutrophils | 50–70% |
| Eosinophils | 1–4% |
| Lymphocyte | 20–40% |
| Monocyte | 2–8% |
| Basophils | 0–1% |
| Total platelet count | 150,000–400,000/$mm^3$ |
| Reticulocyte count | 0.5–1% of red cells |
| ESR (Westergren method) | |
| Men | 3–5 mm at the end of 1 h |
| Women | 5–12 mm at the end of 1 h |

### 2. Coagulation studies

| Test | Normal value |
|---|---|
| Bleeding time (Duke method) | 1–5 min |
| Clotting time (capillary tube method) | 2–8 min |
| Fibrinogen | 200–400 mg% |
| Fibrin degradation product | 10 µg/dl |
| Activated partial thromboplastin time (APTT) | 25–40 sec |
| Thrombin time | 15–20 sec |
| Clot retraction time | 50% by 1 h |
| Whole blood clot lysis time | > 24 h |

### 3. Gases

| Test | Normal value |
|---|---|
| $PO_2$ | |
| Arterial blood | 75–100 mmHg |
| Venous blood | 25–40 mmHg |

| | |
|---|---|
| $PCO_2$ | |
| Arterial blood | 35–45 mmHg |
| Venous blood | 40–50 mmHg |
| **4. pH** | 7.35–7.45 |

## B. Serum

| | |
|---|---|
| Bilirubin | |
| Adult | 0.2–0.8 mg % |
| Newborn | 0.5–5 mg % |
| At 3 days after birth | 1–10 mg % |
| Creatinine | 0.6-1.8 mg % |
| Calcium | 8–11 mg/dl |
| Iron | 50–150 μg/dl |
| Plasma glucose (fasting) | 70–110 mg/dl |
| Electrolytes | |
| Sodium | 135–145 meq/L |
| Potassium | 3.5–5 meq/L |
| Chlorides | 100–110 meq/L |
| Phosphorus (inorganic) | 2.5–4.5 mg/dl |
| Cholesterol | 120–220 mg/dl |
| Osmolality | 280–295 mosm/kg of water |

## C. Urine

| | |
|---|---|
| Glucose | |
| Qualitative | absent |
| Quantitative | 16–300 mg/24 h |
| Protein | |
| Qualitative | absent |
| Quantitative | 10–150 mg/24 h |
| Bilirubin | absent |
| Hemoglobin | absent |
| Creatine | 0–200 mg in 24 h |
| Uric acid | 600–700 mg/24 h |
| Urobilinogen | 0.05–3.5 mg/24 h |
| Sodium | 10–150 meq/24 h |
| Potassium | 25–100 meq/24 h |
| Chloride | 120–240 meq/24 h |
| Calcium (normal diet) | 0.05–0.30 meq/kg body weight/24 h |
| Osmolality | 50–1200 mosm/L |
| pH | 4.6–8.0 (average 6) |

## D. Cerebrospinal fluid

| | |
|---|---|
| Glucose | 45–75 mg/dl |
| Protein | 15–45 mg/dl |
| Bilirubin | absent |
| Cells | 0–5/$mm^3$ (usually lymphocytes) |
| Chloride | 600–700 mg/dl |

| | |
|---|---|
| Pressure | 7–20 cm of water |
| pH | 7.34–7.43 |

**E. Semen**

| | |
|---|---|
| Liquefaction | completes at 15 min |
| Morphology | minimum 60% normal |
| Motility | minimum 75% motile |
| pH | 7.2–8.0 |
| Count | 50 million/ml |
| Volume | 2–5 ml |

**F. Synovial fluid**

| | |
|---|---|
| Cells | 200 cells/$mm^3$ |
| Glucose | same as serum |
| Hyaluronic acid | 2.5–4 g/dl |
| Proteins | 2.5 g/dl |
| pH | 7.32–7.64 |
| Crystals | absent |

**G. Stool**

| | |
|---|---|
| Fat | 3–5 g/day |
| Nitrogen | 2.2 g/24 h |
| Stercobilinogen | 40–280 mg/24 h |
| Corpoporphyrin | 15–500 mg/24 h |

# Bibliography


## Hematology

Beutler E, Lichtman MA, Coller BS, Kipps TJ and Seligsohn U. 2014. *William's Hematology;* sixth edition. London: McGraw-Hill.

Firkin F, Chesterman C, Penington P and Rush B (eds.). 2012. *de Gruchy's Clinical Hematology in Medical Practice;* seventh edition. London: Science.

Freeman JA and MF Beeler. 2011. *Laboratory Medicine: Urinalysis and Medical Microscopy;* second edition. Philadelphia: Lea and Febiger.

Lewis SM, Dacie JV, Bain BJ and Bates I. 2015. *Practical Hematology;* eleventh edition. London: Churchill Livingstone.

Linne, JJ and Ringsrud KM. 1992. *Basic Techniques in Clinical laboratory Science;* third edition. New York: Mosby Year Book.

Mukherjee KL et al. (ed.). 2010. *Medical Laboratory Technology.* London: Tata McGraw-Hill.

## Human Practicals

Alberto M. Heart rate variability: From bench to bedside. *Europ J Int Med* 2005; 16(1): 12–20.

Bannister R and Mathews CJ (ed). 2003. *Autonomic Failure: A Textbook of Clinical Disorders of the Autonomic Nervous System;* fourth edition. London: Oxford University Press.

Berne RM and Levy MN. 2004. *Physiology;* fifth edition. New York: CV Mosby Co.

Bouchier IAD, Ellis H and Fleming PR (eds.). 1996. *French's Index of Differential Diagnosis;* thirteenth edition. London: Butterworth-Heinemann.

Ganong WF. 2005. *Review of Medical Physiology;* twenty-second edition. New York: Prentice Hall Inc.

Johnson EW and Pease WS (eds.). 1997. *Practical Electromyography;* third edition. London: Williams and Wilkins.

Kasper DL, Braunwald E, Fauci AS, Longo DL, Hauser SL and Jameson JL (eds.). 2015. *Harrison's Principles of Internal Medicine;* nineteenth edition. New York: McGraw-Hill.

Mishra UK and Kalita J. 1991. *Clinical Neurophysiology.* New Delhi: BI Churchill Livingstone.

Ogilvie C. 1980. *Chamberlain's Symptoms and Signs in Clinical Medicine;* tenth edition. London: John Wright and Sons Ltd.

Pal GK. 2011. Spectral analysis of heart rate variability. *Textbook of Medical Physiology;* second edition. New Delhi: Ahuja Publications. pp. 222–226.

Sahu D. 1983. *Critical Approach to Clinical Medicine.* New Delhi: Vikas Publishing House Pvt Ltd.

Sainani GS et al (ed.). 1992. *API Textbook of Medicine;* fifth edition. New Delhi: Association of Physicians of India.

Schamroth C (ed.). 1990. *An Introduction to Electrocardiography;* seventh edition. London: Blackwell Science.

Swash M. 1995. *Hutchison's Clinical Methods;* twentieth edition. London: WB Saunders.

Task Force of the European Society of Cardiology and the North American Society of Pacing and Electrophysiology. Heart rate variability. Standard and measurement, physiological interpretation and clinical use. *Circulation* 1996; 93: 1043–1065.

Tierney LM Jr, Me Phee SJ and Papadakis MA (eds.). 2004. *Current Medical Diagnosis and Treatment;* forty-third edition. New York: Prentice Hall Inc.

Vakil RJ and Golwala AF. 1990. *Physical Diagnosis;* sixth edition. Mumbai: Media Promoters and Publishers Pvt. Ltd.

## Experimental Physiology

Bell GH. 1959. *Experimental Physiology.* London: Churchill Livingstone.

Ghosh MN. 1984. *Fundamentals of Experimental Pharmacology;* second edition. Kolkata: Scientific Book Agency.

Gray WI. 1965 . *Methods of Animal Experimentation.* London: Academic Press.

Levedahl BH, Barber AA and Grinnel A. 1971. *Laboratory Experiments in Physiology;* eighth edition. New York: CV Mosby Co.

Tuttle WW and Schottelius BA. 1963. *Physiology Laboratory Manual.* New York: CV Mosby Co.

# Index